Introduction to
Basic Cardiac
Dysrhythmias

Introduction to

Basic Cardiac Dysrhythmias

Fourth Edition

Sandra Atwood, RN, BA

Cheryl Stanton, RN

Jenny Storey-Davenport, RN, BSN, BC

Original illustrations by Jenny Storey-Davenport, RN, BSN, BC
Modified versions by Mark Wieber

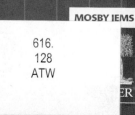

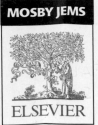

11830 Westline Industrial Drive
St. Louis, Missouri 63146

INTRODUCTION TO BASIC CARDIAC DYSRHYTHMIAS   ISBN: 978-0-323-05225-2

Notice

Library of Congress Control Number: 2007939676

Executive Editor: Linda Honeycutt
Developmental Editor: Katherine Tomber
Publishing Services Manager: Julie Eddy
Project Manager: Celeste Clingan
Design Direction: Amy Buxton

Printed in China

Last digit is the print number: 9 8 7 6 5 4 3 2 1

*We lovingly dedicate this book
to our husbands
Phil, Ken, and Tracy,
and
to our children
Lee, Alicia, Melynda, Michael, and Jim*

Preface

Introduction to Basic Cardiac Dysrhythmias was originally written to help the beginning learner unravel the mysteries of those squiggly lines seen on the monitor and rhythm strip. Our intent is to explain what happens inside the heart when a dysrhythmia is seen, as well as how the dysrhythmia appears on a monitor or rhythm strip.

Although the text is designed for students without a medical background, the learner with cardiac knowledge should also find it helpful as a review of dysrhythmias and treatment.

The term dysrhythmia is used in the title and throughout the text because we believe it is an accurate description of the information presented.

We have used simple medical terminology whenever feasible; numerous illustrations are also included to make learning as easy as possible.

The hearts found in the illustrations are not drawn to scale; the atria, atrioventricular junction, and septum are drawn larger than normal, to show the conduction pathway of the heart clearly. A sequential approach is used, following the normal electrical conduction pathway of the heart.

Most rhythm strips appear as from a Lead II placement and all reflect examples of cardiac rhythms found in the adult patient.

- **Chapter 1** covers the basic anatomy and physiology of the cardiac, pulmonary, and vascular systems, with corresponding illustrations for additional clarification. Medical terms are introduced with simple explanations and definitions.
- **Chapter 2** explains the equipment and supplies used in telemetry, the components of a cardiac complex, and information for interpreting rhythm strips.
- **Chapters 3 to 7** explain basic cardiac dysrhythmias, following the normal, sequential conduction pathway of the heart (i.e., atrial, junctional, and ventricular dysrhythmias), as well as heart blocks, aberrant and escape beats, followed by pacemaker rhythms.
- **Chapter 8** offers a concise review of all dysrhythmias discussed in the book, providing sample rhythm strips and brief explanations of the criteria involved in identifying each dysrhythmia.
- **Chapter 9** focuses on the treatment of basic dysrhythmias and follows current American Heart Association Standards.
- **Chapter 10** includes at least one example of each dysrhythmia shown in the book, as well as space for the reader to evaluate the measurements of each component, describe abnormal complexes, and identify the dysrhythmia
- **Chapter 11** provides various case studies/scenarios for additional review of dysrhythmias and treatment.

Review questions can be found at the end of Chapters 1 to 7, as well as review rhythm strips after Chapters 2 to 7, to assist readers in measuring their progress in learning. Crossword and word puzzles are included throughout the book to assist in learning and "for fun." An answer section, glossary, abbreviations, index, and two sections of flashcards can be found at the end of the book, along with a review of rhythm strips and medical animations on CD.

We gratefully acknowledge the efforts of others who were so instrumental in the completion of this text. Many thanks to all of our nursing friends, physicians, and other colleagues for their encouragement and to all the nurses and monitor technicians who attended our courses and provided such valuable feedback about our original study guide. Also, many thanks again to all the students for their continued comments and evaluations of the book.

Last, but certainly not least, our loving thanks to our families for their patience, understanding, and encouragement.

Introduction to the Fourth Edition

We have made several changes in the fourth edition of *Introduction to Basic Cardiac Dysrhythmias*. These changes include the complete revision of the medication review and treatment guidelines in Chapter 9, based on the 2005 Emergency Cardiovascular Care Guidelines.

These changes and additions also include the following new information:
- Updated illustrations and materials
- Updated definitions of terminology at the beginning of each chapter
- Additional information on complex components (P, T, ST and QT)
- Updated information on artificial pacemakers, ICDs and AEDs
- Updated and additional crossword puzzles
- Additional word puzzles to aid in terminology recognition.
- Updated case studies in Chapter 11
- Revised medication flashcards for review of drug treatments
- Expanded and updated glossary and index
- Abbreviation list updated to current standards of The Joint Commission
- Addition of a CD with Rhythm Strip Review and Medical Animations
- Updated Heart Rate Review

Note to the Reader:
Although the authors and the publisher have made every attempt to check the accuracy of this text, the possibility of error can never be eliminated. At the time of publication, the information presented here represents accepted practices in the United States, but is not offered as a standard of care. It is the reader's responsibility to learn and follow the protocols of their locality, and to follow the direction of a licensed physician. It is also the reader's responsibility to stay informed of procedural changes and new drugs used in emergency cardiac care.

Acknowledgments

The editors wish to acknowledge and thank the many reviewers of this book, who devoted countless hours to intense review. Their comments were invaluable in helping develop and fine-tune the manuscript

Kathleen A. Ballman, RN, MSN, ACNP, CEN, EMT-P, EMSI
Director
Bethesda Hospital Paramedic Training Program
Nurse Practitioner
Heart Failure Services
Bethesda North Hospital
Cincinnati, Ohio

Steven Dralle, LP, BA, EMSC
General Manager
American Medical Response—South Texas
San Antonio, Texas

Mark Goldstein, RN, BSN, EMT-P I/C
EMS Coordinator
William Beaumont Hospital
Royal Oak, Michigan

Joanne McCall, RN, MA, CEN, CFN, SANE-A
Senior Education Specialist
St. John—Providence Park Hospital
Novi, Michigan

Michelle M. McLean, MD, EMT-P
Medical Doctor, Paramedic
Covenant Emergency Care Center, Covenant Hospital
Saginaw, Michigan

Lynn Pierzchalski-Goldstein, BSP, PharmD
Emergency Medicine Pharmacy Specialist
William Beaumont Hospital
Royal Oak, Michigan

Larry Richmond, AS, NREMT-P, CCEMT-P
EMS Education Manager
Mountain Plains Health Consortium
Fort Meade, South Dakota

Contents

8 DYSRHYTHMIA REVIEW, 187

9 MEDICATION REVIEW and ADULT TREATMENT GUIDELINES, 213

10 DYSRHYTHMIA INTERPRETATION PRACTICE, 239

11 CASE STUDIES, 309

ANSWER SECTION, 339

GLOSSARY, 379

ABBREVIATION LIST, 387

REFERENCE LIST, 389

INDEX, 391

FLASHCARDS

DYSRHYTHMIA REVIEW

MEDICATION REVIEW

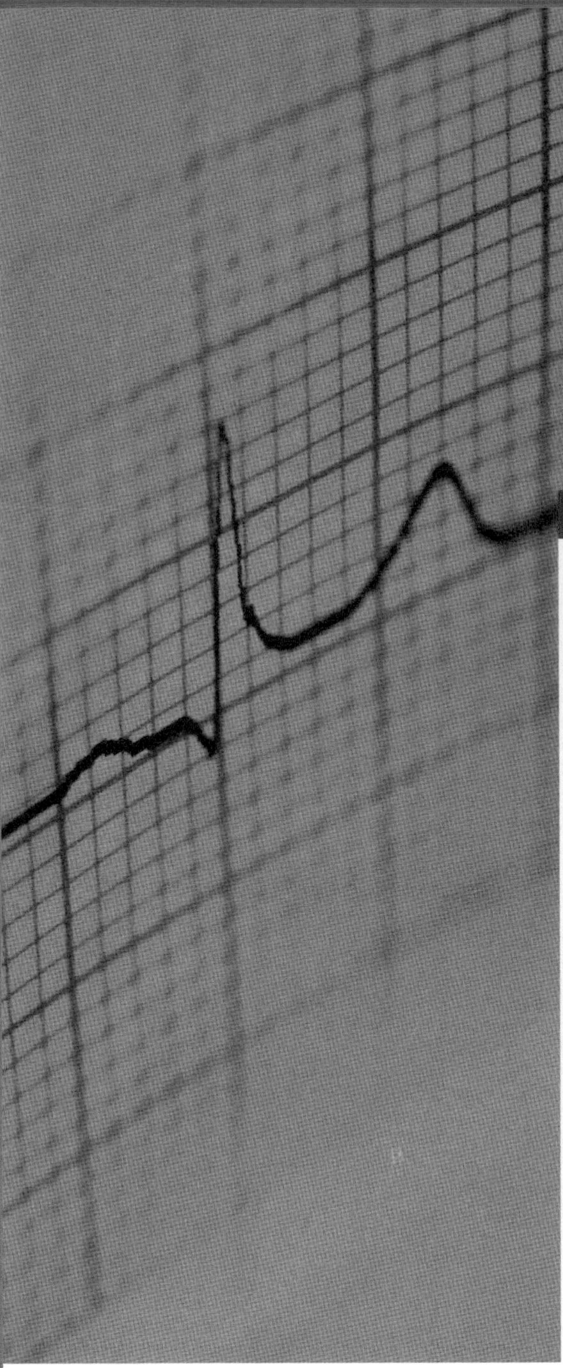

On completion of this chapter, the reader should be able to:

1 List the two main organs of the cardiopulmonary system.
2 Identify the four heart chambers, three cardiac muscle layers, and four main heart valves.
3 Explain the basic function of the lungs.
4 Describe the three main types of blood vessels.
5 Explain the possible causes and four common symptoms of myocardial infarction.
6 Describe the flow of a drop of blood from the vena cava through the heart and lungs to the aorta.
7 Explain how to measure cardiac output.
8 Explain the four common characteristics of cardiac cells.
9 Define the following terms: *polarization*, *depolarization*, and *repolarization*.
10 Describe the movement of an electrical impulse, following the normal cardiac conduction pathways.
11 Explain the actions of the sympathetic and parasympathetic nervous systems on the heart rate.

Anatomy and Physiology

DEFINITIONS

Automaticity—Ability of cardiac cells to initiate or generate an electrical impulse

Autonomic Nervous System—Part of the nervous system that regulates many organs, such as the heart and blood vessels

Cardiac—Pertaining to the heart

Cardiac Output—Amount of blood pumped by the left ventricle in 1 minute

Conductivity—Ability of cardiac cells to transmit an electrical impulse

Contractility—Ability of cardiac cells to respond to an electrical impulse by contracting

Cyanosis—Bluish-gray color of the lips, skin, and nail beds, caused by a lack of oxygen

Depolarization—Conduction of an electrical impulse through the heart muscle; normally causes a cardiac contraction

Dyspnea—Difficult or painful breathing

Excitability—Ability of cardiac cells to respond to an electrical impulse

Heart—Muscular organ that pumps blood to the body cells

Heart/Lung Circulation—Transportation of blood from the body cells, through the heart and lungs, and back to the body cells

Hypotension—Decreased blood pressure; below patient's normal blood pressure

Lungs—Two organs that remove carbon dioxide from the blood, replacing it with oxygen

Polarization—Cardiac ready state; the cells are ready to receive an electrical impulse

Pulmonary—Pertaining to the lungs

Repolarization—Cardiac recovery phase; the cells are returning to the ready state

ANATOMY

The main organs of the cardiopulmonary system are the heart and lungs. These organs work together to circulate oxygenated blood through blood vessels to all body cells.

Heart

The adult heart is a hollow, muscular organ that is located in the chest cavity, between the sternum (breastbone) and the spinal column. The normal adult heart weighs about 1 lb (0.45 kg) and is approximately the size of an adult fist (Figure 1-1).

The heart functions as a double-sided pump. The pumping action of the right and left sides occurs when the muscular walls of each heart chamber contract (squeeze), causing blood to be forced out of the chambers.

> **NOTE:** The following hearts are drawn for simplicity and ease of illustration. They are **not** drawn to scale.

Heart Chambers

The heart has four chambers: right atrium, left atrium, right ventricle, and left ventricle (Figure 1-2). The *atria* (plural for atrium) are thin-walled, upper chambers that function as reservoirs, or holding areas, for blood. *Ventricles* are the lower chambers of the heart. The right ventricle has a thin muscular wall. The muscle of the left ventricular wall is much thicker, because it has to pump blood throughout the body, to all body cells.

The heart is further divided by a muscular wall called the *septum*. The septum separates the atria (*interatrial septum*) and ventricles (*interventricular septum*) into right and left sides (Figure 1-3). The right ventricle pumps blood to the lungs, while the left ventricle pumps blood throughout the body.

The atria contract at the same time, followed by the ventricles contracting at the same time. These contractions usually occur in a rhythmic beat. The pumping action of the left ventricle produces a *pulse*, or wave of pressure, which can be counted.

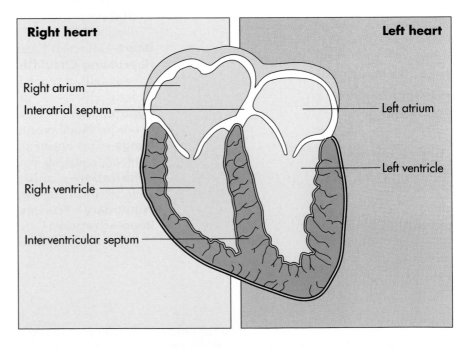

Right heart

Left heart

Right atrium

Interatrial septum

Left atrium

Left ventricle

Right ventricle

Interventricular septum

Figure 1-1 Adult heart.

This pulse is called the heart rate (HR) and usually is measured as heartbeats per minute.

Heart Muscle

The heart is made of specialized muscle tissue that is not found anywhere else in the body. This specialized tissue forms the cardiac wall and has three main layers. The inner layer of the cardiac wall is called the *endocardium* and lines the chambers of the heart and covers the valves.

The middle layer of the cardiac wall is the *myocardium*. This layer is the heart muscle and provides the pumping action needed to circulate blood. The *epicardium* is the outer layer of the cardiac muscle and is a thin, protective membrane that covers the outside of the heart.

The heart is contained in a loose-fitting membrane called the *pericardial sac* (Figure 1-4). A small amount of fluid (10 to 30 ml) can be found in the space

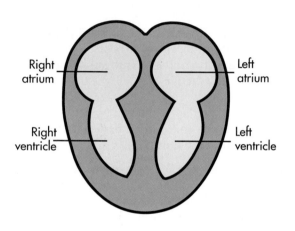

Right atrium

Left atrium

Right ventricle

Left ventricle

Figure 1-2 The four chambers of the heart.

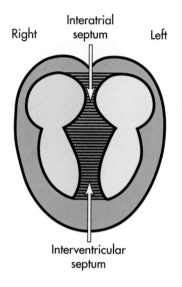

Right

Interatrial septum

Left

Interventricular septum

Figure 1-3 Septum divides the right and left sides of the heart.

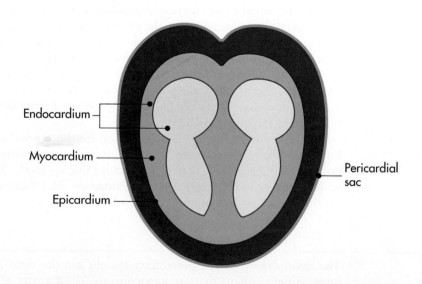

Endocardium

Myocardium

Epicardium

Pericardial sac

Figure 1-4 Three layers of cardiac tissue and pericardial sac.

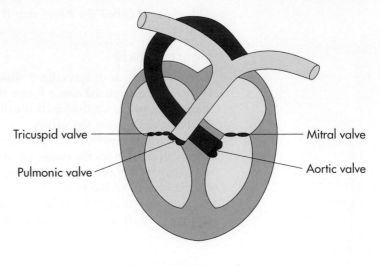

Figure 1-5 Heart valves.

between the epicardium and pericardium. This fluid (*pericardial fluid*) acts as a lubricant, allowing the heart to move within the sac as it beats.

The myocardium and pericardium are further divided into sub-layers, which are discussed in 12-Lead electrocardiogram (ECG) courses.

Heart Valves

The heart has four valves that are covered with endocardial tissue. These four valves are located in the following areas of the heart (Figure 1-5):

Tricuspid valve—Between the right atrium and the right ventricle
Pulmonic valve—Between the right ventricle and the pulmonary artery
Mitral valve—Between the left atrium and the left ventricle
Aortic valve—Between the left ventricle and the aorta

These valves are flaplike structures that open and close in response to the pumping action of the heart. The opening and closing of the heart valves permit the flow of blood in a forward direction and prevent blood from flowing backward.

For example, in the left side of the heart, as the blood enters the empty left atrium, the blood causes increased pressure against the atrial walls. When the atrial pressure becomes greater than the ventricular pressure, the mitral valve opens, allowing most of the blood to flow into the left ventricle. The atrium then gives a mild contraction (atrial kick), emptying the remaining blood into the left ventricle.

As the left ventricle contracts, the mitral valve closes and the aortic valve opens. The closed mitral valve prevents the flow of blood back into the left atrium. The open aortic valve allows the blood to be pumped from the heart and then carried throughout the body, to all body cells.

The "lub dub, lub dub" noises caused by the normal closing of the valves are known as *heart sounds*. In an adult, a *murmur* is an abnormal sound made by blood flowing through a valve that is not functioning correctly. This sound can be heard when listening to the heart with a stethoscope. Heart murmurs are usually caused by an improperly functioning mitral valve.

Lungs

The main organs of the pulmonary system are the right and left lungs. They are large, spongy organs that are located in the chest cavity, slightly behind and on either side of the heart. Each lung is encased in a protective sac called the *pleural sac*.

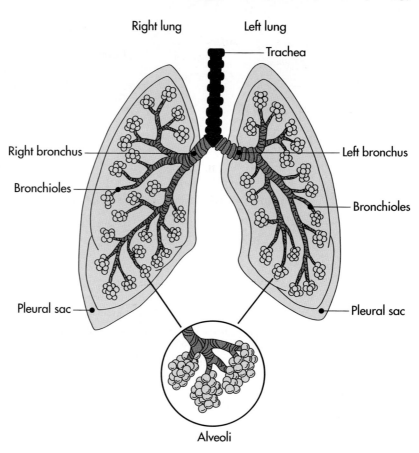

Figure 1-6 Lungs and air pathways from trachea to alveoli.

The main function of the lungs is to remove carbon dioxide from the blood and to replace it with oxygen (Figure 1-6).

This exchange begins when air, containing oxygen, is inhaled through the nose or mouth into the trachea. The *trachea* is a hollow tube that extends downward for approximately 4½ inches, where it then divides into two slightly smaller tubes, called *bronchi,* one for each lung. After the bronchi enter the lungs, each bronchus further divides into smaller tubes, called the *bronchioles.* The air continues traveling through the bronchioles, as they further divide into smaller and smaller tubes and finally end in the *alveoli* (see Figure 1-6).

The alveoli are tiny sacs of tissue that are arranged in grapelike clusters. The alveoli are surrounded by very small blood vessels called *capillaries.* The actual exchange of carbon dioxide from the capillary blood for oxygen from the inhaled air takes place in these tiny sacs. Because the walls of both the alveoli and the capillaries are only one cell thick, the exchange of carbon dioxide for oxygen takes place easily.

Blood Vessels

Blood vessels are hollow tubes composed of smooth muscle, which are located throughout the body. Their primary purpose is transportation. They carry oxygenated blood to all body cells and then transport blood with carbon dioxide from the body cells to the lungs.

The three main types of blood vessels are *arteries, veins,* and *capillaries* (Figure 1-7). Arteries carry blood away from the heart, and veins carry blood to the heart. The exchange of nutrients and waste products for the body cells takes place in the capillaries.

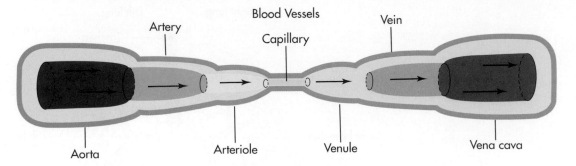

Figure 1-7 Gradual change in the size of blood vessels and vessel walls.

Arteries

Arteries are blood vessels that carry oxygenated blood away from the heart to all parts of the body. Arteries have the thickest walls of all blood vessels because they must withstand the pumping pressure of the heart. The *aorta* is the largest artery in the body.

The arteries divide into arterioles, which are smaller blood vessels with thinner walls. The *arterioles* connect arteries to capillaries.

Veins

Veins are vessels that carry blood with carbon dioxide from the body cells back to the heart. The venous walls are thinner than the arterial walls. *Peripheral veins* (in the arms and legs) contain tiny valves, similar to cardiac valves, which prevent the backward flow of blood. The *inferior* and the *superior vena cava* are the largest veins in the body and do not have these types of valves. The smallest veins are called *venules*, and they connect veins to capillaries.

> **NOTE:** A major exception to the definition of arteries and veins is found in the heart/lung circulation. The pulmonary arteries carry blood with carbon dioxide to the lungs, and the pulmonary veins carry blood with oxygen to the heart.

Capillaries

Capillaries, the smallest blood vessels in the body, also have the thinnest walls of any blood vessel. The exchange of oxygen and waste products between the blood and the body cells takes place through the capillary walls, which are only one cell thick.

Coronary Arteries

The heart muscle receives its blood supply from *coronary arteries*. These special arteries branch off the aorta and supply oxygenated blood to each portion of the heart muscle.

For example, the right coronary artery divides into the marginal artery and the right anterior and right posterior descending arteries, which again divide into smaller arteries (Figure 1-8). Therefore, the right coronary artery and its branches are able to provide oxygenated blood to the muscle tissue of the right atrium, the left ventricle, and the right ventricle. The left coronary artery branches (divides) into the left anterior descending artery and the circumflex artery, which both divide into smaller arteries. The left coronary artery and its branches provide oxygenated blood to the muscle tissue of the left atrium, the left ventricle, and the right ventricle. Most of this oxygenated blood flows to the cardiac muscle between heartbeats (contractions) while the myocardium is resting.

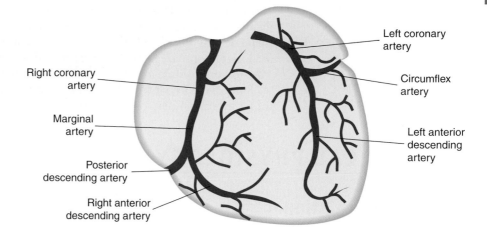

Figure 1-8 Coronary vessels: arteries that supply oxygen and nutrients to cardiac muscle cells.

Myocardial Infarction

Coronary arteries may become partially or completely blocked by blood clots or from a buildup of cholesterol inside the artery walls. A spasm of the blood vessel wall may also cause a temporary blockage of the artery. When a blockage occurs in a coronary artery, the cardiac muscle that is usually nourished by that artery does not receive enough oxygen. This decreased supply of oxygen to tissue is called *ischemia*, while a total lack of oxygen in the cells is known as *hypoxia*.

Cardiac ischemia often causes chest pain, known as *angina pectoris* (angina), which may be mild or severe. Angina may occur after physical exercise, after eating a large meal, in stressful situations, or when exposed to extreme temperatures. The symptoms of angina may be described as a vague, dull ache; indigestion (heartburn); pressure "like an elephant sitting on my chest"; or crushing, squeezing tightness in the chest "like having a tight belt around my chest." Angina may remain centered in the chest or may travel to the left shoulder, either arm, jaw, or upper back. There may also be shortness of breath *(SOB)*, or a feeling of not being able to get enough air.

Stable angina usually starts with physical exertion and is relieved by rest. Medication, such as nitroglycerin, may be used to relieve the pain. If the episodes of chest pain increase in frequency or severity, stable angina becomes *unstable angina (UA)*.

Unstable angina is not relieved by rest, may be more painful than usual, and may also cause nausea, vomiting, difficulty breathing, and sweating. Unstable angina is a serious symptom that may indicate an increase in the myocardial ischemia, or a decrease in the patient's ability to tolerate the ischemia. Angina that is not diagnosed and treated usually leads to *myocardial infarction* (death of cardiac tissue). The death of cardiac tissue may decrease the ability of the cardiac muscle to contract and pump blood effectively.

> **NOTE:** *Acute coronary syndrome (ACS)* is a term used to describe either unstable angina or myocardial infarction.

A myocardial infarction (MI, heart attack, or coronary) can affect any area of the heart muscle. The location of the MI may cause an interruption in the cardiac electrical conduction pathways. This interruption may cause *dysrhythmias* (abnormal cardiac rhythms), which are discussed in Chapters 3 through 7.

Symptoms of an MI, which usually last longer than 20 to 30 minutes, may include chest pain or pressure that is described as a heavy feeling, a dull ache, a crushing sensation, or indigestion that is not relieved by antacids. The patient may deny that he or she is having a heart attack, saying, "It's just something I ate." The discomfort, pain, or pressure may radiate (move) down the left arm or up into the neck, jaw, shoulders, or back. Other symptoms may include nausea, vomiting, difficulty breathing, shortness of breath, anxiety, a feeling of impending doom, ashen (pale or grayish colored) skin, light to extreme sweating, extreme fatigue, confusion, or loss of consciousness. Chest pain or discomfort with other symptoms may indicate either unstable angina or an MI and usually requires treatment.

Some patients, such as those with heart transplants, severe diabetes, different types of paralysis, women, or the elderly, may have very mild to no symptoms at all.

MECHANICAL PHYSIOLOGY

Heart/Lung Circulation

The right side of the heart receives blood from the inferior and superior vena cava and sends this blood to the lungs. The lungs filter carbon dioxide from the blood and exchange it for oxygen. The oxygenated blood then flows to the left side of the heart, which pumps the blood into the aorta. Blood is circulated through the heart and lungs in the following order (Figure 1-9):

inferior and superior vena cava → right atrium → tricuspid valve → right ventricle → pulmonic valve → pulmonary arteries → lungs → pulmonary veins → left atrium → mitral valve → left ventricle → aortic valve → aorta → rest of the body, including the heart

Cardiac Output

One method of measuring how efficiently the heart is pumping and circulating blood to the body cells is by determining the cardiac output (CO). CO is the amount of blood pumped by the left ventricle in 1 minute.

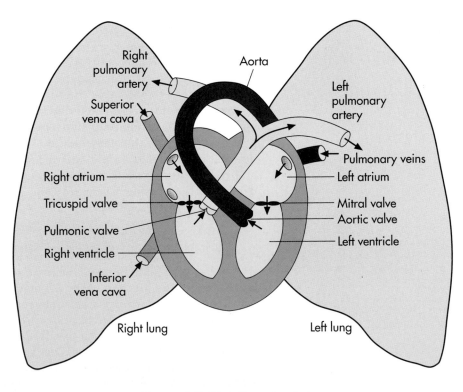

Figure 1-9 Heart/lung circulation.

CO is measured by multiplying the heart rate (HR) by the stroke volume (SV), which is the amount of blood pumped by the left ventricle with each beat. The formula is CO = SV × HR.

> CO—Cardiac output is the amount of blood pumped by the left ventricle in 1 minute. The normal amount is usually 4000 to 8000 ml, depending on body size, age, and gender.
>
> SV—Stroke volume is the amount of blood pumped by the left ventricle with each contraction or beat, approximately 70 ml.
>
> HR—Heart rate is the number of times the left ventricle contracts in 1 minute; the normal rate is 60 to 100.

Example: CO = SV × HR; the stroke volume is 70 ml and the heart rate is 80: CO = 70 × 80 = 5600 ml = normal cardiac output.

When the CO is abnormal, the heart will try to balance it by changing either the SV or the HR. For example, if a person exercises and becomes physically fit, the SV usually increases because the heart muscle is stronger and pumps more blood with each beat. The HR then decreases to keep the CO within the normal range.

Example: CO = SV × HR; with an increased SV of 90 ml and a decreased HR of 60: CO = 90 × 60 = 5400 ml = normal CO

The opposite is also true. When the heart cannot pump the usual amount of blood because of injury or disease, the SV decreases. The HR then increases to maintain a normal CO.

Example: CO = SV × HR; with a decreased SV of 50 ml and an increased HR of 110: CO = 50 × 110 = 5500 ml = normal CO

If the heart is unable to increase the SV or the HR, the CO will decrease.

Example: CO = SV × HR; with a decreased SV of 50 ml and a HR of 60: CO = 50 × 60 = 3000 ml = decreased CO

A decreased (poor) cardiac output may cause damage to major organs such as the heart and brain. This damage occurs because there is not enough blood being circulated to carry oxygen to the body cells.

Poor cardiac output may be indicated by any combination of the following signs and symptoms:

- Pale, cool, clammy (damp) skin
- Nausea and vomiting (N/V)
- Dizziness, weakness, faintness
- Shortness of breath (SOB)
- Hypotension (decreased blood pressure)
- Dyspnea (difficulty breathing)
- Tachycardia (rapid heart rate)
- Diaphoresis (excessive sweating)
- Mild to severe chest pain
- Confusion or disorientation
- Cyanosis (bluish-gray color to skin)
- Decreased urinary output
- Unresponsiveness

ELECTROPHYSIOLOGY

All muscle tissue contracts in response to an electrical stimulus or impulse. For example, skeletal muscle will contract after receiving stimulation from a nerve. However, *cardiac muscle* is unique; not only can it respond to an electrical impulse, cardiac muscle also has *pacemaker cells* that can generate electrical impulses.

The following definitions explain four common characteristics of cardiac cells:

Automaticity—Ability of cardiac pacemaker cells to generate or initiate their own electrical impulses

Excitability— Irritability; the ability of cardiac cells to respond to an electrical stimulus; when a cardiac cell is highly irritable, less stimulus is required to cause a contraction

Conductivity—Ability of cardiac cells to transmit an electrical stimulus to other cardiac cells

Contractility—Ability of cardiac cells to shorten, causing cardiac muscle contraction in response to an electrical stimulus

Contractility is a mechanical function of the heart. Automaticity, excitability, and conductivity are electrical functions.

Depolarization and Repolarization

The following terms explain the phases of the normal electrical activity of the heart:

Polarization—Phase of readiness; the muscle is relaxed and the cardiac cells are ready to receive an electrical impulse

Depolarization—Phase of contraction; the cardiac cells have transmitted an electrical impulse, usually causing the cardiac muscle to contract

Repolarization—Recovery phase; the muscle has contracted and the cells are returning to a ready state

All tissue, including cardiac muscle, is made of many single cells that contain chemicals such as potassium and sodium. The cells normally have *potassium* (K+) on the inside of the cell and *sodium* (Na+) on the outside, making the cells negatively charged. These cells are *polarized*, or in the ready state (Figure 1-10, *A*).

When a pacemaker cell generates an electrical impulse to a polarized cardiac cell, most of the potassium moves to the outside of the cell and most of the sodium moves to the inside of the cell, making the cells positively charged. This movement of the potassium and sodium through the cell wall causes a "spark" of electricity. The electrical spark is then conducted to the remaining cells in that part of the heart, causing *depolarization* (Figure 1-10, *B*). While in this state, the cardiac cells contract. They cannot respond to any further electrical impulses until they have repolarized and become negatively charged again.

After the electrical impulse has passed through the cells, the potassium reenters the cells and the sodium leaves, causing *repolarization* (Figure 1-10, *C*). However, not all cells repolarize at the same time. Therefore, some cardiac cells are able to conduct an additional electrical impulse sooner than others.

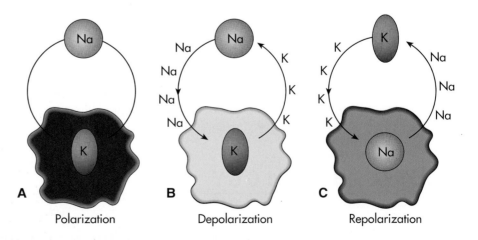

A	B	C
Polarization	Depolarization	Repolarization

Figure 1-10 A to C, Electrical conduction within cardiac cells showing exchange of sodium and potassium.

Electrical Conduction Pathways

Although any cardiac pacemaker cell is capable of initiating an electrical impulse, the normal pacemaker is the *sinoatrial (SA) node*. The normal electrical conduction pathway of the heart occurs in the following order (Figure 1-11):

sinoatrial node (SA node) → intraatrial and internodal pathways → atrioventricular node (AV node) → bundle of His → bundle branches → Purkinje's fibers → ventricular muscle.

Sinoatrial node (SA node)	The SA node is located in the upper portion of the right atrium and is called the *pacemaker of the heart*. The SA node initiates an electrical impulse that travels downward, throughout the muscle of both atria. This impulse travels through the atrial muscles by way of the *intraatrial conduction pathways*, causing depolarization of the atrium. The same impulse is also transmitted from the SA node to the atrioventricular (AV) node through the *internodal conduction pathways*. The SA node usually generates 60 to 100 electrical impulses per minute.
Atrioventricular node (AV node)	The AV node is located in the general area of the lower right atrium near the septum. The AV node continues transmitting the impulse from the atria to the bundle of His. If the SA node fails to function, pacemaker cells between the atria and the AV node *(AV junction)* are capable of functioning as a *secondary pacemaker*. This area of the electrical conduction system usually generates 40 to 60 electrical impulses per minute.
Bundle of His	The bundle of His, located below the AV node, continues transmitting the electrical impulse to the bundle branches.
Bundle branches (BB)	The lower portion of the bundle of His divides into a *right bundle branch* (leading into the right ventricle) and a left bundle branch (leading into the left ventricle). The bundle branches continue transmitting the electrical impulse to the Purkinje's fibers.
Purkinje's fibers	Extending from the bundle branches into the muscular walls of the ventricles, the Purkinje's fibers conduct the electrical impulse from the bundle branches to cells of the ventricular muscle.

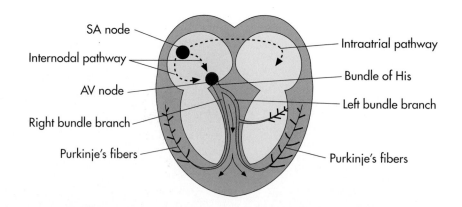

Figure 1-11 Normal electrical conduction pathway of the heart.

Ventricular muscle   The cells of the ventricular muscle receive an electrical stimulus from the Purkinje's fibers and contract. If the SA node **and** the AV junction do not initiate an electrical impulse, an impulse can be generated from any pacemaker cell in the ventricles, including the Purkinje's fibers or the bundle branches. Impulses initiated below the AV node are usually generated at a rate of 20 to 40 impulses per minute.

Autonomic Nervous System

The electrical conduction system of the heart is affected by the *autonomic nervous system*. The function of the autonomic nervous system is to maintain the body in a normal state by controlling several organs, including the heart, as well as the blood vessels. This control is done automatically, without a person being aware it is happening.

The autonomic nervous system is divided into two parts: the *sympathetic* and the *parasympathetic* systems.

The sympathetic nervous system prepares the body to react in times of stress or emergencies, increasing cardiac output by increasing the heart rate, blood pressure, and force of cardiac contractions. This is known as the "fight or flight response." The sympathetic nerves can be stimulated by anger, pain, fright, caffeine, and some drugs.

The parasympathetic nervous system affects the heart in the opposite way by decreasing the rate of cardiac contractions. This reaction usually occurs after the stress or emergency is over, allowing the body to restore energy. The parasympathetic nerves can be stimulated by straining to have bowel movement, a urinary bladder that is too full, vomiting, and some drugs.

Medications are available to reverse the effects of the sympathetic and parasympathetic nervous systems on the heart, when necessary. For example, when the parasympathetic nerves have been stimulated and decrease the heart rate too much, drugs such as atropine block the parasympathetic nerves. This allows the heart rate to increase to a more normal rate, in order to maintain adequate cardiac output.

REVIEW QUESTIONS

True	**False**	1. The main organs of the cardiopulmonary system are the heart and blood vessels.
True	**False**	2. The parasympathetic nervous system decreases the rate of cardiac contractions.
True	**False**	3. The ventricles function as reservoirs for blood.
True	**False**	4. Contractility is an electrical function of the heart.

5. The upper chambers of the heart are known as the _____, and the lower chambers of the heart are known as the_____.

6. List the three main layers of cardiac muscle.

   a. _____

   b. _____

   c. _____

7. Identify the four valves of the heart.

   a. _____

   b. _____

   c. _____

   d. _____

8. a. What type of blood vessels carry blood away from the heart?

   _____

   b. What type of blood vessels carry blood back to the heart?

   _____

   c. What type of blood vessels allow the exchange of oxygen and nutrients for waste products at the cellular level?

   _____

9. The layer of the heart that contracts to pump blood to the lungs and throughout the body to all body cells is the _____ layer.

   a. endocardial

   b. myocardial

   c. epithelial

   d. epicardial

10. Cardiac muscle tissue receives its blood supply from the

   a. pulmonary arteries

   b. coronary arteries

   c. myocardial arteries

   d. coronary veins

11. In the lungs, the exchange of oxygen from inhaled air and carbon dioxide from capillary blood takes place inside tiny sacs called _____.

Continued

12. Cardiac output is determined by
    a. stroke volume multiplied by the respiratory rate
    b. stroke volume divided by the heart rate
    c. heart rate divided by the stroke volume
    d. heart rate multiplied by the stroke volume

13. Automaticity is the ability of cardiac pacemaker cells to
    a. contract
    b. respond to an electrical impulse
    c. regenerate themselves
    d. initiate an electrical impulse

14. The sympathetic nervous system
    a. increases cardiac output and blood pressure
    b. decreases heart rate and blood pressure
    c. controls the autonomic nervous system
    d. increases heart rate, blood pressure, and the force of cardiac contractions

15. The ability of cardiac cells to transmit an electrical impulse is
    a. excitability
    b. conductivity
    c. contractility
    d. automaticity

16. Explain the following terms.
    a. depolarization

    _____

    _____

    _____

    b. repolarization

    _____

    _____

    _____

17. Trace a drop of blood from the inferior vena cava to the aorta:
    Inferior and superior vena cava →

    _____

    _____

    _____

    _____

18. Trace the normal electrical conduction pathway system of the heart:

_____

_____

_____

_____

19. Define the following terms.

    a. Ischemia _____

    b. Myocardial infarction _____

    c. Stable angina _____

    d. Unstable angina _____

20. List four common symptoms of a myocardial infarction (MI):

    a. _____

    b. _____

    c. _____

    d. _____

CROSSWORD PUZZLE CLUES

Across

1 One of the lower chambers of the heart.

3 Ability of cardiac cells to initiate an electrical impulse.

6 Divides the right and left sides of the heart.

8 Lack of oxygen in any of the body's cells.

9 SV × HR = _____.

10 Difficult or painful breathing.

14 Abnormal heart sound.

15 The _____ node is the normal pacemaker of the heart.

16 The heart is enclosed in a(n) _____ sac.

17 Middle layer of heart muscle.

20 Ability of cardiac cells to respond to an electrical impulse.

21 Main organs of the pulmonary system.

23 Feeling of choking, suffocation, or crushing pressure and pain.

25 Ability of cardiac cells to transmit an electrical impulse to other cardiac cells.

27 Phase of readiness.

28 Tiny sacs of lung tissue where exchange of carbon dioxide and oxygen takes place.

Down

2 Decreased supply of oxygen to tissue.

4 The superior and inferior _____ _____ are the largest veins in the body.

5 Upper chambers of the heart.

7 Ability of cardiac cells to shorten, causing myocardium to contract.

11 Part of nervous system that raises heart rate and blood pressure: fight-or-flight response.

12 Heart sounds are the noises caused by the normal closing of heart _____.

13 Pertaining to the heart.

17 The _____ valve is located between the left atria and the left ventricle.

18 The bundle of ___ transmits the electrical impulse from the atria to the bundle branches.

19 Bluish discoloration of skin, nail beds, and lips due to lack of oxygen.

22 The _____ _____ is the secondary pacemaker of the heart.

24 Largest artery in the body.

26 Heart attack.

The solution to this crossword puzzle is in the answer section.

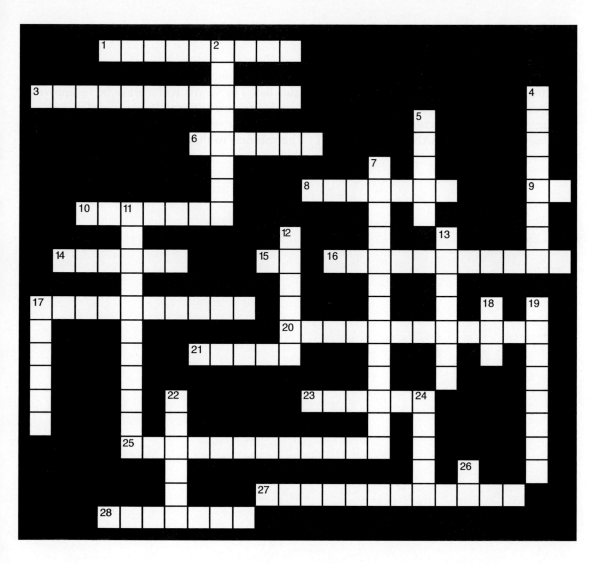

WORD PUZZLE

This word puzzle is designed to help familiarize you with some of the new terminology found in this chapter. Have fun finding all the words on this list. The words will always be in uppercase and found in a straight line. The words may be spelled forward (normal), backward, up, down, or diagonally in any direction. Phrases will not have any spaces between the words; for example, SA node will appear as SANODE. Good luck! **The solution to this word puzzle is in the answer section.**

```
B E N K L G P E R I C A R D I A L S A C N N
F X S M A M N Y L V G F T L V K I P I M V Q
Q C A U R L V O P U L M O N A R Y X T Q W P
G I N T J W V M I K H D M K J N C U O R M J
Y T O P T Q H E L T T N Y L Q Y P L B P J M
I B E S B K M J N L B R R K U M U R N K Y H
C I L G Q R W T B R I M A O L N N C D T X E
I L M N L X Q K K Y X P C F G P O B L N A L
T I A I M E H C S I C A A S N N G L E C T B
A T H M Y O C A R D I U M T D I R B B O R A
M Y V R P L J F P D T V R U H Q D M R R O T
O K P D T P N F R Q P N C B T W Q W A O A S
T V K C Y H P A T D M T R V L M A J N N K N
U L R J H S C K A L I G E J K P M Y C A Z U
A T T R H N P V W V R N T G N N J L H R X K
R L K W K K A N I C T A V N O D E K E Y J W
K B J Q K C X T E R K G R V W T A Z S E T G
T N B T A W Y G I A N I G N A Q K I V N W B
K C O N T R A C T I L I T Y M G K L R X X H
V Z E L N L L K L L D F C M R Q A L K T N C
N V G N H E Y K C M K N R X R V Z X C W A M
```

ALVEOLI	CORONARY	PATHWAY
ANGINA	DYSPNEA	PERICARDIAL SAC
AORTA	EXCITABILITY	PULMONARY
ATRIA	HR	SA NODE
AUTOMATICITY	HYPOXIA	SEPTUM
AV NODE	INFARCTION	UNSTABLE
BUNDLE BRANCHES	ISCHEMIA	VALVE
CARDIAC OUTPUT	LUNGS	VENA CAVA
CONDUCTIVITY	MI	VENTRICLE
CONTRACTILITY	MYOCARDIUM	

OBJECTIVES

On completion of the chapter, the reader should be able to:

1 Define the terms *monitor, electrodes, leads, Lead II, baseline, rate, rhythm,* and *artifact.*

2 Describe the importance of using Lead II and MCL$_1$ for cardiac monitoring.

3 Identify the components of a cardiac cycle.

4 Define the terms *refractory period, absolute refractory period,* and *relative refractory period.*

5 List five questions to ask when evaluating P waves or QRS complexes.

6 List two questions to ask when evaluating PR intervals.

7 Describe a normal and a prolonged QT interval.

8 Describe an elevated and a depressed ST segment and T wave.

9 Describe the use of calipers when measuring the rhythm (regularity) of a cardiac rhythm.

10 Explain how to calculate the heart rate using either the 3-second rhythm strip method, or the 6-second rhythm strip method, and two division methods.

11 List three causes of artifact.

CHAPTER 2

Monitoring and Telemetry

OUTLINE

DEFINITIONS

Absolute Refractory Period—The period of time when the cardiac cells have not completed repolarization and cannot contract again

Artifact—Interference or static seen on the monitor

Biphasic (Diphasic)—Going in two opposite directions; describes a complex component that is both above and below the baseline

Complex Components—Set of waves seen on a monitor, which represent an electrical impulse traveling through the electrical conduction pathway of the heart; it includes P, Q, R, S, and T waves

Electrode—Adhesive pads that are attached to the patient's skin

leads—Wires that connect the electrodes to the monitor or telemetry unit, also called lead wires

Leads—Specific placement of electrodes on the patient's skin

Monitor—A TV-like screen that shows the conduction of electrical impulses as they travel through the electrical conduction pathway of the heart

P to P Interval—Length of time between one P wave and the next P wave

Rate—Number of electrical impulses conducted in 1 minute

Refractory Period—Time between depolarization and repolarization

Relative Refractory Period—The period of time when cardiac cells have repolarized enough that some cells can be stimulated to depolarize

Rhythm—Regularity of the appearance of the complex components

R to R Interval—Length of time between one R wave and the next R wave

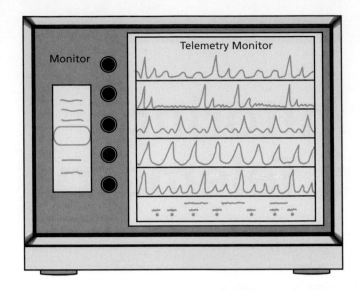

Figure 2-1 Monitor screen.

Telemetry refers to the process of monitoring cardiac electrical activity by transmitting the information to a monitor or telemetry unit. This process includes a machine, graph paper, the identification of complex components, and the interpretation of rhythm strips.

MONITORS AND TELEMETRY UNITS

The movement of electrical impulses through the heart can be seen by using a machine that is called an *electrocardiograph* or *monitor*. The monitor shows the electrical impulses as a pattern of waves on the monitor screen (Figure 2-1).

These wave patterns can also be transferred to graph paper for a printed record of the electrical impulses as they travel through the heart. This printed record is called a *rhythm strip* (Figure 2-2).

Many monitors feature a *freeze mode* to stop the action on the screen. A *delay* mode may also be available to print a specific part of the wave pattern that has already been seen. These special features allow the observer to study the wave pattern more closely.

> **NOTE:** Remember that the monitor does **not** show the actual **contraction** of the cardiac muscle, only the conduction of the electrical impulses through the heart. Cardiac contractions can only be confirmed by the presence of a pulse.

Electrodes and Leads

The monitor receives electrical impulses from the patient's heart through a system of electrodes placed on the body. *Electrodes* are adhesive pads that contain a conductive gel and are attached to the patient's skin.

Electrodes are connected to the monitor by clearly marked and color-coded wires called *leads* (lead wires) (Figure 2-3). A positive (red), a negative (white), and a ground lead must be used for the monitor to receive a clear picture of the cardiac electrical impulses.

The leads from the electrodes may be connected either directly to a monitor or to a telemetry unit. The *telemetry unit* is a small, battery-operated box that is approximately the size of a cell phone. It transmits the electrical impulses to a monitor at a nursing station or other central location (Figure 2-4).

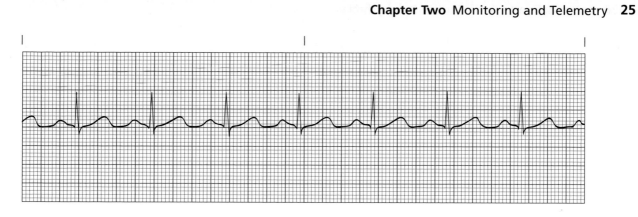

Figure 2-2 Rhythm strip.

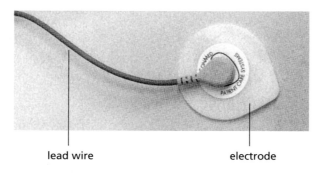

lead wire   electrode

Figure 2-3 Monitor lead wire and electrode.

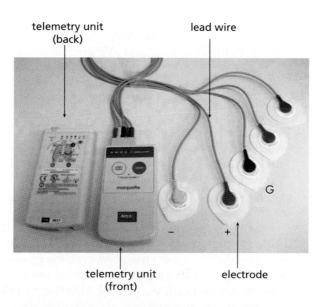

telemetry unit   lead wire
(back)

G

−   +

telemetry unit   electrode
(front)

Figure 2-4 Telemetry unit with lead wires and electrodes.

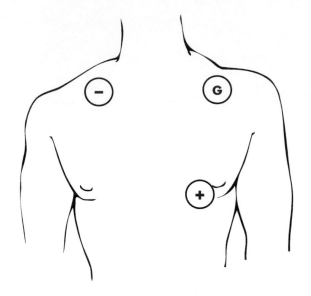

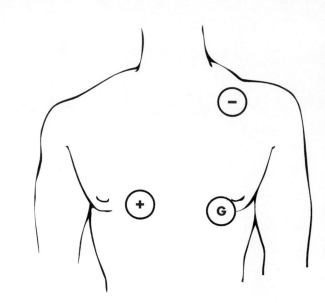

Figure 2-5 Placement of electrodes for Lead II monitoring.

Figure 2-6 Placement of electrodes for modified chest Lead I (MCL$_1$) monitoring.

Lead Placement

The placement of the electrodes on the patient's body determines the angle at which the electrical impulses are received and therefore the part of the heart being observed. The 12-Lead *electrocardiogram (ECG)* "looks" at the heart from 12 different viewing angles. However, most patients are monitored using only one or two "viewing angles." The patterns of the electrodes on the patient are called *Leads*.

> **NOTE:** The term *leads* is used in two different ways:
> 1. The wires leading from electrodes to the monitor. The word "leads" is not capitalized in this definition.
> 2. The different types of electrode placements. In this definition, the word "Leads" is capitalized.

The standard ECG leads are I, II, III, aVR, aVL, aVF, V$_1$, V$_2$, V$_3$, V$_4$, V$_5$, and V$_6$. Leads I, II, III, aVR, aVL, and aVF are known as limb or peripheral Leads. Leads V$_1$, V$_2$, V$_3$, V$_4$, V$_5$, and V$_6$ are known as *chest* or *precordial* Leads. In limb Leads, electrodes are placed on the arms and legs or outer areas of the chest. In chest Leads, electrodes are attached to very specific areas of the chest.

The placement of electrodes for the chest Leads is sometimes changed slightly to "see" a specific area of the heart more clearly. The chest Leads (V$_1$ through V$_6$) are then referred to as *modified chest Leads* (MCL) and become MCL$_1$ through MCL$_6$. These leads are discussed in more detail in a 12-Lead ECG course.

Patients are usually monitored in Lead II or MCL$_1$. Lead II shows the movement of the electrical impulse (depolarization) through the ventricles most clearly, and MCL$_1$ shows the depolarization of the atria.

In Lead II, the negative electrode is placed on the patient's right upper chest and the positive electrode on the left lower chest. The ground electrode is usually positioned on the left upper chest; however, the ground lead may be placed anywhere on the body because its purpose is to reduce static (Figure 2-5).

In the MCL$_1$ Lead, the positive electrode is placed on the patient's mid-chest to the right of the sternum and the negative electrode on the left upper chest. The ground electrode may be applied anywhere on the body, but is usually positioned on the left lower chest (Figure 2-6).

Most current telemetry units are capable of monitoring two or more leads at the same time.

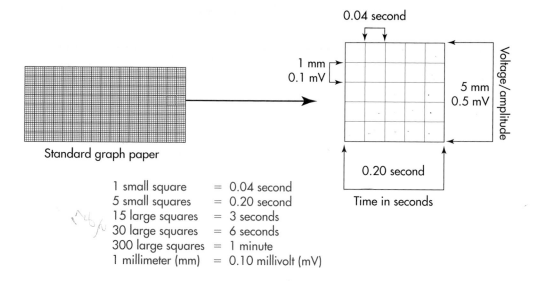

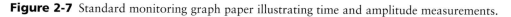

1 small square	= 0.04 second
5 small squares	= 0.20 second
15 large squares	= 3 seconds
30 large squares	= 6 seconds
300 large squares	= 1 minute
1 millimeter (mm)	= 0.10 millivolt (mV)

Figure 2-7 Standard monitoring graph paper illustrating time and amplitude measurements.

"How To" place the color-coded leads is usually described on the back of the telemetry unit.

NOTE: Most rhythms included in this book are described as they appear in Lead II or MCL$_1$ on an adult patient.

Graph Paper

The rhythm strip provides a printed record of cardiac electrical activity and is printed on ruled *graph paper*. Graph paper is divided into small squares that are 1 mm in height and width. The paper is further divided by darker lines every fifth square, both vertically (top to bottom) and horizontally (side to side). Each large square is 5 mm high and 5 mm wide.

Graph paper measures both time and amplitude. *Time* is measured on the horizontal line. Each small square is equal to **0.04 second,** and each large square (five small squares) is equal to **0.20 second.** These squares measure the length of time it takes an electrical impulse to pass through a specific part of the heart (Figure 2-7).

The force of the electrical impulse is measured by *amplitude.* Amplitude is measured on the vertical line. Each small square on the graph paper is equal to **0.1 millivolt** (mV), and each large square (five small squares) is equal to **0.5 mV.**

COMPLEX COMPONENTS

Each wave seen on the graph paper or monitor screen represents an electrical impulse in a specific part of the heart. (Wave components used in this book are described as they appear in Lead II.)

Baseline

The *baseline,* or *isoelectric line,* is the straight line, without any waves, that can be seen on either the monitor or the graph paper. It represents the absence of electrical activity in the cardiac tissue. All waves begin and end at the baseline. A *deflection* (wave) above the baseline is positive (+) and indicates electrical flow **toward** a

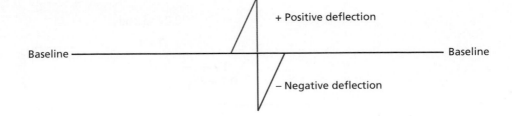

Figure 2-8 Baseline (isoelectric line) with positive and negative deflections.

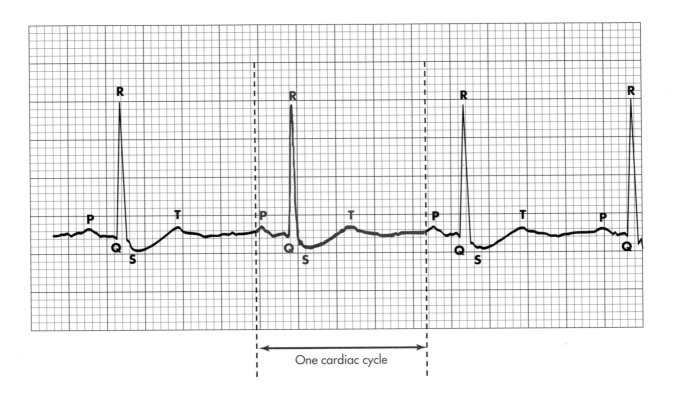

Figure 2-9 Cardiac cycle with P, Q, R, S, T waves, and baseline.

positive electrode. A deflection below the baseline is negative (−) and indicates an electrical flow **away from** a positive electrode (Figure 2-8).

The conduction of an electrical impulse for a single heart beat normally contains five major waves: P, Q, R, S, and T. The combination of these five waves, plus the baseline, represents a single heartbeat, or one *cardiac cycle*. A cardiac cycle is measured from the beginning of one P wave to the beginning of the next P wave (Figure 2-9).

P Wave

The *P wave* is the first positive (upward) deflection before the QRS complex. The P wave represents the depolarization of both the right and the left atria (Figure 2-10, *A* through *E*). The repolarization of the atria is not usually seen on the rhythm strip because the wave that shows the recovery of the atrial cells is buried in the QRS complex.

A normal P wave is well rounded and two small boxes or less in height. P waves can also be described as peaked (more than two small boxes in height), notched ("m" shaped), inverted (negative deflection below the baseline), absent, and biphasic or diphasic (both above and below the baseline).

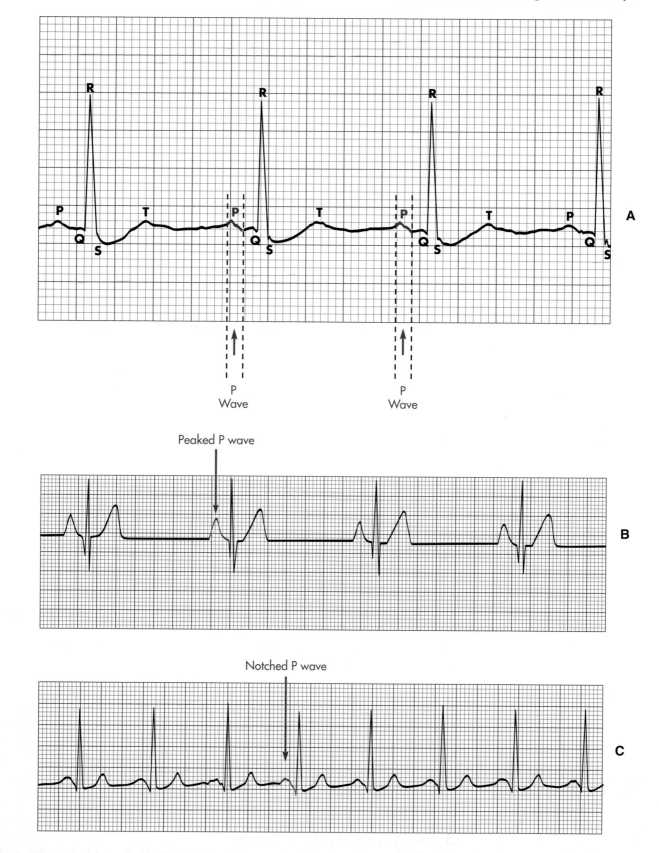

Figure 2-10 P waves. **A,** Normal shaped P waves. **B,** Peaked P waves, greater than 2 small boxes in height. **C,** Notched P waves, "m" shaped.

Continued

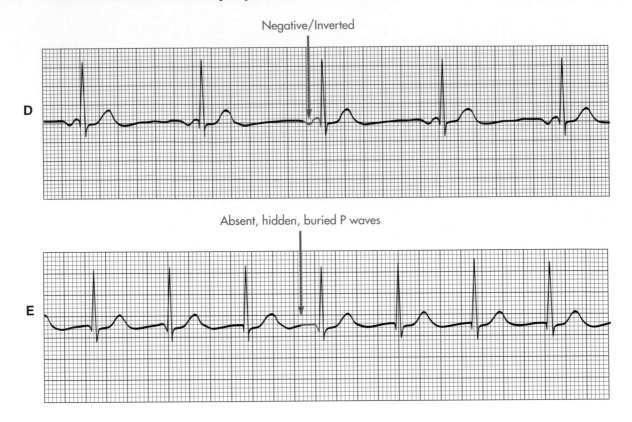

Figure 2-10, cont'd P waves. **D,** Negative/inverted P waves, below the baseline. **E,** Absent, hidden, buried P waves. (Both D and E are seen when the electrical impulse is initiated from the AV junctional area.)

These changes in P waves could be evidence of the following:

- *Peaked P waves* may indicate enlargement of the right atria.
- *Notched P waves* may signify enlargement of the left atria.
- *Negative/inverted and absent P waves* are usually a sign of electrical conduction that is initiated from the AV junction.
- *Biphasic or diphasic P* waves may indicate enlargement of both atria, seen only with a 12 lead ECG.

PR Interval

The *PR interval (PRI)* represents the time it takes an electrical impulse to be conducted through the atria and the atrioventricular node until the impulse begins to cause ventricular depolarization. The PR interval is measured from the beginning of the P wave to the beginning of the next deflection of the baseline. The normal PRI is **0.12 to 0.20 second,** or three to five small squares on the graph paper (Figure 2-11). An abnormal PRI indicates a disturbance in the electrical conduction pathway.

QRS Complex

The *QRS complex* usually contains three waves: the Q, R, and S. The *Q wave* is the first negative (downward) deflection following the PRI. The *R wave* is the first positive deflection after the P wave. The *S wave* is the first negative deflection that follows the R wave (Figure 2-12). Although the Q wave may not be present in all Leads, this combination of waves is still called a **QRS complex.**

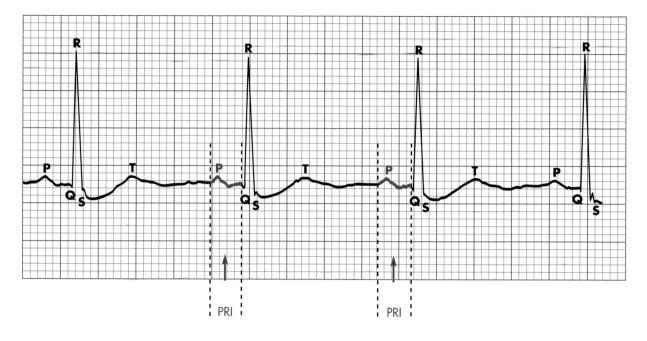

Figure 2-11 PR intervals.

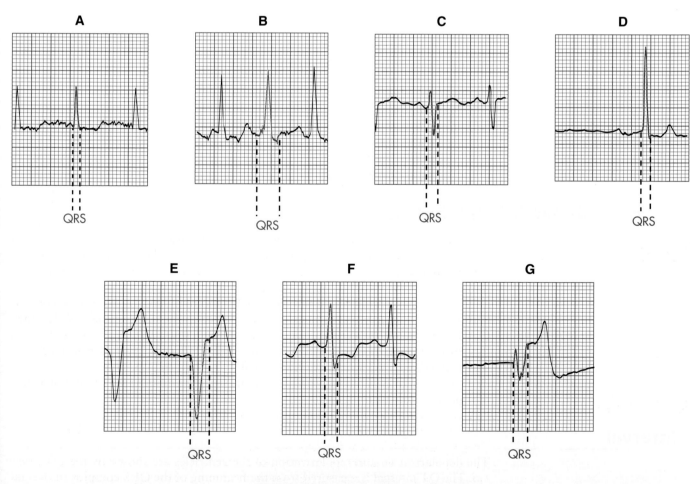

Figure 2-12 A to G, QRS complexes.

The QRS complex represents ventricular depolarization, or the conduction of an electrical impulse from the bundle of His through the ventricular muscle.

The measurement of the QRS complex starts at the beginning of the Q wave (or the R wave if the Q wave is not present). The QRS measurement ends where the S wave meets the baseline, or where the S wave would meet the baseline if it did not curve into the ST segment.

The QRS complex normally measures less than **0.12 second**, or less than three small squares on the graph paper. A QRS complex that measures greater than 0.12 second indicates a disturbance in the electrical conduction pathway.

ST Segment

The portion of the line that leads from the end of the S wave to the beginning of the T wave is the *ST segment* (Figure 2-13, *A*). The ST segment may be normal (flat), elevated (more than one small box above the baseline), or depressed (more than one small box below the baseline) (Figure 2-13, *B* and *C*). The baseline may be easiest to identify either immediately before the P wave or before the QRS wave. The beginning of the T wave may be difficult to determine in elevated ST segments.

Changes in the ST segment, as little as one small box (0.1 mV) above or below the baseline, may indicate cardiac problems, such as ischemia (decreased supply of oxygen) or cardiac disease. However, these changes can be used to diagnose a cardiac problem only when seen in a 12-Lead ECG.

T Wave

The *T wave* follows the ST segment and indicates the repolarization of the ventricular myocardial cells (Figure 2-14, *A*). The T wave may be either above or below the baseline (isoelectric) line.

A T wave greater than half the height of the QRS complex is *elevated* (peaked) and may indicate new ischemia of the cardiac muscle (Figure 2-14, *B*). A *depressed* (inverted) T wave follows an upright QRS complex, is below the isoelectric line, and looks upside down (Figure 2-14, *C*). An inverted T wave is frequently an indication of previous cardiac ischemia.

A T wave that is seen both above and below the baseline is called biphasic or diphasic, while a T wave that cannot be seen is identified as *flat* (Figure 2-14, *D*). These variations could also be evidence of heart muscle ischemia or of changes in the blood level of potassium.

P to P Intervals and R to R Intervals

The P to P interval is the length of time from one P wave to the next P wave. It is usually measured from the beginning of the P wave to the beginning of the next P wave. However, any part of the P wave can be used for measurement, as long as the identical part of each P wave is used.

The R to R interval is the length of time from one R wave to the next R wave. It is usually measured from the peak of one R wave to the peak of the next R wave. However, as when measuring P waves, any point on the R wave may be used, as long as the identical point is used on each R wave. These intervals can be measured by using either calipers or paper and pencil (see "Rhythm," p 39).

The measurements of these intervals are used to determine if the rhythm of a strip is regular or irregular.

QT Interval

The depolarization and repolarization of the ventricles are shown by the *QT interval*. The QT interval is measured from the beginning of the QRS complex to the end of the T wave.

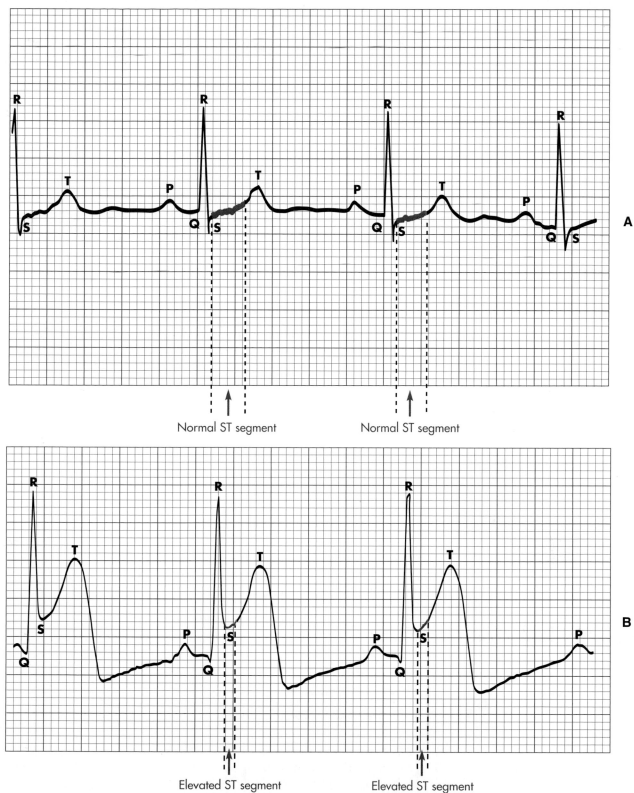

Figure 2-13 **A,** Normal ST segments. **B,** Elevated (peaked) ST segments.

Continued

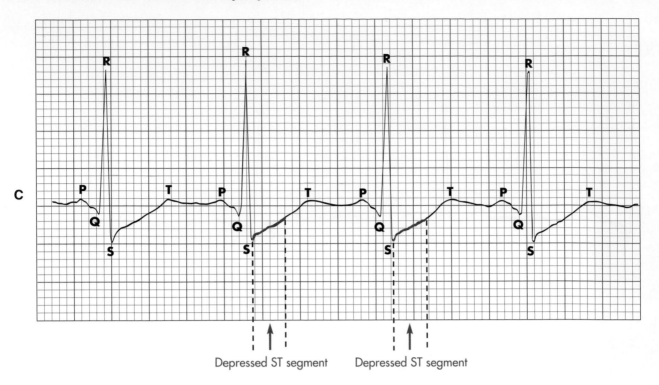

Figure 2-13, cont'd C, Depressed ST segments.

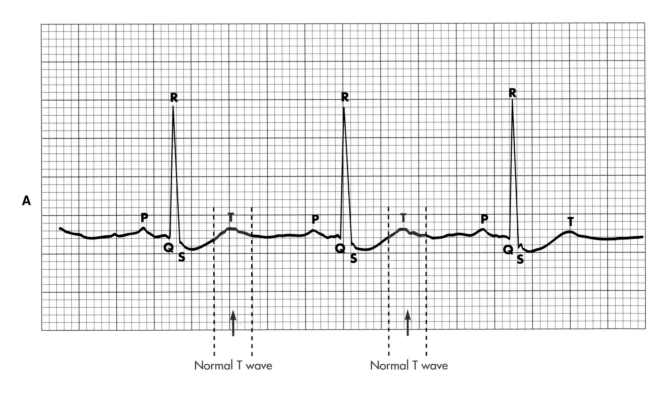

Figure 2-14 A, Normal T waves.

Continued

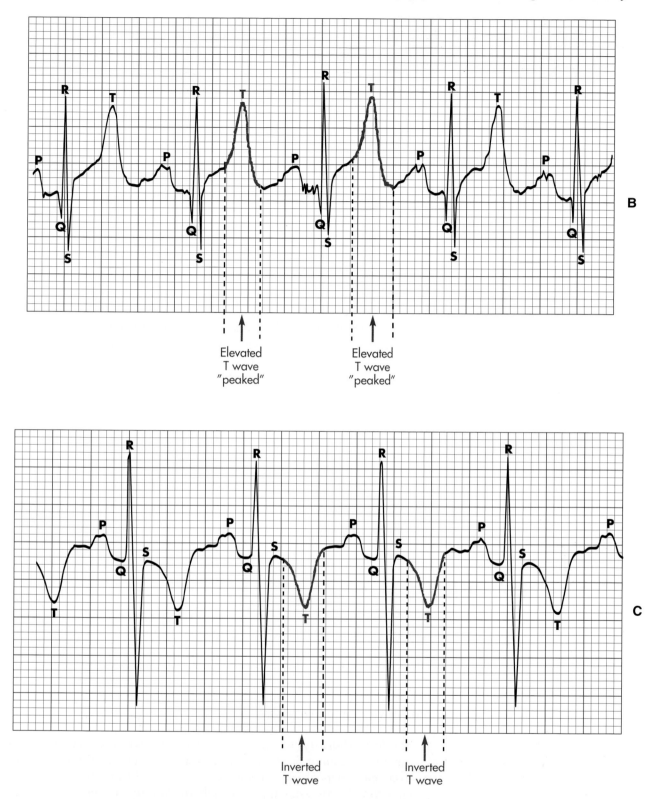

Figure 2-14, cont'd B, Elevated T waves. C, Depressed (inverted) T waves.

Continued

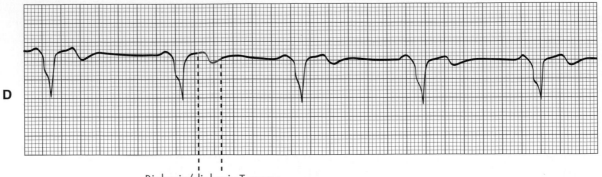

Biphasic/diphasic T waves

Figure 2-14, cont'd D, Biphasic or diphasic T waves.

QT intervals are either normal or prolonged. A normal QT interval is less than one-half the R to R interval of that complex and the R wave of the following complex (Figure 2-15, *A*). The QT interval can also be measured by counting the number of small boxes between the beginning of the QRS and the end of the T wave, multiplied by 0.04 second. In most cases, a QT interval of less than 0.44 second is considered normal. (This method of measurement is discussed in further detail in 12-Lead ECG courses and Advanced Life Support classes.)

A QT interval that is either greater than one-half the R to R interval of that complex and the R wave of the following complex or greater than 0.44 second is *prolonged* (Figure 2-15, *B*). A prolonged QT interval usually indicates a problem within the electrical conduction pathway of the heart.

> **NOTE:** The rhythm strip represents **only** the conduction of electrical impulses through the myocardial cells. Normally, it also represents the contraction of the heart muscle. However, this is not always true, so **you must treat the patient** and any symptoms that are present, **not the monitor.**

REFRACTORY PERIODS

In addition to identifying wave and complex formations, it will be helpful to understand refractory periods.

The *refractory period* is the time between depolarization and the return of the cardiac cells to the ready or polarized state. While the cells are recovering, the atria and ventricles are refilling with blood, preparing to contract again. The refractory period is divided into two phases:

1. *Absolute refractory period*—The cardiac cells have not completed repolarization and **cannot** be stimulated to conduct an electrical impulse and contract again (depolarize). This period is measured from the beginning of the QRS complex through approximately the first half of the T wave.
2. *Relative refractory period*—The cardiac cells have repolarized to the point that **some** cells can again be stimulated to depolarize, if the stimulus is strong enough. However, if these cells are stimulated during this period, they will probably conduct the electrical impulse in a slow, abnormal pattern. This period is measured from the end of the absolute refractory period (approximately the first half of the T wave) to the end of the T wave. The relative refractory period is also known as the *vulnerable period of repolarization* (Figure 2-16).

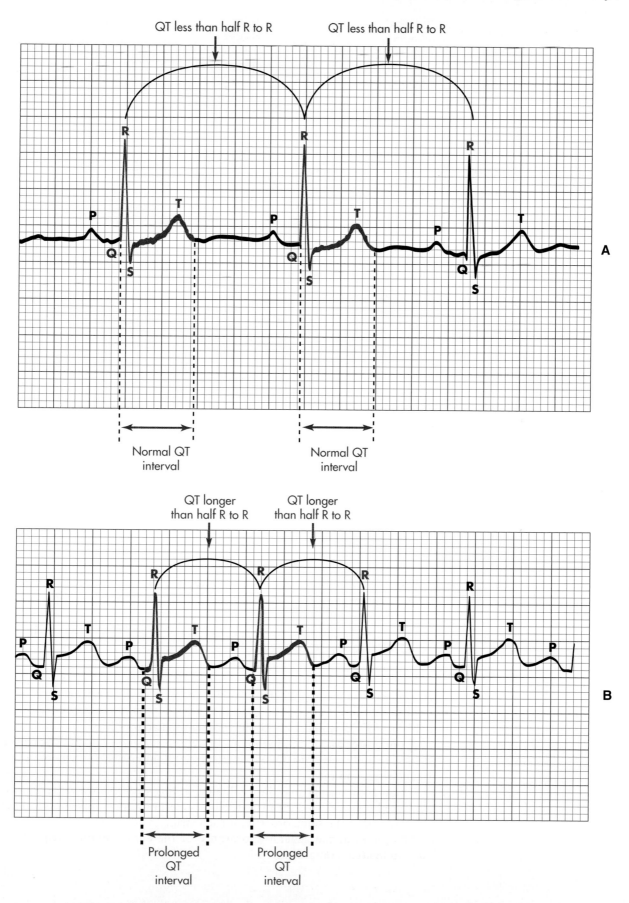

Figure 2-15 A, Normal QT intervals. B, Prolonged QT intervals.

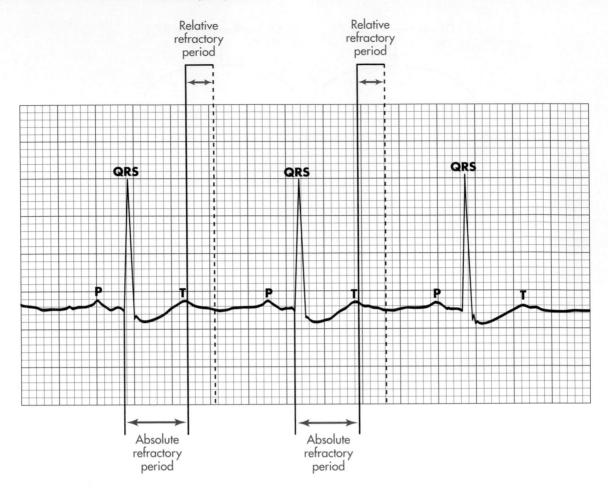

Figure 2-16 Absolute and relative refractory periods.

This information allows more accurate interpretation of dysrhythmias, particularly those involving premature ventricular contractions (see Chapter 6).

INTERPRETING A RHYTHM STRIP

A *rhythm strip* is a tool that assists the observer in the interpretation of a patient's cardiac rhythm. It also is useful to monitor changes in the cardiac cycle. However, a 12-Lead ECG is necessary to diagnose a cardiac problem.

To interpret a cardiac rhythm accurately, you must evaluate P waves (including the ratio of P waves to QRS complexes), PR intervals, QRS complexes, rhythm (regularity), and rate.

These components may be evaluated in any order; however, they must all be evaluated on every rhythm strip. Rhythm interpretation is easier if each component is examined in the same order with each strip.

First, look at the general appearance of the entire rhythm strip; then examine each individual component.

Complex Formation

The **appearance** of the P, Q, R, S, and T waves and the **ratio** of P waves to QRS complexes should be evaluated. Examine each cardiac cycle from the beginning to its end.

1. *P waves*—Examine each P wave.
   a. Are P waves present?
   b. Are they all upright?
   c. Do all P waves look alike?
   d. Is there a P wave before every QRS complex?
   e. Are the P to P intervals equal?
2. *PR intervals*—Measure each PRI.
   a. Are PRIs present?
   b. Are all PRIs equal?
   c. Are all PRIs within the normal range of 0.12 to 0.20 second?
3. *QRS complexes*—Examine and measure each QRS complex.
   a. Are QRS complexes present?
   b. Do all QRS complexes look alike?
   c. Is there a QRS complex after every P wave?
   d. Are the R to R intervals equal?
   e. Are all QRS complexes within the normal range of less than 0.12 second?

The shape and measurement of ST segments, T waves, and QT intervals are not required for the interpretation of cardiac rhythms. However, they can be important as indicators of changes in a patient's cardiac condition, such as new ischemia. Therefore, any abnormal change in the P wave, ST segment, T wave, or QT interval should be included in the interpretation of a cardiac rhythm strip.

Rhythm

The term *rhythm* is used to describe how regularly the complexes occur. To determine if the complexes occur regularly, measure the R to R intervals and the P to P intervals (if P waves are present). If the R to R intervals are equal, the ventricular rhythm is regular (Figure 2-17). If the P to P, R to R, or both intervals vary by less than 0.06 second (1.5 small squares), the rhythm can be considered regular. If the intervals vary by more than 0.06 second, the rhythm is irregular. The P to P intervals are also measured to determine if the atrial rhythm is regular.

Calipers provide the most accurate method of measuring rhythm. Place the point of one caliper leg on the top of an R wave (Figure 2-18, *A*). Adjust the caliper so the point of the second caliper leg is on the top of the next R wave. Then twist the caliper so that the point of the first leg is going toward the third R wave. If the rhythm is regular, the second caliper point will be on the top of the third R wave (Figure 2-18, *B*). Continue moving the calipers across the rhythm strip, measuring the distance between each two R waves, to check the regularity of the R waves (Figure 2-18, *C*). The rhythm is irregular if the measurement differs by more than 0.06 second. The P to P rhythm can be checked in the same way using P waves instead of R waves.

When calipers are not available, an acceptable alternative involves the use of a blank piece of paper and a pencil. Place the paper over the rhythm strip so only the tips of the R waves are showing. Mark small dots on the paper where the first two R waves occur. Then move the paper so the first dot is now on the second R wave. If the rhythm is regular, the second dot will fall on the next R wave. Continue moving the paper across the rhythm strip in this manner to check the regularity of each R wave. The P to P rhythm can be checked in the same way (Figure 2-19, *A* through *C*).

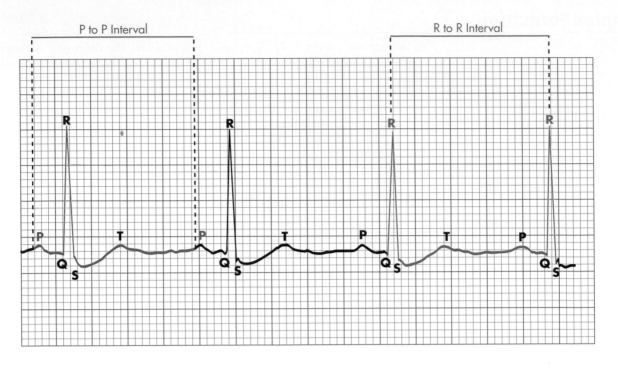

Figure 2-17 P to P interval and R to R interval.

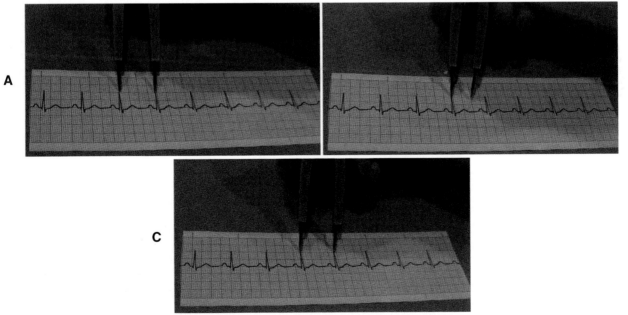

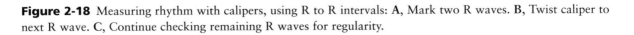

Figure 2-18 Measuring rhythm with calipers, using R to R intervals: **A**, Mark two R waves. **B**, Twist caliper to next R wave. **C**, Continue checking remaining R waves for regularity.

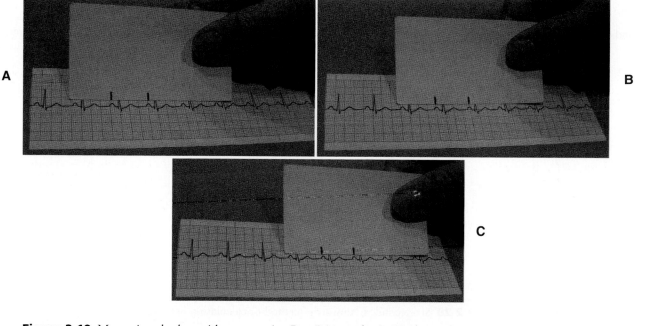

Figure 2-19 Measuring rhythm with paper, using P to P intervals. A, Mark two P waves. B, Move paper to next P wave. C, Continue checking remaining P waves for regularity.

Rate

Rate is the number of electrical impulses conducted through the myocardium in 1 minute. **Atrial rate** is determined by the number of P waves seen, while the **ventricular rate** is determined by the number of R waves. The ventricular rate <u>should</u> be the same as the patient's pulse, if the myocardium is contracting with each QRS complex and if the cardiac output is within normal limits.

Many methods of calculating rate exist, but the following are the methods used most frequently.

1. *Calculation by a 6-second rhythm strip.* The graph paper may have small indicator lines (vertical lines) in the top margin of the paper, which measure 1-second intervals. Every 3 seconds, the indicator line is longer or darker. The space between three long lines equals 6 seconds. To calculate the heart rate, count the number of R waves in a 6-second rhythm strip and multiply that number by 10. If a QRS complex falls directly under the beginning or ending indicator line, it is included in the total number of R waves counted. This calculation gives an *approximate* heart rate per minute (Figure 2-20). If the graph paper does not have 1- or 3-second interval lines, you can:
   a. Measure 6 inches of the paper to get a 6-second strip, because 1 inch of graph paper equals 1 second. Then count the number of R waves in the strip and multiply that number by 10.
   b. Count the number of R waves in 30 large squares and multiply that number by 10, because 30 large squares equal 6 seconds.

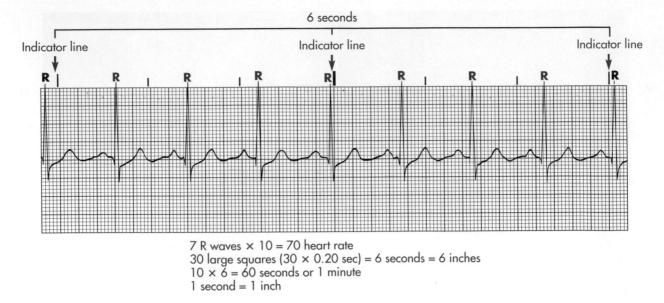

7 R waves × 10 = 70 heart rate
30 large squares (30 × 0.20 sec) = 6 seconds = 6 inches
10 × 6 = 60 seconds or 1 minute
1 second = 1 inch

Figure 2-20 Six-second rhythm strip method of calculating heart rate.

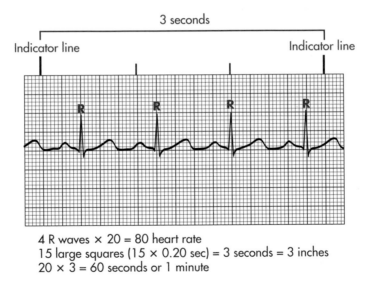
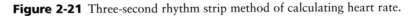

4 R waves × 20 = 80 heart rate
15 large squares (15 × 0.20 sec) = 3 seconds = 3 inches
20 × 3 = 60 seconds or 1 minute

Figure 2-21 Three-second rhythm strip method of calculating heart rate.

2. *Calculation by a 3-second rhythm strip.* The space between two long indicator lines equals 3 seconds (3 inches). Count the number of R waves between the two long lines and multiply by 20, or count the number of R waves in 15 large squares and multiply by 20. This calculation gives an *approximate* heart rate per minute (Figure 2-21).

3. *Calculation by division.* This method is more precise than the first two methods; however, **it should only be used when the rhythm is regular.** To use this method, count the number of large squares between two R waves and divide 300 by this number to determine the heart rate. For example, 300 divided by 3 (number of large squares between two R waves) equals 100. The heart rate is 100.

   When counting the number of large squares between two R waves, if part of a large square is included, count each small square as 0.2. Add the number of large and small squares and then divide 300 by that number. For example, 4 large and 4 small squares equal 4.8 squares; 300 divided by 4.8 equals 62.5. The heart rate is approximately 63 (Figure 2-22).

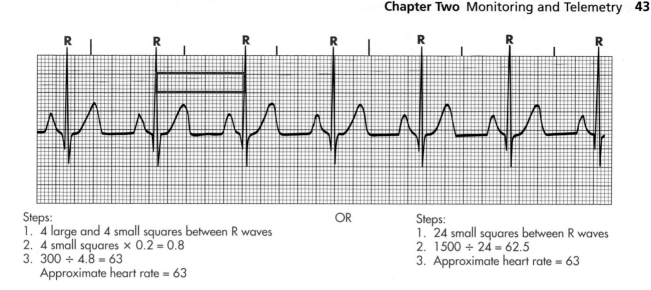

Steps:
1. 4 large and 4 small squares between R waves
2. 4 small squares × 0.2 = 0.8
3. 300 ÷ 4.8 = 63
   Approximate heart rate = 63

OR

Steps:
1. 24 small squares between R waves
2. 1500 ÷ 24 = 62.5
3. Approximate heart rate = 63

Figure 2-22 Two division methods of calculating heart rate.

An additional method using calculation by division involves counting the number of small squares between two R waves. Then divide 1500 by that number to determine the rate. For example, in Figure 2-22, 24 small squares are between the two R waves: 1500 divided by 24 equals 62.5, or a heart rate of approximately 63.

4. *Calculation by a 1-minute rhythm strip.* This method is the most accurate for calculating rate. Count the number of R waves in a 1-minute rhythm strip. This method is rarely used because it requires a relatively long period of time to perform.

All heart rates in this book have been calculated by the 6-second rhythm strip method unless stated otherwise and are only approximate rates.

Take time to practice identifying the various components of many rhythm strips. These components are the *basic building blocks* needed for future identification of rhythms and dysrhythmias. The more you practice, the easier it will become to identify each component.

ARTIFACT

Artifact is interference or static seen on the monitor screen or rhythm strip. This interference may be caused by the electrode losing contact with the patient's skin, patient movement or shivering, a broken cable or lead wire, or improper grounding.

One type of artifact is *60-cycle interference,* which appears as a fuzziness of the baseline. The P wave may not be seen because of this interference, but the QRS is usually visible (Figure 2-23).

The 60-cycle interference is usually seen when the electrodes have lost contact with the patient's skin. This situation may result from excessive chest hair, sweaty skin, or the loss of conductive gel.

> **NOTE:** The conductive gel of the electrodes may dry out with prolonged use or improper storage. Be sure that the conductive gel is still moist and the electrodes are firmly attached to the patient's skin.

The 60-cycle interference also may be caused by either the patient or the lead cable touching a metal object, such as a bed rail. A blanket between the metal object and the patient or lead wire should correct the interference.

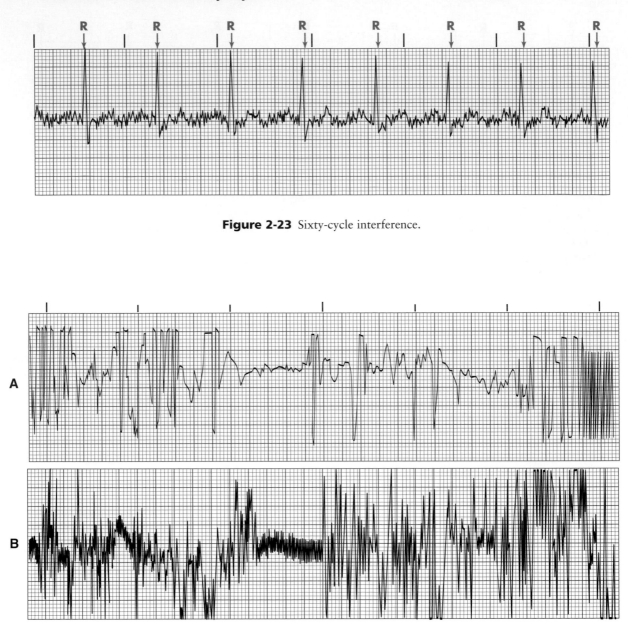

Figure 2-23 Sixty-cycle interference.

Figure 2-24 A, Artifact: rhythm not measurable. B, Artifact: rhythm not visible.

Outside the hospital setting, 60-cycle interference may be caused by electrical equipment, such as refrigerators, window air conditioners, or large fans.

Artifact that completely hides both the P wave and the QRS complex may be caused by either a loose lead or patient movement (Figure 2-24, *A* and *B*). Patient assessment is very important because this artifact can mimic a *lethal* (death-producing) dysrhythmia on the monitor or rhythm strip.

Patient movement or deep, rapid breathing also may cause an artifact in which the baseline moves up and down rapidly on the monitor screen or rhythm strip. This type of artifact is called a *wandering baseline* and is usually corrected when the patient lies still or when the electrode placement is changed (Figure 2-25).

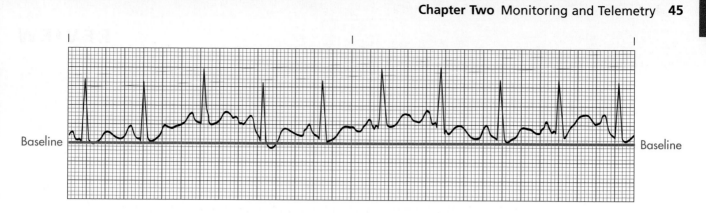

Figure 2-25 Wandering baseline.

REVIEW QUESTIONS

True   **False**   1. The monitor shows the conduction of the electrical impulses through the heart, not the actual contraction of the heart muscle.

True   **False**   2. Leads are color-coded wires that connect the telemetry unit to the patient's cardiac muscle.

True   **False**   3. Lead II and MCL1 are the two Leads most often used to monitor patients.

True   **False**   4. It is important to check complex formation, rhythm, and rate when interpreting a rhythm strip.

5. The P wave represents the depolarization of both the right and left

    a. ventricles

    b. atria and ventricles

    c. valves

    d. atria

6. The normal PR interval measures

    a. 0.04 to 0.12 second

    b. 0.4 to 0.12 second

    c. 0.12 to 0.20 second

    d. 0.04 to 0.20 second

7. The measurement of a normal QRS complex is

    a. 0.4 to 0.12 second

    b. 0.12 to 0.20 second

    c. 0.4 to 0.20 second

    d. 0.04 to 0.12 second

8. Identify the components and intervals included in one complete cardiac cycle.

    a. _____

    b. _____

    c. _____

    d. _____

    e. _____

    f. _____

    g. _____

9. The T wave represents

    a. depolarization of the ventricles

    b. repolarization of the atria

    c. polarization of all cardiac cells

    d. repolarization of the ventricles

10. A normal QT interval measures

_____

_____

_____

_____

11. Explain how to calculate heart rate using the 6-second rhythm strip method.

_____

_____

_____

_____

12. Calculate the heart rate using both of the division methods when the distance between two R waves is:

a. Three large squares

_____

_____

_____

_____

b. Four large and two small squares:

_____

_____

_____

_____

13. List two facts about PR intervals that are important to measure when you are interpreting a rhythm strip.

a. _____

_____

b. _____

_____

14. List five facts about QRS complexes that are important to evaluate when you are interpreting a rhythm strip.

a. _____

_____

b. _____

_____

c. _____

_____

d. _____

_____

e. _____

_____

15. Three common causes of artifact are

    a. patient movement; low amplitude; 60-cycle interference

    b. patient movement; slow respirations; loose leads

    c. patient movement; chest Leads; 60-cycle interference

    d. patient movement; loose leads; 60-cycle interference

16. Explain the difference between relative and absolute refractory periods.

    _____

    _____

    _____

    _____

17. Match each component with the correct description:

    _____ peaked p wave

    _____ normal p wave

    _____ notched p wave

    _____ biphasic wave

    _____ prolonged QT interval

    _____ depressed ST segment

    _____ elevated ST segment

    _____ depressed T wave

    _____ elevated T wave

    a. greater than one-half the height of the QRS complex

    b. a wave that is both above and below the baseline

    c. more than one small box above the baseline

    d. "m"-shaped wave

    e. follows an upright QRS and looks upside down

    f. well rounded; less than two small boxes in height

    g. absent or not seen

    h. more than one small box below the baseline

    i. more than two small boxes in height

    j. greater than one-half the R to R interval of that complex and the R wave of the following complex

RHYTHM STRIP REVIEW

Example

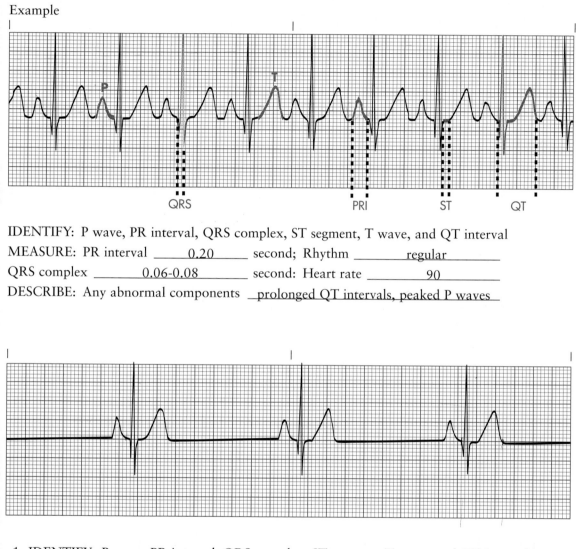

QRS   PRI ST QT

IDENTIFY: P wave, PR interval, QRS complex, ST segment, T wave, and QT interval

MEASURE: PR interval _____0.20_____ second; Rhythm _____regular_____

QRS complex _____0.06-0.08_____ second: Heart rate _____90_____

DESCRIBE: Any abnormal components __prolonged QT intervals, peaked P waves__

1. IDENTIFY: P wave, PR interval, QRS complex, ST segment, T wave, and QT interval

   MEASURE: PR interval _____ second; Rhythm _____

   QRS complex _____ second: Heart rate _____

   DESCRIBE: Any abnormal components _____

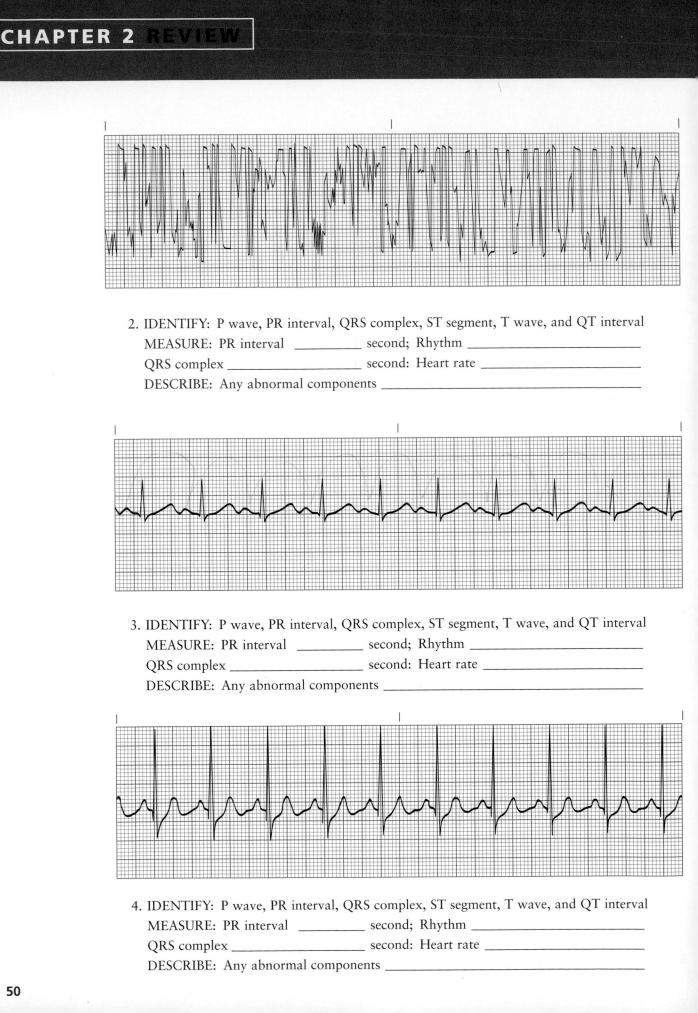

2. IDENTIFY: P wave, PR interval, QRS complex, ST segment, T wave, and QT interval
   MEASURE: PR interval _____ second; Rhythm _____
   QRS complex _____ second: Heart rate _____
   DESCRIBE: Any abnormal components _____

3. IDENTIFY: P wave, PR interval, QRS complex, ST segment, T wave, and QT interval
   MEASURE: PR interval _____ second; Rhythm _____
   QRS complex _____ second: Heart rate _____
   DESCRIBE: Any abnormal components _____

4. IDENTIFY: P wave, PR interval, QRS complex, ST segment, T wave, and QT interval
   MEASURE: PR interval _____ second; Rhythm _____
   QRS complex _____ second: Heart rate _____
   DESCRIBE: Any abnormal components _____

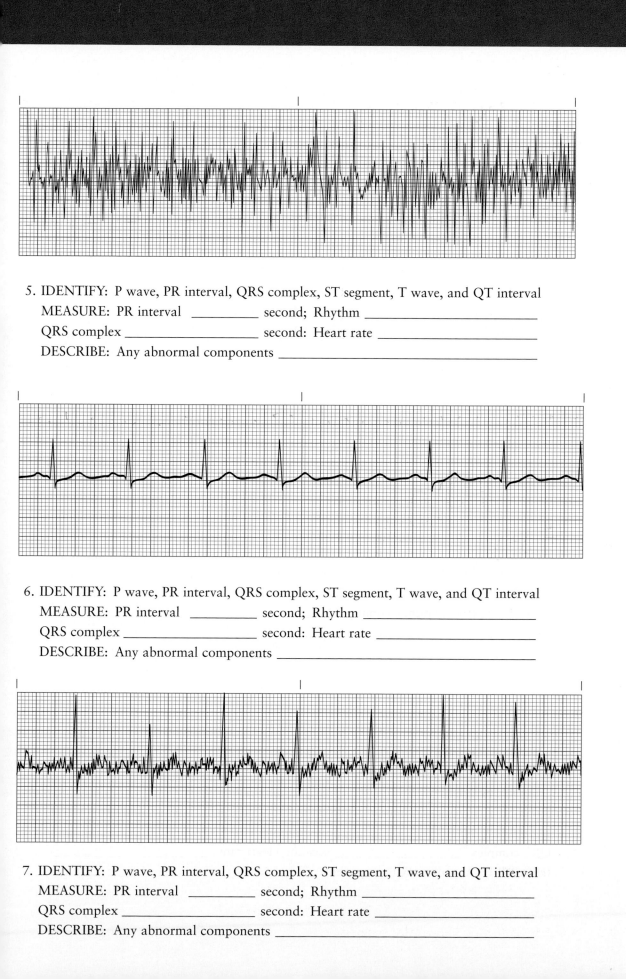

5. IDENTIFY: P wave, PR interval, QRS complex, ST segment, T wave, and QT interval
   MEASURE: PR interval _____ second; Rhythm _____
   QRS complex _____ second: Heart rate _____
   DESCRIBE: Any abnormal components _____

6. IDENTIFY: P wave, PR interval, QRS complex, ST segment, T wave, and QT interval
   MEASURE: PR interval _____ second; Rhythm _____
   QRS complex _____ second: Heart rate _____
   DESCRIBE: Any abnormal components _____

7. IDENTIFY: P wave, PR interval, QRS complex, ST segment, T wave, and QT interval
   MEASURE: PR interval _____ second; Rhythm _____
   QRS complex _____ second: Heart rate _____
   DESCRIBE: Any abnormal components _____

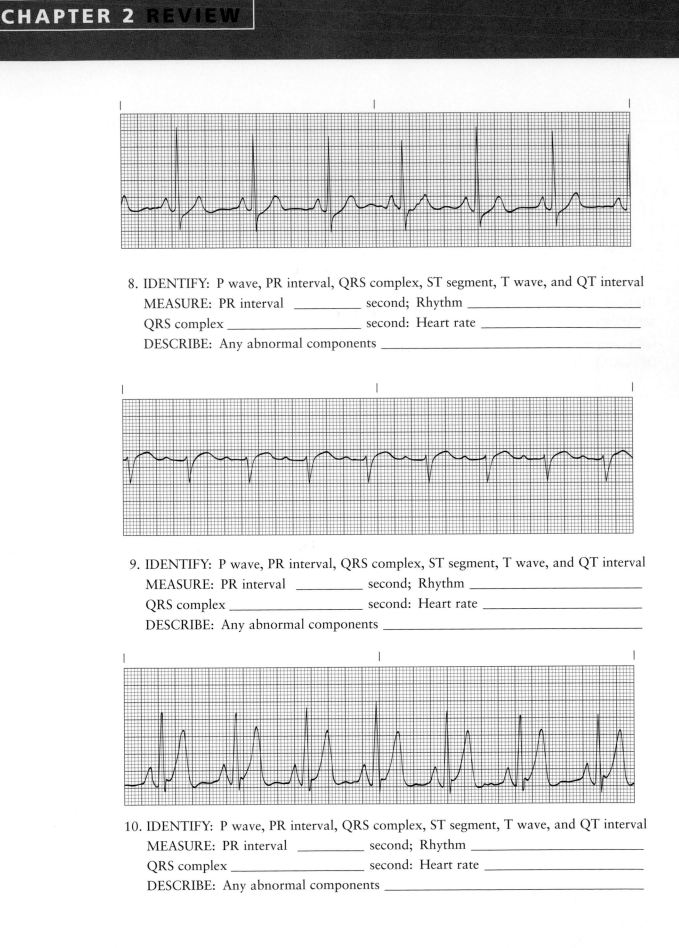

8. IDENTIFY: P wave, PR interval, QRS complex, ST segment, T wave, and QT interval
   MEASURE: PR interval _____ second; Rhythm _____
   QRS complex _____ second: Heart rate _____
   DESCRIBE: Any abnormal components _____

9. IDENTIFY: P wave, PR interval, QRS complex, ST segment, T wave, and QT interval
   MEASURE: PR interval _____ second; Rhythm _____
   QRS complex _____ second: Heart rate _____
   DESCRIBE: Any abnormal components _____

10. IDENTIFY: P wave, PR interval, QRS complex, ST segment, T wave, and QT interval
    MEASURE: PR interval _____ second; Rhythm _____
    QRS complex _____ second: Heart rate _____
    DESCRIBE: Any abnormal components _____

CROSSWORD PUZZLE CLUES

Across

1 The _____ rate is determined by the number of R waves seen in 1 minute.

4 The ____ ____ represents repolarization of the ventricles.

8 Interference or static seen on monitor.

9 Inverted T wave.

10 Above and below the baseline; moving in two opposite directions.

11 An ST segment above the baseline is _____.

17 A set of waves seen on monitor, which represents an electrical impulse traveling through the cardiac muscle.

18 Each _____ box on graph paper equals 0.04 second horizontally, and 0.1 mV vertically.

19 0.12 to 0.20 second is normal.

21 The number of P waves seen in 1 minute determines the _____ rate.

23 Depolarization of the atria.

24 Adhesive, conductive pad that connects patients to a telemetry monitor or electrocardiograph machine.

Down

2 Refractory period when cardiac cells have repolarized enough that some cells can respond to electrical impulse and depolarize.

3 Number of electrical impulses conducted through the myocardium in 1 minute.

5 Force of an electrical impulse is measured by _____.

6 Depolarization of the ventricles.

7 Baseline or _____ line.

12 Process of monitoring cardiac electrical activity.

13 ____ ____ measures both time and amplitude of cardiac electrical activity.

14 QT interval greater than one-half the R-to-R interval or greater than 0.44 second is _____.

15 Time between depolarization and repolarization of cardiac cells.

16 Refractory period when cardiac cells have not repolarized and cannot contract.

20 Describes how regular the complexes occur.

22 Different types of electrode placements on the patient's body; I, II, III, aVR, aVL, etc.

The solution to this crossword puzzle is in the answer section.

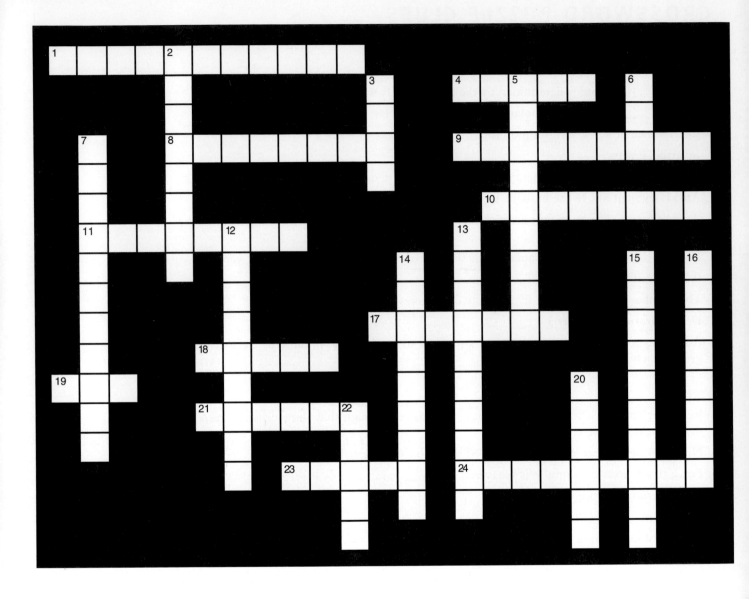

WORD PUZZLE

This word puzzle is designed to help familiarize you with some of the new terminology found in this chapter. Have fun finding all the words on this list. The words can be spelled forward (normally), backward, up, down, or diagonally in any direction. The words will always be in uppercase and found in a straight line. Good luck! **The solution to this word puzzle is in the answer section.**

```
P  G  C  D  E  P  O  L  A  R  I  Z  A  T  I  O  N  M  P  K  J  K
L  K  R  H  P  K  R  H  N  T  V  M  Y  Z  X  V  R  R  J  Z  N  T
C  L  K  A  J  R  R  M  B  X  L  A  V  R  E  T  N  I  T  Q  I  X
Q  E  C  G  P  G  I  J  H  J  Y  R  T  E  M  E  L  E  T  M  F  M
R  N  A  T  Y  H  N  N  F  K  X  Q  H  R  S  P  L  C  E  W  Y  Q
S  M  M  W  M  N  P  G  T  Q  N  L  B  T  R  K  M  K  G  N  V  F
C  R  P  L  N  Z  L  A  L  E  G  G  S  L  L  F  N  V  F  Q  U  M
O  E  L  S  Q  K  C  X  P  X  R  E  N  I  L  E  S  A  B  Y  L  K
M  F  I  E  L  N  B  I  L  E  G  V  M  H  T  Y  H  R  R  B  N  R
P  R  T  R  M  F  D  D  R  M  R  X  A  M  L  D  G  D  T  Q  E  M
L  A  U  I  L  K  N  E  E  T  M  Y  B  L  M  E  K  B  H  Z  R  X
E  C  D  W  F  L  E  N  G  H  C  Q  G  E  R  K  T  J  L  R  A  B
X  T  E  D  L  T  T  D  T  N  B  E  V  B  B  A  Y  K  O  T  B  R
N  O  T  A  I  G  C  R  O  F  O  A  L  N  C  E  K  T  Y  L  L  F
F  R  C  E  M  P  E  A  R  R  W  L  N  E  H  P  I  V  V  O  E  Z
Y  Y  P  L  M  V  H  K  F  T  T  P  O  M  O  N  D  L  W  V  P  C
T  P  Z  R  A  T  T  A  T  I  G  C  J  R  O  S  T  W  Q  I  E  V
J  E  J  W  C  Y  M  F  S  K  T  N  E  M  P  F  I  T  R  L  R  L
H  R  P  B  W  N  Z  Z  W  I  J  R  K  L  L  M  L  A  C  L  I  R
J  I  W  X  R  L  M  G  J  Y  C  P  A  B  E  C  T  N  K  I  O  D
J  O  T  N  R  D  K  W  M  B  V  J  W  T  L  E  B  G  L  M  D  N
T  D  H  C  H  R  J  T  J  B  I  P  H  A  S  I  C  J  R  M  V  N
```

AMPLITUDE	PR INTERVAL
ARTIFACT	PROLONGED
BASELINE	P WAVE
BIPHASIC	QRS COMPLEX
DEPOLARIZATION	QT INTERVAL
DIPHASIC	RATE
ECG	REFRACTORY PERIOD
ELECTRODE	RHYTHM
GRAPH PAPER	ST SEGMENT
ISOELECTRIC	TELEMETRY
LEAD WIRES	TIME
MILLIVOLT	T WAVE
MONITOR	VULNERABLE PERIOD

On completion of this chapter, the reader should be able to:

1 Describe the conduction of a normal electrical impulse from the sinoatrial node to the ventricular muscle.

2 Describe a normal sinus rhythm, including measurements of the components.

3 Identify sinus bradycardia, sinus tachycardia, and sinus arrhythmia.

4 Explain the differences between a sinus exit block and a sinus arrest, including measurements of the components.

5 Describe the appearance of a premature atrial complex, including measurements of the components.

6 Explain the primary difference between paroxysmal atrial tachycardia and supraventricular tachycardia.

7 Describe the appearance of atrial flutter, including measurements of the components and types of blocks/ratios.

8 Describe atrial fibrillation, including measurements of the components.

9 Describe Wolff-Parkinson-White syndrome, including measurements of the components.

CHAPTER 3

Sinus and Atrial Dysrhythmias

OUTLINE

DEFINITIONS

Accessory Pathway—Additional or abnormal electrical conduction pathway; the bundle of Kent (Kent bundle) is one accessory pathway

Antegrade—Downward movement of an electrical impulse from atria to ventricles

Atrial Dysrhythmia—Rhythm that is initiated from any pacemaker site in the atria, when the sinoatrial (SA) node fails to initiate an electrical impulse

Bradycardia—Heart rate slower than 60 electrical impulses per minute

Compensatory Pause—A pause in the rhythm that measures 2 times the R to R interval of the underlying rhythm

Delta Wave—Extra "bump" seen in the slurred section at the beginning of a QRS complex; seen in Wolff-Parkinson-White syndrome

Dysrhythmia—Abnormal cardiac rhythm; may be used interchangeably with the term arrhythmia

Inherent Heart Rate—Normal rate at which electrical impulses are generated; the inherent heart rate for the sinoatrial node is 60 to 100 heartbeats per minute

Noncompensatory Pause—A pause in the rhythm that measures less than 2 times the R to R interval of the underlying rhythm

Normal Electrical Conduction Pathway—Sinoatrial (SA) node to atrioventricular (AV) node, through the bundle of His and bundle branches, to the Purkinje's fibers, ending in the ventricular muscle

Paroxysmal—Sudden, intermittent start and stop of symptoms or dysrhythmias; usually used to describe a type of atrial tachycardia

Premature Complex—A complex that occurs earlier than expected in the underlying rhythm

Sinoatrial (SA) Node—Pacemaker of the heart; it usually initiates the electrical impulses that travel through the electrical conduction pathway of the heart

Continued

DEFINITIONS—*cont'd*

Sinus Rhythm—Cardiac rhythm that shows the movement of an electrical impulse traveling from the sinoatrial node to the ventricles, following the normal electrical conduction pathway

Tachycardia—Heart rate faster than 100 electrical impulses per minute

SINUS RHYTHMS

The sinoatrial (SA) node is located in the upper portion of the right atrium and is referred to as the *pacemaker of the heart* (see Chapter 1). The SA node normally initiates the electrical impulse that travels throughout the heart, leading to depolarization of the atria and ventricles (Figure 3-1). If the SA node fails to generate an electrical impulse, any other pacemaker cell within the atria is capable of initiating an impulse.

The SA node, as well as other pacemaker cells in the atria, normally generates 60 to 100 electrical impulses per minute. This is known as the *inherent heart rate of the atria*. In sinus rhythms, the electrical impulse travels from the SA node, through the atria to the atrioventricular (AV) node, continuing through the bundle of His and bundle branches, to the Purkinje's fibers, and ending in the ventricular muscle.

Because the electrical impulse follows the normal pathway throughout the heart, an upright P wave is present, representing atrial depolarization. The PR interval is within the normal limits of 0.12 to 0.20 second. The QRS complex, representing ventricular depolarization, measures less than 0.12 second (Figure 3-2). However, in some sinus rhythms, the length of PR intervals may vary within the normal limits.

Rhythms originating from the SA node are *sinus rhythms* or *sinus dysrhythmias* (abnormal rhythms), and rhythms originating from other atrial sites are *atrial dysrhythmias*. The term *dysrhythmia* is used to describe all cardiac rhythms except normal sinus rhythm.

Sinus dysrhythmias are usually not serious. However, as with any rhythm, **patient assessment** is essential to determine the patient's tolerance of the dysrhythmia.

NOTE: The patient is considered medically unstable if any combination of the following occurs: weakness, faintness, sudden decrease in blood pressure, chest pain, confusion, unresponsiveness, or any other sign or symptom of poor cardiac output.

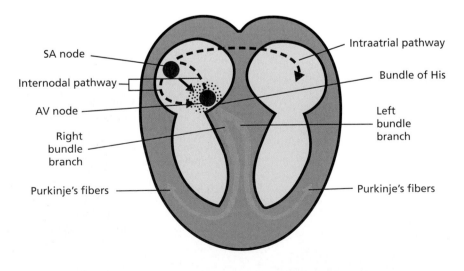

Figure 3-1 Normal cardiac electrical conduction pathway.

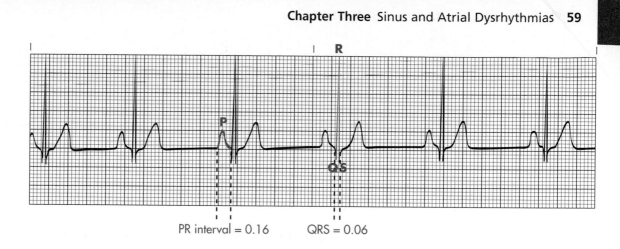

PR interval = 0.16   QRS = 0.06

Figure 3-2 Atrial rhythm strip with PR interval and QRS complex (notice peaked P waves).

Normal Sinus Rhythm

Normal sinus rhythm (NSR) is the ONLY rhythm considered "normal." In this rhythm, the SA node initiates all the electrical impulses that are transmitted throughout the heart. The SA node generates an impulse that travels downward, throughout both the right and the left atria, by means of the intraatrial and internodal pathways, causing atrial depolarization. The impulse is then transmitted through the AV node, the bundle of His, and both bundle branches to the Purkinje's fibers and ends in the ventricular muscle, where it causes ventricular depolarization (Figure 3-3).

Because the electrical impulse follows the normal conduction pathway, an upright P wave precedes every QRS complex. All PR intervals range from 0.12 to 0.20 second, and the QRS complex is less than 0.12 second. All P waves look alike, and all QRS complexes are the same size and shape.

In normal sinus rhythm, both the atria and the ventricles depolarize at regular intervals. Therefore, the P to P intervals and R to R intervals are regular. In addition, the P to P intervals are the same length as the R to R intervals. Normal sinus rhythm is very regular, and the rate is 60 to 100 electrical impulses per minute (Figure 3-4).

> **NOTE:** Rhythms included in this book are described as they appear in Lead II on an adult patient.

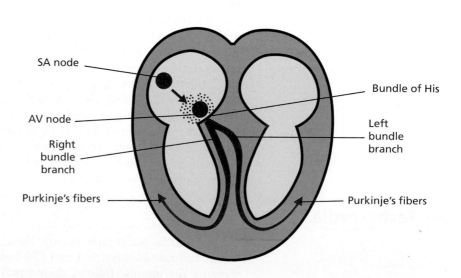

Figure 3-3 Normal electrical conduction pathway.

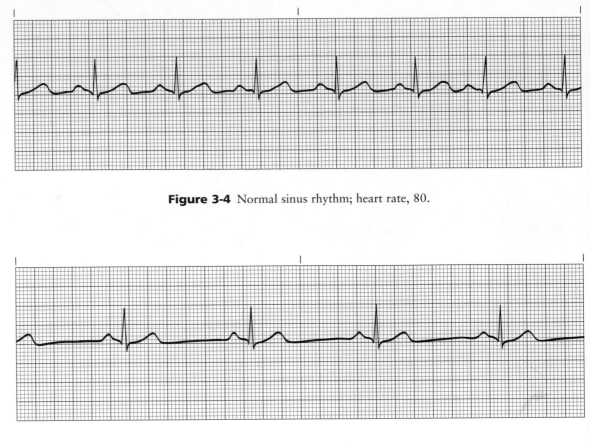

Figure 3-4 Normal sinus rhythm; heart rate, 80.

Figure 3-5 Sinus bradycardia; heart rate, 40.

Sinus Bradycardia

Sinus bradycardia (sinus brady) is a dysrhythmia that occurs when all electrical impulses originate from the SA node and follow the normal conduction pathway. However, the rate is slower than 60 impulses per minute (see Figure 3-3).

An upright P wave occurs before every QRS complex. The PR intervals remain within the normal range of 0.12 to 0.20 second, and the QRS complexes are less than 0.12 second. All P waves look alike, and QRS complexes are the same size and shape. Because the P to P intervals and the R to R intervals are regular and equal in length, the rhythm is regular. The rate can vary, but it must be slower than 60 electrical impulses per minute in sinus bradycardia (Figure 3-5).

Sinus bradycardia may be normal in sleeping individuals and athletes. However, it may become a dangerous dysrhythmia if the rate falls significantly or if the patient begins to show signs of poor cardiac output. These signs and symptoms include any combination of the following: pale, cool, clammy skin; cyanosis; dyspnea; confusion or disorientation; dizziness, weakness, or faintness; sudden decrease in blood pressure; shortness of breath; nausea or vomiting; decreased urinary output; mild or severe chest pain; or unresponsiveness.

Some common causes of sinus bradycardia are vomiting and/or drugs such as digitalis, morphine, and sedatives.

Sinus Tachycardia

Sinus tachycardia (sinus tach) occurs when all electrical impulses originate from the SA node at a rate between 101 and 150 beats per minute (see Figure 3-3).

Because the impulse follows the normal electrical conduction pathway, an upright P wave occurs before every QRS complex. PR intervals remain within the

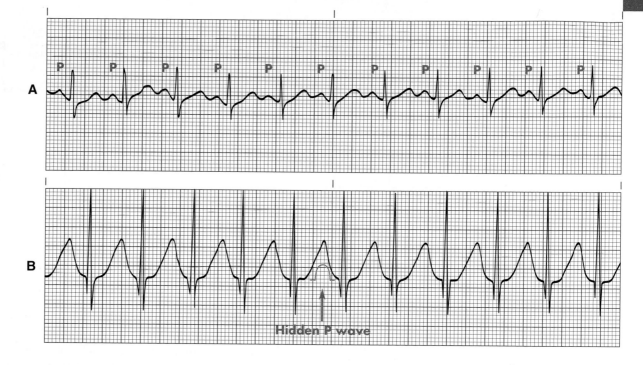

Figure 3-6 Sinus tachycardia. **A,** P waves seen; heart rate, 110. **B,** P waves buried in preceding T waves; heart rate, 110.

normal range of 0.12 to 0.20 second, and QRS complexes are less than 0.12 second (Figure 3-6, *A*). All P waves look alike, and all QRS complexes are the same size and shape.

As the rate of the tachycardia increases, the P waves are frequently hidden in the T wave of the preceding QRS complex, causing a slight change in the appearance of the T wave (Figure 3-6, *B*).

Because the P to P intervals and R to R intervals are usually regular and equal in length, the rhythm usually is regular. The rate can vary, but it usually falls between 101 and 150 electrical impulses per minute.

Sinus tachycardia may become a serious dysrhythmia if the patient becomes *medically unstable* (poor cardiac output).

The most common causes of sinus tachycardia are pain, fever, anemia, dehydration, hemorrhage (sudden loss of a large amount of blood), exercise, fear, sudden excitement, anxiety, or the effects of drugs such as atropine, nicotine, caffeine, or some street drugs.

Sinus Arrhythmia

Sinus arrhythmia occurs when the SA node initiates all the electrical impulses but at irregular intervals. The P to P intervals and the R to R intervals change with respirations, producing an irregular rhythm (see Figure 3-3).

Because the impulses are all generated by the SA node and follow the normal conduction pathway, an upright P wave still occurs before every QRS complex. The PR intervals remain within 0.12 to 0.20 second, and the QRS complexes are less than 0.12 second. All P waves look alike, and the QRS complexes are the same in size and shape.

Because the heart rate increases as the patient inhales and decreases as the patient exhales, the 6-second rhythm strip is a more reliable method of determining heart rate. However, the overall heart rate will usually be 60 to 100 electrical impulses per

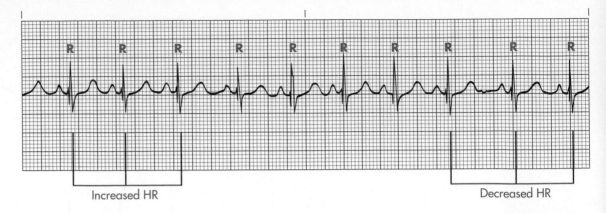

Increased HR · Decreased HR

Figure 3-7 Sinus arrhythmia. Heart rate increases with inspiration and decreases with expiration; overall heart rate, 100 (notice peaked P waves).

minute. P to P and R to R intervals are irregular, causing the rhythm to be irregular. The longest R to R interval will be **less** than twice the length of any of the remaining R to R intervals (Figure 3-7).

Although sinus arrhythmia is normal for infants and young children, it may be a warning of a diseased SA node or coronary artery disease in the adult patient. Sinus arrhythmia is usually not serious unless the patient's cardiac output decreases and the patient becomes medically unstable.

As with any rhythm, **patient assessment** is essential to determine the patient's tolerance of the dysrhythmia.

> **NOTE:** Normal sinus rhythm, sinus bradycardia, sinus tachycardia, and sinus arrhythmia all follow the normal electrical conduction pathway of the heart; only the rate or rhythm varies.

Sinus Exit Block and Sinus Arrest

Sinus exit block (sinus block) occurs when the SA node initiates an electrical impulse that is blocked and **not** conducted to the atria. The atria and ventricles do not depolarize, and a P wave will not be seen until the next conducted complex.

Sinus arrest occurs when the SA node does **not** initiate an electrical impulse. Because an impulse is not generated, depolarization will not occur and the next expected complex will not be seen.

Both dysrhythmias appear similar on the monitor screen or rhythm strip. P waves are absent, and QRS complexes are not seen because an impulse is not conducted to the ventricles to cause depolarization. The lack of both a P wave and QRS complex forms a *pause* on the monitor and rhythm strip.

The length of the pause may help determine whether the dysrhythmia is a sinus exit block or a sinus arrest. The pause of a sinus exit block is equal to **exactly** two or more previous cardiac cycles of the underlying rhythm. For example, the P to P interval of the underlying rhythm will fit into the pause of a sinus exit block exactly 2 times, or exactly 3 times, and so forth (Figure 3-8). The SA node continues to fire at its normal rate, so the rhythm will usually be regular except where the pause occurs.

The pause of a sinus arrest is not equal to exactly two or more cardiac cycles of the underlying rhythm. It will be **more** than 2 times the cardiac cycle of the underlying rhythm. For example, the P to P interval of the underlying rhythm will not fit into the pause of a sinus arrest exactly 2 times, or exactly 3 times, and so forth. Because the SA node is not firing, any pacemaker cell in the heart can begin to initiate electrical impulses. Therefore, the complex that ends the sinus arrest may be either atrial, junctional, or ventricular (Figure 3-9). The rhythm after the sinus arrest may be different than the rhythm before the pause.

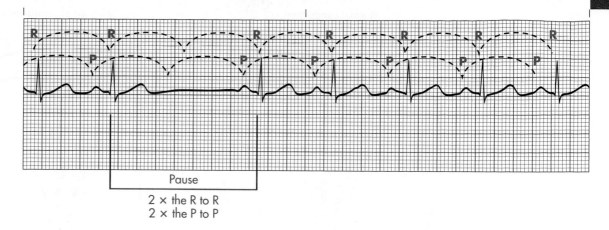

Figure 3-8 Sinus exit block; pause equal to two previous cardiac cycles; overall heart rate, 70.

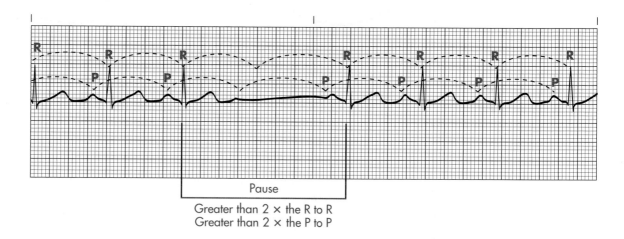

Figure 3-9 Sinus arrest. Pause will be more than 2 times the previous cardiac cycle of the underlying rhythm; overall heart rate, 70.

Both dysrhythmias may be caused by myocardial infarction (MI), ischemia (decrease supply of oxygen to tissues), hypoxia (lack of oxygen in the cells), or drugs such as digitalis or quinidine.

As with any rhythm, **patient assessment** is essential to determine the patient's tolerance of the dysrhythmia. Treatment should be started if the patient is medically unstable (i.e., if the patient has any combination of the following signs and symptoms: pale, sweaty skin; weakness; sudden change in blood pressure; chest pain, or any other symptoms of poor cardiac output).

> **NOTE:** *Sick sinus syndrome* (SSS) or *sinus pause* has been used in the past to describe a sinus rhythm with a pause. However, sick sinus syndrome is currently used to refer to any dysrhythmia caused by a disruption in the electrical conduction pathway of the atria.

ATRIAL DYSRHYTHMIAS

When the SA node fails to generate an electrical impulse, any other pacemaker site within the atria is capable of initiating the impulse. Cardiac rhythms originating from atrial sites are *atrial dysrhythmias*.

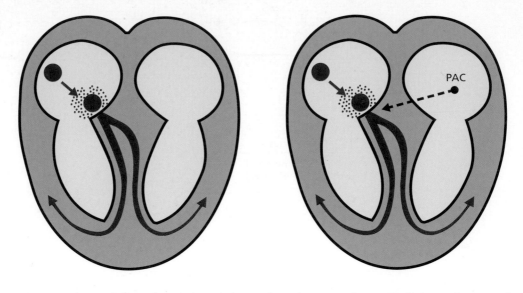

Figure 3-10 *Left heart* shows normal electrical conduction pathway. *Right heart* shows conduction pathway of a premature atrial complex (PAC).

In atrial dysrhythmias, the electrical impulse travels through the atria to the AV node, continues through the bundle of His and bundle branches to the Purkinje's fibers, and ends in the ventricular muscle. Although the depolarization of the atria will vary, depending on the atrial dysrhythmia, the ventricles usually depolarize in a normal manner.

Most atrial dysrhythmias are usually not *lethal* (death producing). However, as with any rhythm, **patient assessment** is essential to determine the patient's tolerance of the dysrhythmia.

Premature Atrial Complex

A *premature atrial complex (PAC),* formerly known as a premature atrial contraction, is an individual complex that occurs earlier than the next expected complex of the underlying rhythm. It originates from any atrial site outside the SA node (Figure 3-10). PACs usually occur in an underlying sinus rhythm, which may be regular except for the PAC.

> **NOTE:** Although the term **contraction** is sometimes used with a PAC, remember this complex represents electrical activity of cardiac muscle and may **not** reflect an actual contraction.

A PAC usually has the same characteristics as other atrial complexes. However, the P wave may appear different in size or shape than the P waves of the underlying rhythm, or it may be hidden in the T wave of the preceding complex.

The PAC is followed by a pause before the underlying rhythm returns. Two different types of pauses follow a premature complex: noncompensatory or compensatory. To determine the type of pause on the rhythm strip, measure the R to R intervals before and after the PAC in the following manner:

1. *Noncompensatory pause:* Measure from the R wave of the complex before the PAC to the R wave of the complex after the PAC. This measurement will be **less** than 2 times the R to R interval of the underlying rhythm. A noncompensatory pause could indicate the development of increased irritability in the SA node, causing it to generate an impulse sooner than expected in

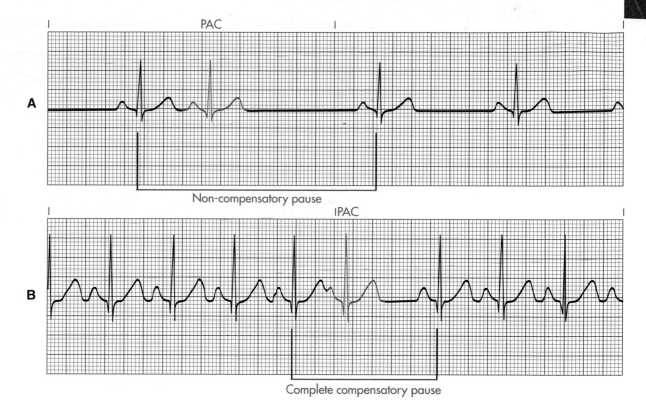

Figure 3-11 A, Premature atrial complex (PAC) with a noncompensatory pause in a sinus bradycardic rhythm; heart rate, 40. B, PAC with a complete compensatory pause in a sinus rhythm; heart rate, 80 to 90.

response to the premature beat. This increase in irritability could lead to sinus tachycardia. (This type of pause may also be called an *incomplete compensatory pause.*)

2. *Compensatory pause:* Measure from the R wave of the complex before the PAC to the R wave of the complex after the PAC. This measurement will **equal** at least 2 times the R to R interval of the underlying rhythm. In a compensatory pause, the SA node does not respond to the premature beat. Therefore there is no change in the rate or regularity of the underlying rhythm. (This type of pause may also be called a *complete compensatory pause.*)

A PAC is usually followed by a noncompensatory pause.

The underlying rhythm **must** also be identified when interpreting rhythm strips containing a PAC. Although a premature atrial complex may occur in any rhythm, it is easier to identify in a sinus rhythm or any rhythm with a bradycardia rate (Figure 3-11, *A* and *B*). When determining the rate of a rhythm containing a PAC, the R wave of the PAC is included in the total count of R waves.

A PAC represents increased irritability of the atria. Increased irritability indicates that the cardiac cells are able to respond to even a mild electrical stimulus and may depolarize in an unpredictable rate or manner. PACs may be caused by pain, fever, fear, anxiety, sudden excitement, exercise, or the effects of drugs such as digitalis, atropine, nicotine, caffeine, and some street drugs.

A PAC by itself is not a serious dysrhythmia. However, PACs are frequently monitored, because they may lead to a more serious dysrhythmia, such as paroxysmal atrial tachycardia.

Although a PAC is **not** a true atrial dysrhythmia but rather an individual complex, it is included in this chapter because it originates from the atria.

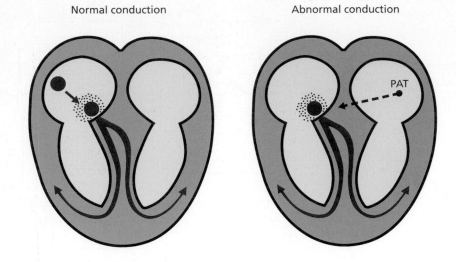

Figure 3-12 *Left heart* shows normal electrical conduction pathway. *Right heart* shows conduction pathway of paroxysmal atrial tachycardia/paroxysmal supraventricular tachycardia.

Paroxysmal Atrial Tachycardia/Paroxysmal Supraventricular Tachycardia

Paroxysmal atrial tachycardia (PAT) is the sudden onset of a tachycardia with a rate greater than 150 electrical impulses per minute. The most recent term for this dysrhythmia is *paroxysmal supraventricular tachycardia (PSVT)*. PAT/PSVT frequently is triggered by a PAC.

Because PAT/PSVT is usually initiated by an irritable site in the atria, a P wave occurs before every QRS complex (Figure 3-12). However, because of the rapid rate of PAT/PSVT, the P wave may be hidden in the T wave of the preceding complex. If P waves are seen, the PR intervals range from 0.12 to 0.20 second and the QRS complexes are usually less than 0.12 second.

The rhythm is regular because the P to P intervals and R to R intervals are regular and equal in length. The rate may vary from 151 to 250, or more, electrical impulses per minute. Because the rate is so rapid, the ventricles do not have time to fill completely before each contraction, causing a decrease in cardiac output.

Because most of the blood flow through the coronary arteries occurs between heartbeats, the rapid heart rate of a PAT/PSVT may also decrease the amount of oxygenated blood circulated to the heart muscle (myocardium).

The patient may complain of symptoms such as weakness, dizziness, palpitations, or a feeling that the heart is doing "flip-flops." PAT/PSVT may stop as suddenly as it starts, or it may require medical treatment if the patient becomes medically unstable.

A paroxysmal atrial tachycardia is not a lethal dysrhythmia but should be monitored closely, because this rapid rate cannot be tolerated for long periods of time.

To interpret a PAT/PSVT, the **beginning** of the PAT/PSVT **must** be seen, and the underlying rhythm that precedes the PAT/PSVT must be identified (Figure 3-13). If the onset of the PAT/PSVT is not seen, the dysrhythmia is called *supraventricular tachycardia*, providing it fits the other characteristics of PAT/PSVT.

A PAT/PSVT may be caused by stimulants such as caffeine, nicotine, or some street drugs.

Supraventricular Tachycardia

Supraventricular tachycardia (SVT) is the term used when a dysrhythmia fits all the characteristics of a PAT/PSVT but the beginning of the dysrhythmia is not seen. SVT is a general term that refers to **any** dysrhythmia that cannot be identified by other

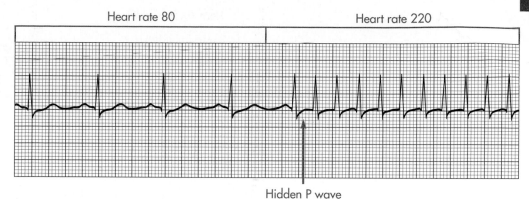

Hidden P wave

Figure 3-13 Normal sinus rhythm (NSR) progressing to paroxysmal atrial tachycardia/ paroxysmal supraventricular tachycardia; NSR: heart rate, 80; PAT/PSVT: heart rate, 220.

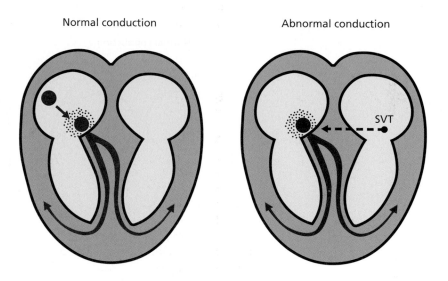

Figure 3-14 *Left heart* shows normal electrical conduction pathway. *Right heart* shows conduction pathway of supraventricular tachycardia (SVT).

means, originates from an irritable site **above the bundle of His,** and has a rate **greater** than 150 (Figure 3-14).

A P wave usually occurs before every QRS complex. However, the P wave may be hidden in the T wave of the preceding complex because of the rapid rate of the SVT. If P waves are seen, the PR intervals usually range from 0.12 to 0.20 second, and the QRS complexes usually measure less than 0.12 second. Any P waves that can be seen usually look alike, and the QRS complexes are usually the same size and shape. The P to P intervals and R to R intervals are regular and equal in length, and the rhythm is regular (Figure 3-15).

The rate of the SVT varies from 151 to 250, or more, electrical impulses per minute. A rhythm resembling SVT but with a heart rate less than 151 is called *sinus tachycardia.*

SVT usually is triggered by an irritable site within the atria. This irritability can be caused by stimulants such as caffeine, nicotine, or some street drugs.

SVT is treated if the patient becomes medically unstable. This dysrhythmia is usually not lethal, but the patient should be assessed frequently because the rapid rate cannot be tolerated for long periods of time.

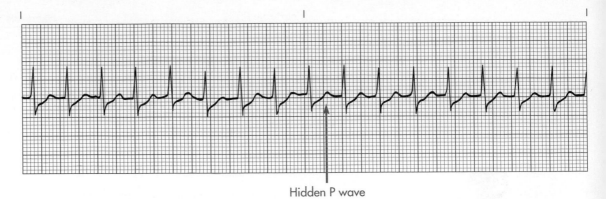

Hidden P wave

Figure 3-15 Supraventricular tachycardia (SVT): P waves hidden in preceding T waves; onset not seen; depressed ST segment; prolonged QT intervals; heart rate, 160.

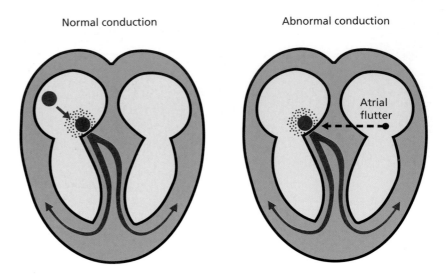

Figure 3-16 *Left heart* shows normal electrical conduction pathway. *Right heart* shows conduction pathway of atrial flutter.

Atrial Flutter

Atrial flutter occurs when a single irritable site in the atria initiates many electrical impulses at a rapid rate (Figure 3-16). The electrical impulses are conducted throughout the atria so rapidly that normal P waves are not produced. Instead of P waves, flutter waves *(F waves)* are formed.

Flutter waves have a typical "saw-toothed" or jagged appearance on the rhythm strip. They may not all look exactly the same, because some F waves may be buried in the QRS complex, ST segment, or T wave.

The negative (downward) stroke of the F wave represents atrial depolarization conducted through an abnormal electrical pathway. The positive (upward) stroke of the F wave indicates atrial repolarization.

During atrial flutter, the atria depolarize more rapidly than normal, but the AV node delays some of the electrical impulses, allowing the ventricles to depolarize at a normal rate. Therefore, every atrial impulse cannot be conducted to the ventricles, and a QRS complex is not present for every F wave.

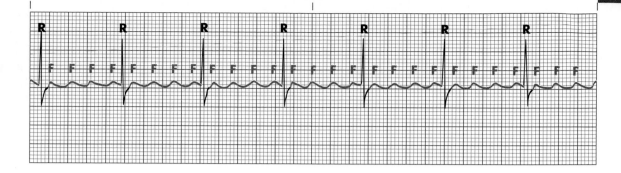

Figure 3-17 Atrial flutter: atrial heart rate, 280; ventricular heart rate, 70.

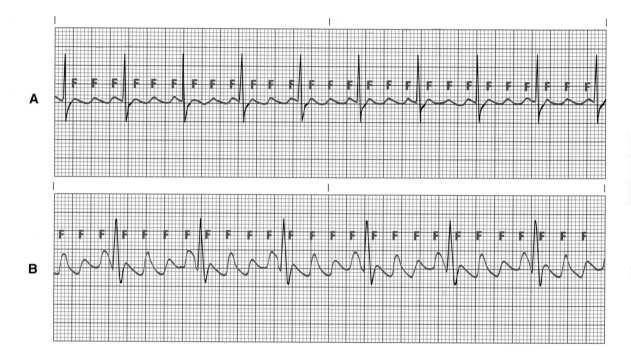

Figure 3-18 Atrial flutter. **A,** Atrial flutter with an atrial heart rate of 270, if counting F waves (or 300 if calculated by 3 × 100); ventricular heart rate of 100, 3:1 block/ratio. **B,** Atrial flutter with an atrial heart rate of 260, if counting F waves (or 240 if calculated by 4 × 60); ventricular heart rate of 60, 4:1 block/ratio.

The ventricles usually depolarize and repolarize at regular intervals, allowing them to respond to the atrial impulse at a regular rate, which may result in a regular ventricular rhythm.

The QRS complexes typically measure less than 0.12 second and usually occur at regular intervals. The ventricular rate, as measured by the number of QRS complexes, is usually 60 to 100 electrical impulses per minute. However, the atrial rate (F waves) usually ranges from 250 to 350 impulses per minute (Figure 3-17).

When an atrial flutter has a ventricular rate of less than 60 impulses per minute, it is called *atrial flutter with a slow ventricular response.* When the ventricular rate is 101 to 150 impulses per minute, it is called *atrial flutter with a rapid ventricular response.*

Because the ratio of flutter waves to each QRS complex further describes the dysrhythmia, it is important to determine the number of flutter waves for every QRS complex (Figure 3-18, *A* and *B*).

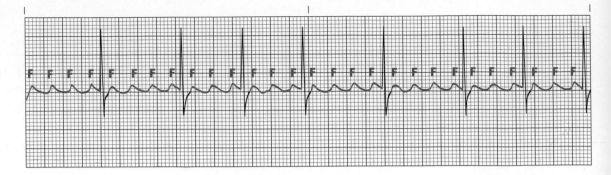

Figure 3-19 Atrial flutter with variable block/ratio; atrial heart rate of 280, if counting F waves (or 250 to 350 if using range); ventricular heart rate, 80.

Example: Two F waves with one QRS complex = 2:1 block/ratio
Three F waves with one QRS complex = 3:1 block/ratio
Four F waves with one QRS complex = 4:1 block/ratio
Five F waves with one QRS complex = 5:1 block/ratio

NOTE: The terms *block* and *ratio* may be used interchangeably.

If the number of flutter waves is the same before every QRS complex, the R to R intervals are equal throughout, and the rhythm is regular. When the number of F waves before each QRS complex varies, the R to R interval is irregular, and the rhythm is called *atrial flutter with a variable ventricular response* (Figure 3-19).

It is not always necessary to determine the actual atrial rate in atrial flutter. However, when an atrial rate does need to be calculated, there are two common methods that can be used:

1. Count the number of F waves in a 6-second strip and multiply that number by 10.
2. Multiply the number of F waves in the block/ratio by the ventricular heart rate, for example:
   a. In a 3:1 block/ratio, with a ventricular rate of 100, use the following shortcut:
      3 F waves (3:1 block/ratio) × 100 (ventricular heart rate) =
      300 F waves or an atrial heart rate of 300
   b. In a 4:1 block/ratio, with a ventricular rate of 60:
      4 F waves (4:1 block/ratio) × 60 (ventricular heart rate) =
      240 F waves or an atrial heart rate of 240

The second method of calculating atrial heart rate in atrial flutter can be used **only** if the block/ratio does not vary.

Atrial flutter may be caused by heart disease, myocardial infarction, or drug toxicity. This dysrhythmia is usually not lethal. However, it is frequently treated because it indicates increased irritability within the atria. This increased irritability may cause the dysrhythmia to progress to a more serious dysrhythmia.

The patient's symptoms vary depending on the cause of the atrial flutter, the ventricular response, and the patient's tolerance of the dysrhythmia.

Atrial Fibrillation

In *atrial fibrillation* (A Fib), an increased irritability of all the cardiac cells in the atria exists. Because of this increased atrial irritability, many sites within the atria attempt to initiate electrical impulses at the same time (Figure 3-20).

Normal conduction   Abnorma

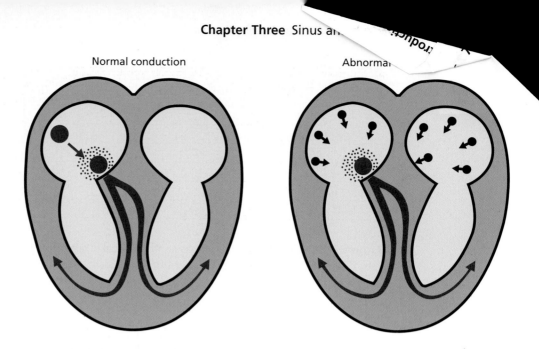

Figure 3-20 *Left heart* shows normal electrical conduction pathway. *Right heart* shows conduction pathway of atrial fibrillation.

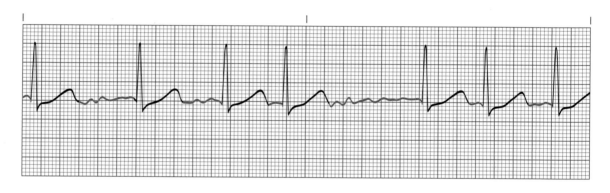

Figure 3-21 Controlled atrial fibrillation; atrial heart rate, 350 to 500; ventricular heart rate, 70.

Because so many electrical impulses are initiated, most of the impulses are not conducted; therefore the atria are not completely depolarized with each impulse. The atria do not contract forcefully; only a quivering movement *(fibrillatory waves)* occurs. These fibrillatory waves (fib waves) appear on the rhythm strip or monitor screen as a wavy baseline between each QRS complex. No true P waves or PR intervals exist.

At irregular intervals, one electrical impulse is conducted through the AV junction and ventricles, resulting in ventricular depolarization and a QRS complex. QRS complexes usually remain within the normal range of less than 0.12 second, and the R to R intervals are irregular throughout the rhythm strip. Frequently, one of the first clues that a dysrhythmia might be atrial fibrillation is seeing R to R intervals that are irregularly irregular (with no pattern to the irregularity).

The atrial heart rate is usually 350 to 500, or more, electrical impulses per minute. However, the AV node delays some of these electrical impulses, allowing the ventricular heart rate to usually remain within the normal limits of 60 to 100 impulses per minute. This dysrhythmia is known as *controlled atrial fibrillation* (Figure 3-21).

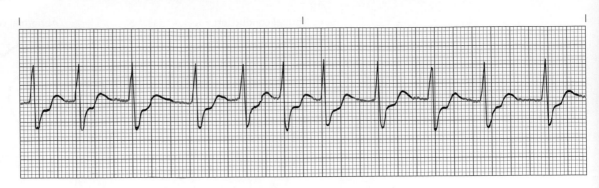

Figure 3-22 Atrial fibrillation with a rapid ventricular response: no distinguishable P waves; atrial heart rate, 350 to 500; ventricular heart rate, 110 (notice depressed ST segments).

Atrial fibrillation with a ventricular rate of less than 60 impulses per minute is called *atrial fibrillation* with a *slow ventricular response*. When this dysrhythmia has a ventricular rate of 101 to 150 impulses per minute, it is called *atrial fibrillation with rapid ventricular response* (Figure 3-22). Atrial fibrillation with a ventricular rate greater than 150 impulses per minute is called *uncontrolled atrial fibrillation*.

Atrial fibrillation is not usually considered lethal and may frequently occur in elderly patients. However, a new occurrence of atrial fibrillation is frequently treated because it indicates an increased irritability within the atria and may progress to a more serious dysrhythmia.

Treatment depends on the patient's tolerance of the dysrhythmia and the patient's symptoms. For example, a patient with atrial fibrillation and a ventricular response of 50 impulses per minute, with stable vital signs, may not require treatment. However, a patient with atrial fibrillation with a ventricular response of 50, who is medically unstable, requires treatment immediately.

Signs and symptoms of a patient who is medically unstable include any combination of the following:

- Pale, cool, clammy (damp) skin
- Nausea and vomiting (N/V)
- Dizziness, weakness, faintness
- Shortness of breath (SOB)
- Hypotension (decrease in blood pressure)
- Dyspnea (difficulty breathing)
- Tachycardia (rapid heart rate)
- Diaphoresis (excessive sweating)
- Mild to severe chest pain
- Confusion or disorientation
- Cyanosis (bluish gray color to skin)
- Decreased urinary output
- Unresponsiveness

Atrial fibrillation may be caused by severe heart disease or myocardial infarction. It may also occur with excessive use of alcohol or caffeine.

1. Atrial fibrillation and atrial flutter may occasionally be combined in the same dysrhythmia on a rhythm strip. It is then called *atrial fib/flutter* or *atrial flutter/fib*. The combination of these two dysrhythmias may indicate a more serious cardiac problem.
2. Atrial fibrillation is usually not a lethal dysrhythmia. However, it **must not** be confused with *ventricular fibrillation*, which **is** a lethal dysrhythmia (see Chapter 6).

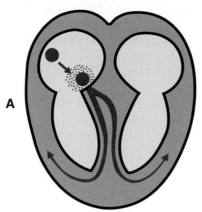

Normal conduction

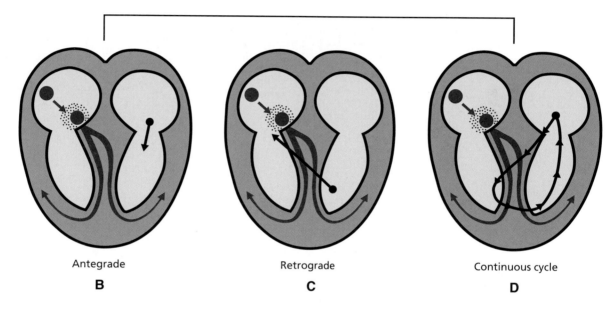

Figure 3-23 Wolff-Parkinson-White (WPW) syndrome. **A,** Normal conduction pathway. **B,** Antegrade conduction pathway. **C,** Retrograde conduction pathway. **D,** Continuous cycle pathway. These show only three of many possible abnormal conduction pathways in WPW syndrome.

Wolff-Parkinson-White Syndrome

Wolff-Parkinson-White (WPW) syndrome is a dysrhythmia that occurs when an electrical impulse follows an additional or abnormal electrical conduction pathway, called the *bundle of Kent* (Kent bundle). Although the normal conduction pathway is working, the impulse from the different pathway, known as an *accessory pathway*, also reaches the ventricles after bypassing the AV node. Electrical impulses can travel through the accessory pathway (bundle of Kent) in any one of the following ways:

1. Downward from the atria to the ventricles (antegrade)
2. Upward from the ventricles to the atria (retrograde)
3. Both downward and upward, in a continuous cycle (Figure 3-23)

Wolff-Parkinson-White (WPW) syndrome is seen on the rhythm strip or monitor screen with the following characteristics:

1. PR interval shorter than 0.12 second, if a P wave is present
2. Usually a widened QRS complex, greater than 0.12 second
3. Delta wave

The PR interval is shorter than normal because the electrical impulse does not travel through the AV node, but goes directly from the atria to the ventricles.

The QRS is usually widened if the electrical impulse travels in a retrograde manner, or in a continuous cycle. The QRS complex is usually within the normal limits of 0.04 to 0.12 second when the electrical impulse travels from the atria to the ventricles. The R wave of the QRS complex usually is "slurred," or curved, at the beginning of the R wave.

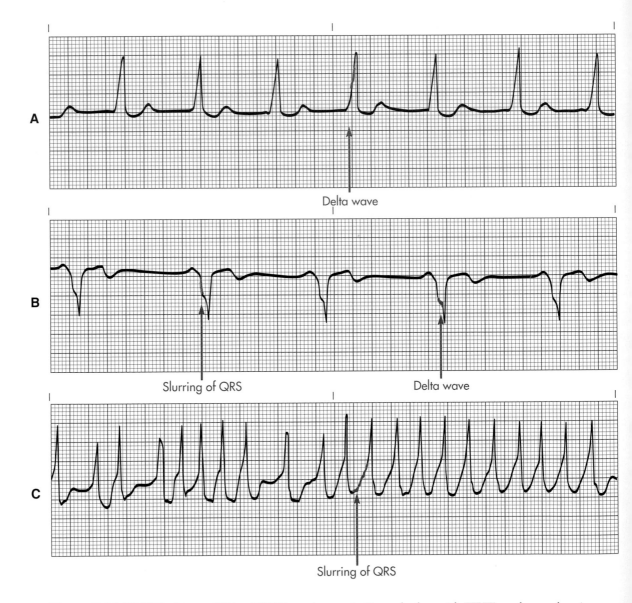

Figure 3-24 Wolff-Parkinson-White (WPW) syndrome. **A,** Sinus rhythm with WPW syndrome showing delta waves; heart rate, 70. **B,** Sinus bradycardia with WPW syndrome showing slurring of QRS and delta waves; heart rate, 50 (notice diphasic T waves). **C,** Uncontrolled atrial fibrillation with WPW syndrome mimicking ventricular tachycardia and showing slurring of QRS; atrial heart rate 350 to 500; ventricular heart rate, 210 (notice depressed ST segments).

The *delta wave* is an extra "bump" seen in the slurred section of the QRS complex. The delta wave is formed by depolarization of the ventricles through the accessory pathway, before the normally conducted electrical impulse can reach the ventricles.

The P to P intervals and R to R intervals of WPW syndrome vary, depending on the underlying rhythm.

The rate of WPW syndrome may also vary, depending on the underlying rhythm. However, because the ventricles are receiving impulses from both the normal and accessory pathways, the ventricles usually depolarize quickly, causing tachycardia (Figure 3-24, *A* through *C*).

This is usually not a dangerous dysrhythmia, and WPW syndrome is often undiagnosed in many patients until it is found on a routine ECG. However, it can become life-threatening if the ventricular rate increases to 200 to 300 beats per minute or greater. WPW syndrome is associated with supraventricular tachycardia and atrial flutter, as well as atrial fibrillation, with uncontrolled ventricular response. It can sometimes mimic *ventricular tachycardia* (see Chapter 6), if the QRS complex is wide and the rate is rapid.

The patient may have no symptoms or may complain of palpitations; racing heart; dizziness, weakness, or faintness; SOB; and/or chest pain.

> **NOTE:** One of the concerns with Wolff-Parkinson-White syndrome, atrial flutter, and especially atrial fibrillation is that clots may form in the atria. The rapid atrial rate may not allow either atrial chamber to empty completely. This could lead to stroke, pulmonary emboli (blockage of an artery in the lungs), and/or MI.

REVIEW QUESTIONS

True   False   1. The SA node normally generates 60 to 100 electrical impulses per minute.

True   False   2. Sinus bradycardia may become dangerous if the heart rate decreases significantly or the patient becomes medically unstable.

True   False   3. The complex that ends a sinus arrest can only be initiated from the SA node.

True   False   4. A PAC is an atrial complex that occurs later than the next expected complex of the underlying rhythm.

True   False   5. In a sinus arrhythmia, the heart rate increases with inspirations and decreases with expirations.

6. The number of electrical impulses in sinus tachycardia is between _____ and _____ per minute.

7. In atrial fibrillation, the QRS complexes usually measure less than _____ second.

8. Sinus exit block occurs when the SA node fails to initiate an electrical impulse for a length of time equal to _____ previous cardiac cycles.

9. If the onset of PAT/PSVT is not seen, the dysrhythmia is called

   a. sinus tachycardia

   b. supraventricular tachycardia

   c. premature atrial tachycardia

   d. atrial tachycardia

10. SVT is a dysrhythmia that originates from an irritable site located

   a. above the bundle of His

   b. within the ventricles

   c. within the bundle branches

   d. below the bundle of His

11. Wolff-Parkinson-White syndrome can be identified by a shortened PR interval and the presence of a(n)

   a. alpha wave

   b. P wave

   c. delta wave

   d. beta wave

12. Atrial flutter has

   a. P waves

   b. Q waves

   c. F waves

   d. T waves

13. Atrial fibrillation has fib waves that are

   a. distinct and regular

   b. notched and regular

   c. wavy and irregular

   d. absent

14. Define "variable ventricular response" in atrial flutter.

_____

_____

_____

15. Trace the path of an electrical impulse from the SA node to the ventricular muscle.

_____

_____

_____

16. Describe the components and intervals of a complex in normal sinus rhythm, including measurements as seen on a rhythm strip.

_____

_____

_____

_____

_____

17. What are the heart rates usually found in
    a. sinus bradycardia? _____
    b. SVT? _____
    c. sinus arrhythmia? _____

18. What is the atrial heart rate in
    a. atrial flutter? _____
    b. atrial fibrillation? _____

19. What is the difference between the pause of a sinus exit block and a sinus arrest, including the length of the pause?

_____

_____

_____

_____

_____

RHYTHM STRIP REVIEW

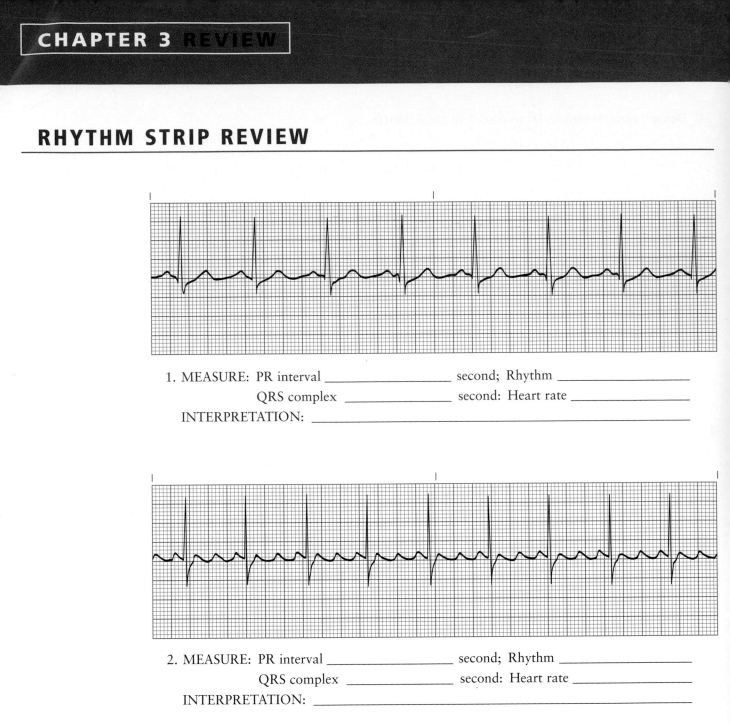

1. MEASURE: PR interval _____ second; Rhythm _____

                  QRS complex _____ second: Heart rate _____

INTERPRETATION: _____

2. MEASURE: PR interval _____ second; Rhythm _____

                  QRS complex _____ second: Heart rate _____

INTERPRETATION: _____

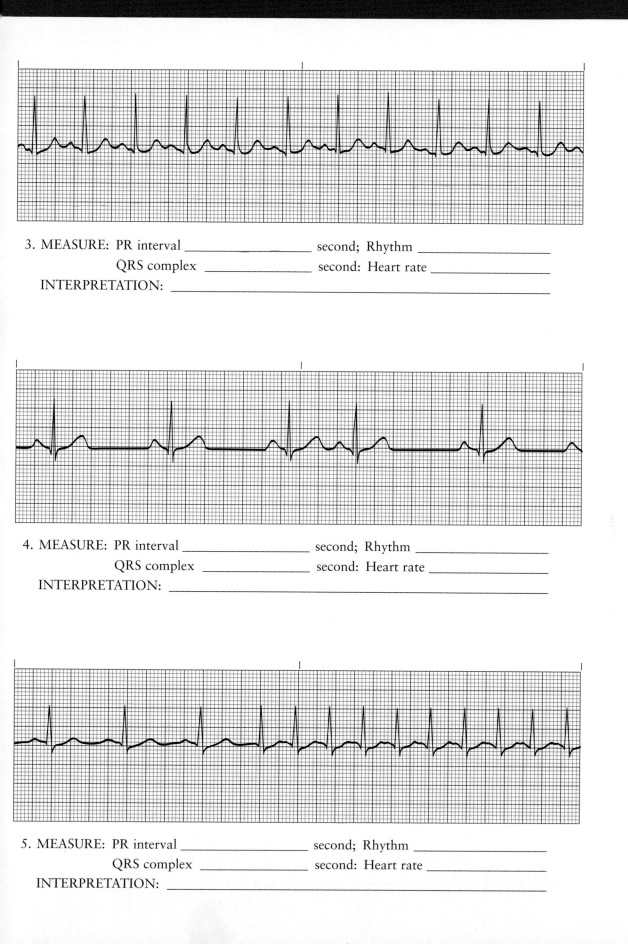

3. MEASURE: PR interval _____ second; Rhythm _____

QRS complex _____ second: Heart rate _____

INTERPRETATION: _____

4. MEASURE: PR interval _____ second; Rhythm _____

QRS complex _____ second: Heart rate _____

INTERPRETATION: _____

5. MEASURE: PR interval _____ second; Rhythm _____

QRS complex _____ second: Heart rate _____

INTERPRETATION: _____

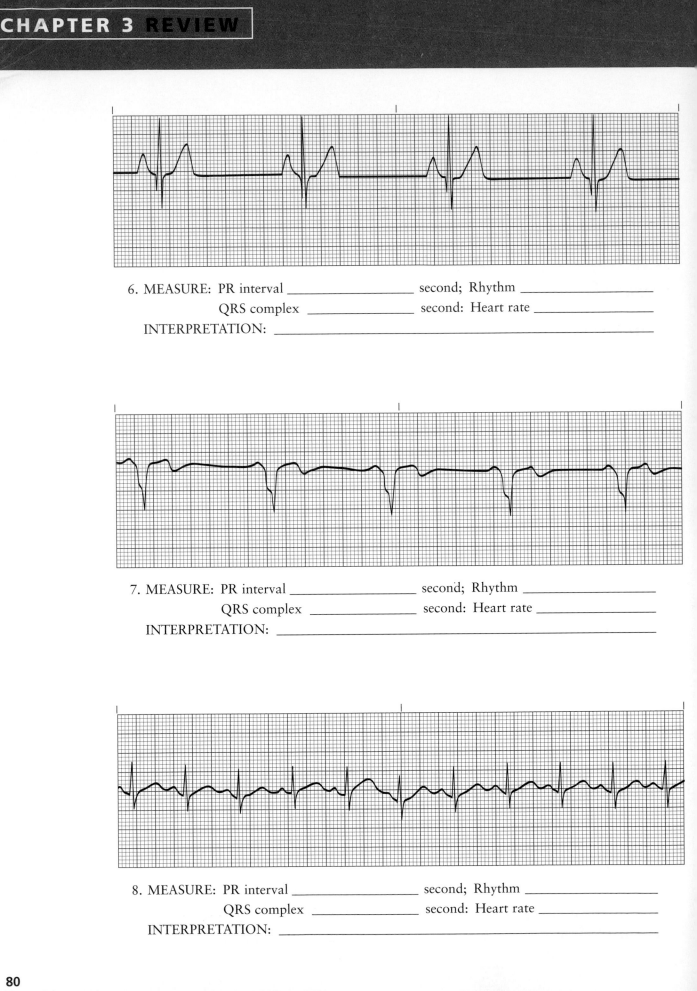

6. MEASURE: PR interval _____ second; Rhythm _____

QRS complex _____ second: Heart rate _____

INTERPRETATION: _____

7. MEASURE: PR interval _____ second; Rhythm _____

QRS complex _____ second: Heart rate _____

INTERPRETATION: _____

8. MEASURE: PR interval _____ second; Rhythm _____

QRS complex _____ second: Heart rate _____

INTERPRETATION: _____

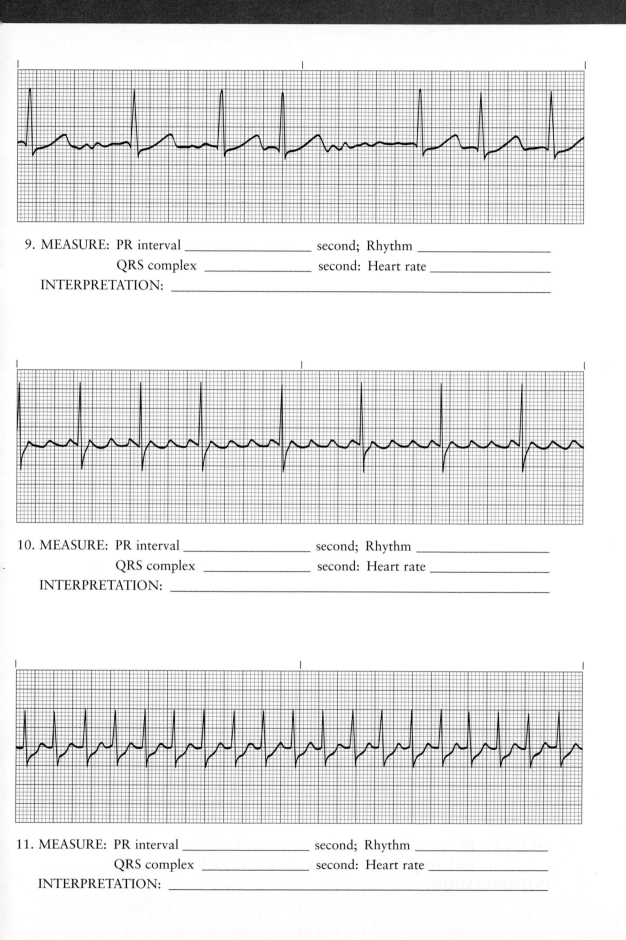

9. MEASURE: PR interval _____ second; Rhythm _____

QRS complex _____ second: Heart rate _____

INTERPRETATION: _____

10. MEASURE: PR interval _____ second; Rhythm _____

QRS complex _____ second: Heart rate _____

INTERPRETATION: _____

11. MEASURE: PR interval _____ second; Rhythm _____

QRS complex _____ second: Heart rate _____

INTERPRETATION: _____

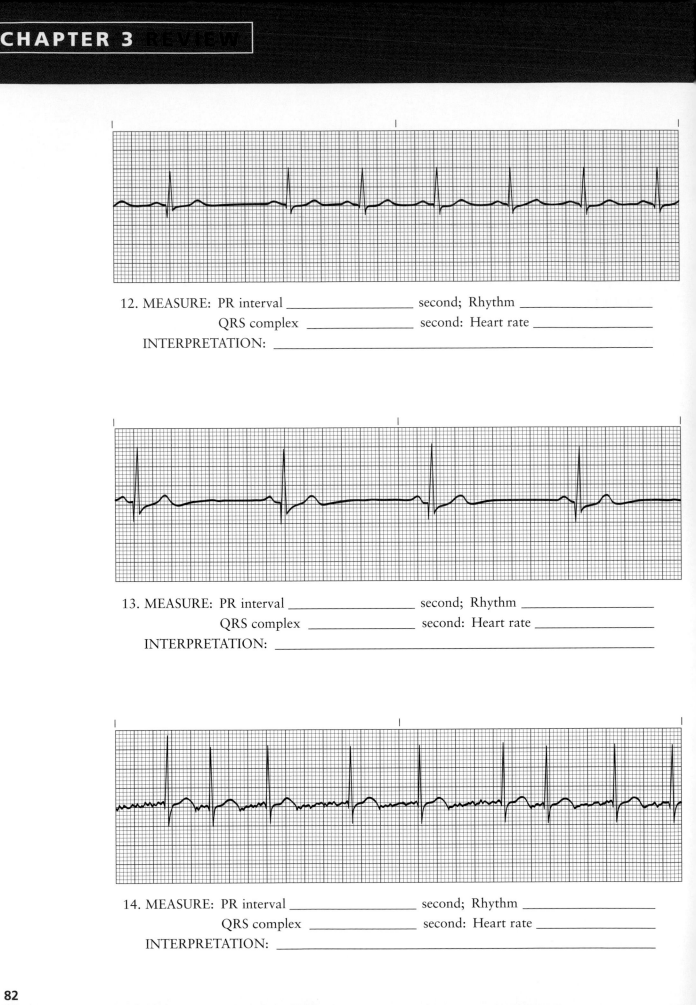

12. MEASURE: PR interval _____ second; Rhythm _____

                 QRS complex _____ second: Heart rate _____

       INTERPRETATION: _____

13. MEASURE: PR interval _____ second; Rhythm _____

                 QRS complex _____ second: Heart rate _____

       INTERPRETATION: _____

14. MEASURE: PR interval _____ second; Rhythm _____

                 QRS complex _____ second: Heart rate _____

       INTERPRETATION: _____

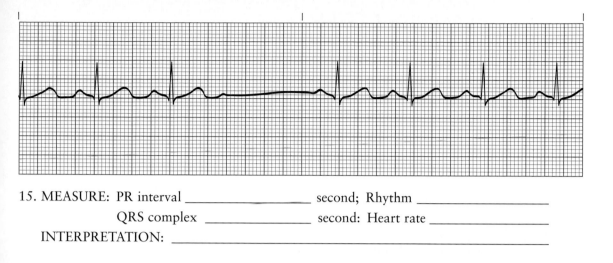

15. MEASURE: PR interval _____ second; Rhythm _____

QRS complex _____ second: Heart rate _____

INTERPRETATION: _____

Suggestion: You may find it helpful reviewing the Chapter 3 rhythm strips on the CD prior to studying the next chapter.

CROSSWORD PUZZLE AND CLUES

Across

1 Occurs when the SA node does not initiate an electrical impulse causing a pause to be seen on the monitor or rhythm strip. [2 words]

8 Occurs earlier than expected.

11 Additional or abnormal electrical conduction pathway.

12 The _____ rate ranges from 250 to 350 electrical impulses per minute in atrial flutter.

14 P to P intervals and R to R intervals change with _____ in a sinus arrhythmia.

16 Dysrhythmia that occurs when an electrical impulse follows an accessory pathway, the bundle of Kent, and bypasses the AV node to reach the ventricles.

18 Only "normal" cardiac rhythm.

19 A noncompensatory _____ measures less than 2 times the R to R interval of the underlying rhythm.

20 The _____ of PAT/PSVT must be seen and the underlying rhythm that precedes the PAT/PSVT must be identified.

22 The dysrhythmia is identifies as atrial flutter with a(n) _____ ventricular response when the number of F waves is different before each QRS complex.

25 Cardiac rhythm or dysrhythmia originating in SA node.

26 Heart rate slower than 60 electrical impulses per minute.

27 Atrial _____ occurs when electrical impulses are initiated by so many atrial sites, no true P waves are produced, only a quivering motion of the atria.

Down

2 Heart rate faster than 100 electrical impulses per min.

3 Pause in the rhythm measuring at least 2 times the R to R interval of the underlying rhythm.

4 _____ is the sudden onset of tachycardia with a rate greater than 150 electrical impulses per minute.

5 Extra "bump" seen in beginning of QRS complex; seen in Wolff-Parkinson-White syndrome. [2 words]

6 The _____ rhythm must be identified when interpreting a rhythm which contains a PAC.

7 Traveling in reverse or backward manner.

8 Occurs earlier than expected; originates from any atrial pacemaker site outside the SA node.

9 "Saw-tooth" F waves produced in atrial flutter instead of P waves. [2 words]

10 Sudden intermittent start and stop of symptoms or dysrhythmias; usually describes a rapid atrial dysrhythmia.

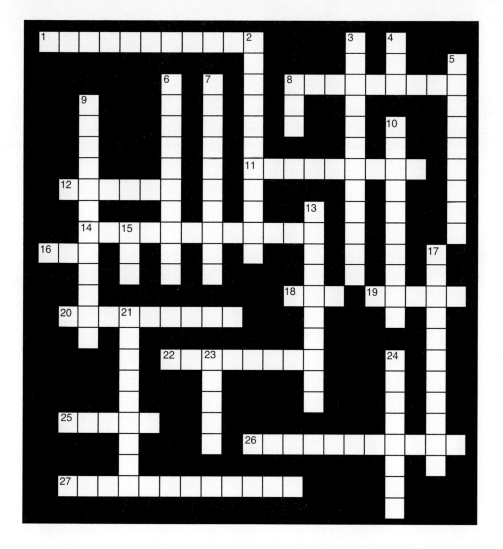

13 Evaluation of patient symptoms or tolerance of any cardiac dysrhythmia.

15 Dysrhythmia that has all the characteristics of PAT/PSVT, but the beginning of the dysrhythmia is not seen.

17 Abnormal cardiac rhythm.

21 The rhythm of atrial fibrillation is _____.

23 The number of F wave to each QRS complex is described as a(n) _____ or block, ie. 2:1; 3:1; 4:1, etc.

24 Normal, natural, or inborn; the _____ rate of the SA node is 60 to 100 electrical impulses per minute.

Note: The solution to this crossword puzzle is in the answer section.

WORD PUZZLE

This word puzzle is designed to help familiarize you with some of the new terminology found in this chapter. Have fun finding all the words on this list. The words will alwyas be in upper case and found in a straight line. The words can be spelled forward (normal), backward, up, down, or diagonally in any direction. Good luck! **The solution to this word puzzle is in the answer section.**

```
M G M L D V K N T C A R D I A C C Y C L E Z G R
V Z L M K C O L B T I X E R L P D L F Y B M N H
Y A T R I A L F L U T T E R W M Q H F N F S I H
M B T M N K M T C P X S P F V W L R X M I R R Z
N T X H R N T V S R X L E L M F M Z L N K B E A
R N C T Y A T A C H Y C A R D I A M U G C B V C
C P M Y Q E L W G W K T Q H R F R S M O M N I C
P A E H H D V U T W L L Y P N A A L M M H Q U E
J T D R K O K L C Q V L M K M R S P D N F P Q S
T I I G L N K C N I N G B C R L E U W R B D K S
G E C N R L Y R F J R K K H N N T R N L W B L O
Q N A I L A G R K J V T Y B S Z C L O I J D Z R
R T L Y R I Z P K H G T N A R L J C F M S D C Y
M A L L G R L R N X H F T E R A K V H W T X D P
H S Y R Q T R W B M R O W R V L D T D V T J T A
L S U E L A A C I I R L E A D A Y Y S G Z K A T
T E N D L O T A M Y F S W W V H R P C G R Y P H
N S S N N N I K P D U A P X R E M P A A H K V W
K S T U S I O A L A W W C S J L S R U C R T F A
D M A K R S U Q P Y R L U W M V N R C S K D P Y
K E B F R S R G M M R N P K Z L L J V Z Y P I Z
W N L Y E D R W L X I J N C R K G W N D J L P A
P T E J Z T G P D S D E L T A W A V E K P W F P
R D N O I T A L L I R B I F N T C N T M C W F H
```

ACCESSORY PATHWAY
A FIB
ATRIAL FLUTTER
BLOCK
BRADYCARDIA
CARDIAC CYCLE
COMPENSATORY PAUSE
DELTA WAVE
EXIT BLOCK
FIBRILLATION

F WAVES
MEDICALLY UNSTABLE
NSR
PAC
PAT
PATIENT ASSESSMENT
PAUSE
PSVT
QUIVERING
RATIO

SINOATRIAL NODE
SINUS ARREST
SINUS ARRHYTHMIA
SINUS RHYTHM
SUPRAVENTRICULAR
SVT
TACHYCARDIA
UNDERLYING RHYTHM
WPW

On completion of this chapter, the reader should be able to:

1 Define the terms *junctional dysrhythmia* and *inherent junctional heart rate.*

2 Describe the three types of P waves seen in a junctional dysrhythmia.

3 Describe the difference between junctional bradycardia dysrhythmia, accelerated junctional dysrhythmia, and junctional tachycardia dysrhythmia.

4 Describe the appearance of a premature junctional complex, including measurements of the components.

5 Describe the appearance of a wandering junctional pacemaker dysrhythmia, including measurements of the components.

6 Describe the appearance of a wandering atrial pacemaker dysrhythmia, including measurements of the components.

Junctional Dysrhythmias

DEFINITIONS

AV Node—Atrioventricular node; part of the normal electrical conduction pathway of the heart; may function as a secondary pacemaker of the heart

Buried P Wave—The P wave is hidden, or buried, within the QRS complex and therefore not seen

Inherent Heart Rate—Normal rate at which electrical impulses are generated; the inherent heart rate for the AV junction is 40 to 60 impulses per minute

Inverted P Wave—Inverted, or upside-down, P wave before the QRS complex

Junctional Dysrhythmia—Cardiac dysrhythmia that is initiated in the AV node (AV junctional area), when the SA node and atrial sites fail to initiate an electrical impulse

Retrograde P Wave—A P wave that is seen after the QRS complex; it is also inverted

JUNCTIONAL DYSRHYTHMIAS

As discussed in Chapter 3, the sinoatrial (SA) node and the atria may fail to generate the electrical impulses needed to begin depolarization for many reasons, such as drug toxicity, myocardial infarction, or heart disease. When this failure occurs, the atrioventricular (AV) node may assume its role of the secondary cardiac pacemaker of the heart (see Chapter 1).

The AV node is located in the general area of the lower right atrium, near the septum. It is an indistinct area and difficult to pinpoint exactly. The cardiac tissue immediately surrounding the AV node is usually called the *AV junction* and is also capable of initiating electrical impulses (Figure 4-1).

Rhythms that start in either the AV node or the AV junctional area are called *junctional dysrhythmias*, or nodal dysrhythmias. The term *nodal* is rarely used today, because *junctional* is more accurate.

Because the AV junction is not the primary pacemaker of the heart, it is not as efficient as the SA node and has a slower rate. The AV junctional rate is 40 to 60 electrical impulses per minute. This rate is also known as *the inherent heart rate* of the AV junctional area.

A junctional dysrhythmia is not usually lethal. However, as with any rhythm, **patient assessment** is essential to determine the patient's tolerance of the dysrhythmia.

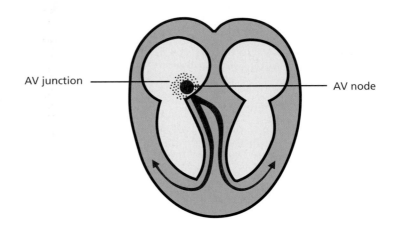

Figure 4-1 Atrioventricular (AV) node and AV junctional area.

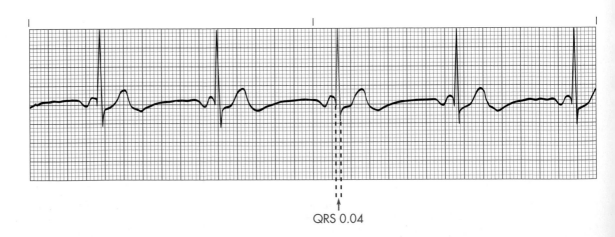

QRS 0.04

Figure 4-2 Junctional dysrhythmia showing normal ventricular depolarization (notice depressed ST segments).

In a junctional dysrhythmia, the electrical impulse travels through the normal conduction pathway from the AV junction, through the bundle of His and bundle branches, to the Purkinje's fibers, ending in the ventricular muscle.

Because the electrical impulse follows the normal conduction pathway through the ventricles, the QRS complex usually measures less than 0.12 second (Figure 4-2).

However, the electrical impulse that depolarizes the atria must travel in a backward, or *retrograde*, motion from the AV junction up through the atria (Figure 4-3). This retrograde motion accounts for all three characteristic changes in the P wave, which identify an AV junctional dysrhythmia: *inverted, buried (hidden),* or *retrograde* (Figure 4-4, *A* through *C*).

Inverted P Wave

If the electrical impulse originates high in the AV junctional area, the atria are depolarized quickly, although in a retrograde manner (Figure 4-5). This retrograde depolarization causes the P wave to be inverted, or upside down (Figure 4-6). It will be seen on the monitor or rhythm strip as an inverted P wave before the QRS complex.

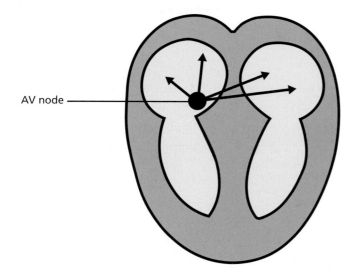

AV node

Figure 4-3 Retrograde electrical conduction pathway from AV node to atria.

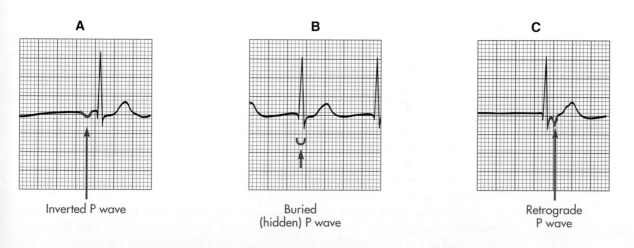

A

Inverted P wave

B

Buried (hidden) P wave

C

Retrograde P wave

Figure 4-4 P waves. **A,** Inverted. **B,** Buried. **C,** Retrograde.

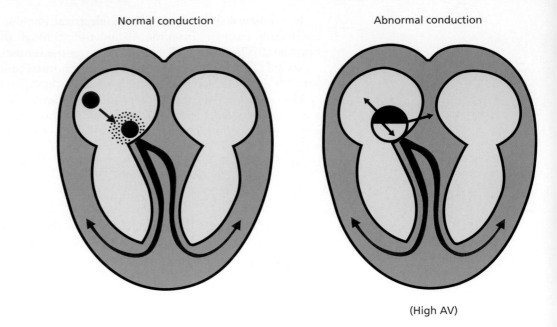

Normal conduction   Abnormal conduction

(High AV)

Figure 4-5 *Left heart* shows normal electrical conduction pathway. *Right heart* shows conduction pathway of high AV junctional area.

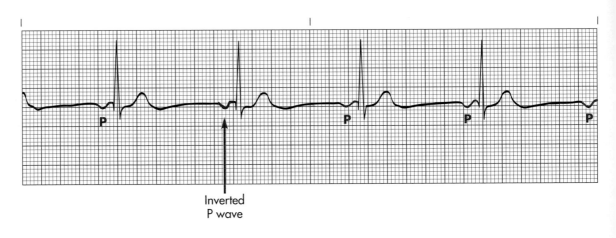

Inverted
P wave

Figure 4-6 Junctional dysrhythmia with inverted P waves.

Because the electrical impulse originates in the AV junction, the distance the impulse must travel to depolarize the ventricles is shorter than normal. The depolarization of the ventricles, reflected by the QRS complex, occurs quickly and may cause a shortened PR interval of less than 0.12 second.

Buried P Wave

When the electrical impulse originates in the mid-AV junctional area, the distance the impulse must travel up through the atria (retrograde) and down through the ventricles is almost the same. This similar distance causes the atria and the ventricles to depolarize at almost the same time (Figure 4-7).

Because the force of the atrial depolarization is less than the force of the ventricular depolarization, the P wave is hidden by the QRS complex. This P wave is described as buried, or hidden, and consequently a P wave and a PR interval are not seen (Figure 4-8).

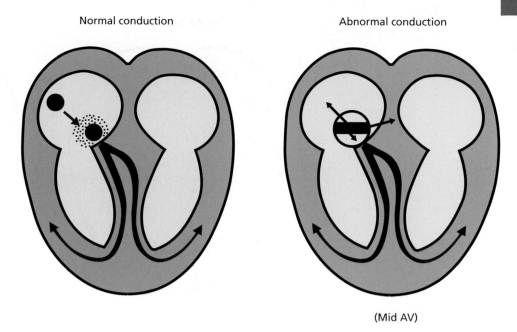

Normal conduction   Abnormal conduction

(Mid AV)

Figure 4-7 *Left heart* shows normal electrical conduction pathway. *Right heart* shows conduction pathway of mid-AV junctional area.

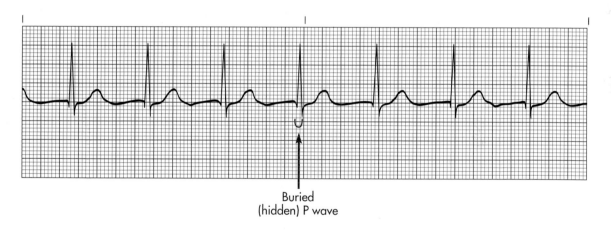

Buried
(hidden) P wave

Figure 4-8 Junctional dysrhythmia with buried (hidden) P waves.

Retrograde P Wave

When the electrical impulse originates in the lower part of the AV junctional area, the distance the impulse must travel to the atria is greater than the distance to the ventricles (Figure 4-9). Therefore the atria depolarize slightly later than the ventricles, producing a retrograde P wave after the QRS complex.

The P wave is said to be retrograde because it appears after the QRS complex; no measurable PR interval is present. The P wave is inverted because the atria are depolarized in a retrograde manner (Figure 4-10).

> **NOTE:** The term *retrograde* is used in two different ways:
> 1. To appear behind or after
> 2. To occur in a backward or reverse motion

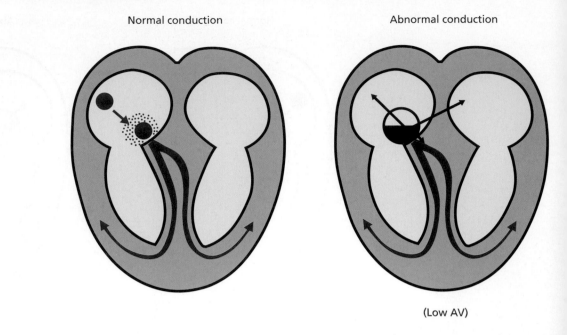

Figure 4-9 *Left heart* shows normal electrical conduction pathway. *Right heart* shows conduction pathway of lower AV junctional area.

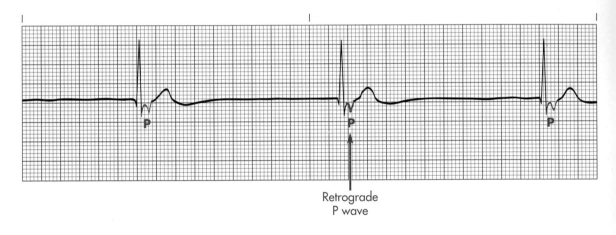

Figure 4-10 Junctional dysrhythmia with retrograde P waves.

JUNCTIONAL BRADYCARDIA DYSRHYTHMIA

Junctional bradycardia dysrhythmia occurs when all the electrical impulses originate from a single site within the AV junctional area, at a rate less than 40 impulses per minute.

The P wave is either inverted, buried, or retrograde. The PR interval, if present, is usually less than 0.12 second. However, the QRS complex usually remains less than 0.12 second. Because the P to P intervals, if seen, and the R to R intervals are regular and equal in length, the rhythm is regular. The rate can vary, but it must be less than 40 electrical impulses per minute (Figure 4-11).

Junctional bradycardia dysrhythmia may be caused by heart disease or drugs such as digitalis, quinidine, or sedatives.

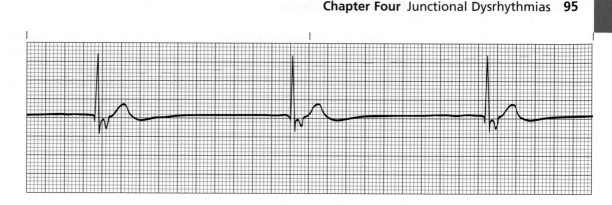

Figure 4-11 Junctional bradycardia dysrhythmia with retrograde P waves; heart rate, 30.

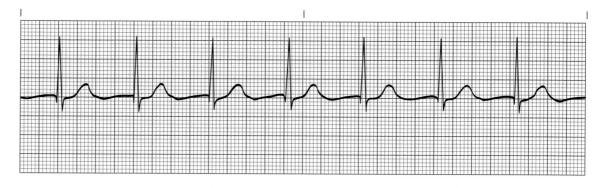

Figure 4-12 Accelerated junctional dysrhythmia with hidden P waves; heart rate, 70.

A junctional bradycardia dysrhythmia may become a serious dysrhythmia if the rate falls significantly or the patient becomes medically unstable.

REMEMBER: Any patient with a heart rate of less than 60 electrical impulses per minute has a bradycardic rate. This is known as an *absolute bradycardia*. However, because the inherent rate of the AV junction is 40 to 60 electrical impulses per minute, only a junctional dysrhythmia with a rate below 40 impulses per minute can be called a junctional bradycardia dysrhythmia.

ACCELERATED JUNCTIONAL DYSRHYTHMIA/JUNCTIONAL TACHYCARDIA DYSRHYTHMIA

Accelerated junctional dysrhythmia occurs when all the electrical impulses originate from a single site within the AV junctional area, at a rate between 61 and 100 impulses per minute.

The P wave is either inverted, buried, or retrograde. The PR interval, if present, is usually less than 0.12 second. Because the electrical impulse follows the normal conduction pathway through the ventricles, the QRS complex usually remains normal, measuring less than 0.12 second.

Because the P to P intervals, if seen, and the R to R intervals are regular and equal in length, the rhythm is regular. The rate can vary, but it must be between 61 and 100 electrical impulses per minute (Figure 4-12).

Any patient with a heart rate greater than 100 electrical impulses per minute has a tachycardic rate. However, only those rhythms that are junctional and have a rate between 61 and 100 impulses per minute can be called accelerated junctional dysrhythmias. A junctional dysrhythmia with a rate between 101 and 150 impulses per minute is called *junctional tachycardia dysrhythmia*.

Both accelerated junctional dysrhythmia and junctional tachycardia dysrhythmia may be caused by heart disease or drugs such as atropine, caffeine, or amphetamines. They also may result from pain, fever, or acute anemia. Exercise or street drugs can also cause these dysrhythmias if heart disease is present.

Either accelerated junctional dysrhythmia or junctional tachycardia dysrhythmia may become a serious dysrhythmia if the rate increases significantly or the patient becomes medically unstable. Assessment is required to determine the patient's tolerance of the dysrhythmia and the appropriate treatment.

PREMATURE JUNCTIONAL COMPLEX

A *premature junctional complex (PJC)*, formerly known as premature junctional contraction, is an individual complex that originates from a single site in the AV junctional area and occurs earlier than the next expected complex of the underlying rhythm (Figure 4-13). PJCs are common and can occur in any rhythm.

Although PJCs are **individual** complexes and **not** true rhythms, they are included in this chapter because they originate from the AV junctional area.

A premature junctional complex has the same characteristics as other junctional complexes. The P wave is either inverted, buried, or retrograde. The PR interval, if seen, may be less than 0.12 second, but the QRS complex is usually normal; less than 0.12 second.

The P to P and the R to R intervals of the underlying rhythm vary, depending on that rhythm. The occurrence of a PJC, in even the most regular rhythm, causes the P to P and the R to R intervals to be irregular.

The premature junctional complex may be followed by a complete compensatory pause, which allows the underlying rhythm to depolarize at its normal rate, as though the PJC had never occurred. The R to R interval from the complex before the PJC to the complex after the PJC is at least 2 times the R to R interval of the underlying rhythm.

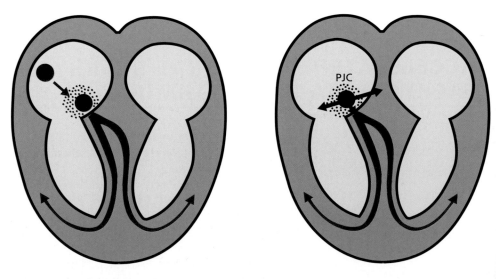

Normal conduction   Abnormal conduction

Figure 4-13 *Left heart* shows normal electrical conduction pathway. *Right heart* shows conduction pathway of a premature junctional complex (PJC).

Although a PJC may occur in any rhythm, it is easier to identify in a sinus or bradycardic rhythm. When determining the rate of any rhythm containing a PJC, the R wave of the PJC is included in the total count of the R waves.

The underlying rhythm must be identified when interpreting a rhythm strip containing a PJC. For example, the underlying rhythm might be a sinus rhythm or a junctional dysrhythmia with PJCs (Figure 4-14).

Premature junctional complexes may be caused by pain, fever, fear, anxiety, sudden excitement, exercise, or the effects of drugs such as digitalis, atropine, nicotine, caffeine, and amphetamines. PJCs also may be caused by an increased irritability of the myocardium. This increased irritability indicates that the cardiac cells are able to respond to even a mild electrical stimulus and may depolarize in an unpredictable rate or manner.

A PJC by itself is not a lethal dysrhythmia. However, it should be monitored closely, because it may trigger a more serious dysrhythmia.

WANDERING JUNCTIONAL PACEMAKER DYSRHYTHMIA

A *wandering junctional pacemaker dysrhythmia* originates from at least **three** sites within the junctional area (Figure 4-15). The size and shape of each complex are determined by the site of origin for each complex.

The individual complexes are characterized by P waves that are inverted, buried, or retrograde. Any PR intervals that are seen are usually less than 0.12 second, but the QRS complexes are usually normal; less than 0.12 second.

The rhythm is irregular with varying P to P intervals and R to R intervals. The rate may also vary but is usually 40 to 60 impulses per minute (Figure 4-16).

This dysrhythmia is not usually lethal. However, it is frequently treated, because it indicates increased irritability within the junctional area that may progress to a more serious dysrhythmia.

A wandering junctional pacemaker dysrhythmia may be caused by heart disease, myocardial infarction, or drug toxicity.

A wandering junctional pacemaker dysrhythmia has three or more **junctional** sites. However, a rhythm that has both atrial and junctional sites is identified as a wandering atrial pacemaker dysrhythmia.

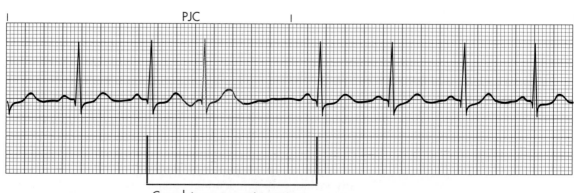

PJC

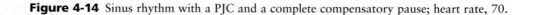

Complete compensatory pause

Figure 4-14 Sinus rhythm with a PJC and a complete compensatory pause; heart rate, 70.

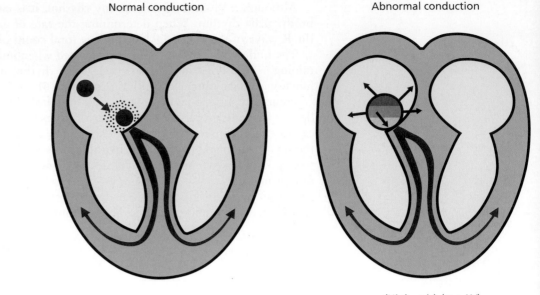

Normal conduction   Abnormal conduction

(High, mid, low AV)

Figure 4-15 *Left heart* shows normal electrical conduction pathway. *Right heart* shows conduction pathway of a wandering junctional pacemaker dysrhythmia.

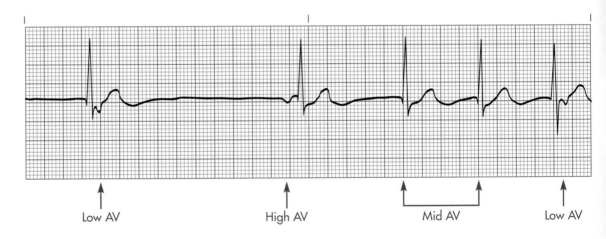

Low AV   High AV   Mid AV   Low AV

Figure 4-16 Wandering junctional pacemaker dysrhythmia originating in the high, middle, and low AV junctional areas; heart rate, 50 (notice depressed ST segments).

WANDERING ATRIAL PACEMAKER DYSRHYTHMIA

A *wandering atrial pacemaker dysrhythmia* originates from at least **three** different sites above the bundle of His. These sites may include the SA node, any pacemaker site in the atria, the AV junction, or a combination of these areas (Figure 4-17). Although this is an atrial dysrhythmia, it is included in this chapter because it usually includes some junctional complexes.

The size and shape of each individual complex are determined by the site of origin for that complex. If the site is from the atria, a P wave occurs, followed by a QRS complex that measures less than 0.12 second. The PR interval is usually 0.12 to 0.20 second, but may vary because the atrial point of origin varies.

Normal conduction

Abnormal conduction

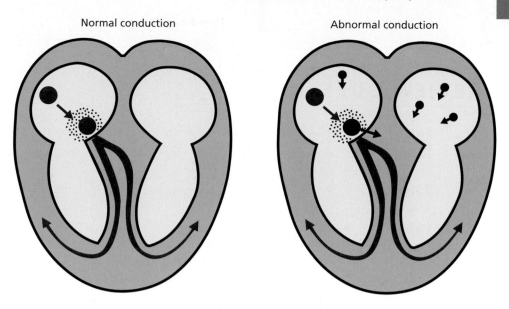

Figure 4-17 *Left heart* shows normal electrical conduction pathway. *Right heart* shows conduction pathway of wandering atrial pacemaker dysrhythmia.

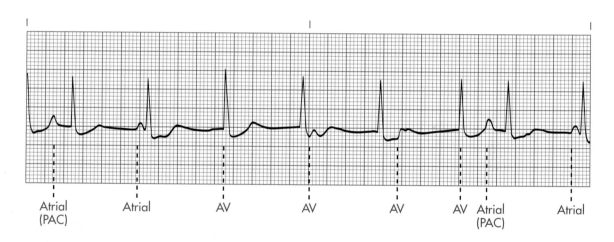

Atrial
(PAC)   Atrial   AV   AV   AV   AV Atrial   Atrial
                                                                                        (PAC)

Figure 4-18 Wandering atrial pacemaker dysrhythmia showing different sites of origin; heart rate, 80 to 90 (notice depressed ST segments).

If the complex is from the AV junctional area, the P waves may be inverted, may be buried, or may follow the QRS complex (retrograde). Therefore, P waves may not be seen before every QRS complex, and the PR intervals may vary or be absent.

The P to P intervals (if present) and R to R intervals vary, producing an irregular rhythm. The rate may also vary but usually remains between 60 and 100 electrical impulses per minute (Figure 4-18).

A wandering atrial pacemaker dysrhythmia may be caused by heart disease, myocardial infarction, or drug toxicity.

This dysrhythmia is usually not lethal. However, it is frequently treated because it indicates increased irritability within the cardiac muscle. This increased irritability may cause the dysrhythmia to progress to a more serious dysrhythmia.

The patient's symptoms vary, depending on the rate of the wandering atrial pacemaker dysrhythmia and the patient's tolerance of the dysrhythmia.

REVIEW QUESTIONS

True   **False**   1. The AV node is located in the lower left atrium, near the septum.

True   **False**   2. A junctional bradycardia dysrhythmia has a heart rate of less than 40 electrical impulses per minute.

True   **False**   3. A wandering junctional pacemaker dysrhythmia originates from both the atria and the AV junctional area.

True   **False**   4. In a junctional dysrhythmia, the P wave will be buried if the electrical impulse is initiated high in the AV junctional area.

5. The inherent heart rate of the AV junctional area is _____ to _____ electrical impulses per minute.

6. The QRS complex in a junctional dysrhythmia usually measures

    a. 0.12 to 0.20 second

    b. 0.4 to 0.12 second

    c. 0.04 to 0.20 second

    d. 0.04 to 0.12 second

7. Junctional tachycardia dysrhythmia has a heart rate of _____ to _____ electrical impulses per minute.

8. What are the two definitions of the term *retrograde,* as used when describing junctional dysrhythmias?

    a. _____

    b. _____

9. A PJC is

    a. a junctional complex that occurs later than the next expected complex of the underlying rhythm

    b. any complex that occurs earlier than the next expected complex of a junctional dysrhythmia

    c. a complex that occurs later than the next expected complex of a junctional dysrhythmia

    d. a junctional complex that occurs earlier than the next expected complex of the underlying rhythm

10. List three types of P waves that can be seen in a junctional dysrhythmia.

    a. _____

    b. _____

    c. _____

11. Where do the electrical impulses originate, which form the three types of P waves found in junctional dysrhythmias?

    a. _____

    b. _____

    c. _____

12. PJCs are usually followed by what kind of a pause?
    a. compensatory
    b. sinus
    c. junctional
    d. noncompensatory

13. Describe a wandering atrial pacemaker dysrhythmia, including measurements.

    _____

    _____

    _____

14. What is the difference between a junctional tachycardia dysrhythmia and an accelerated junctional dysrhythmia?

    _____

    _____

    _____

RHYTHM STRIP REVIEW

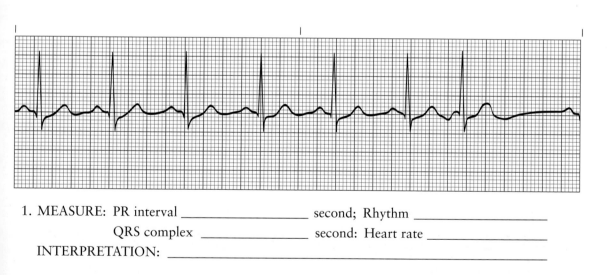

1. MEASURE: PR interval _____ second; Rhythm _____
              QRS complex _____ second: Heart rate _____
   INTERPRETATION: _____

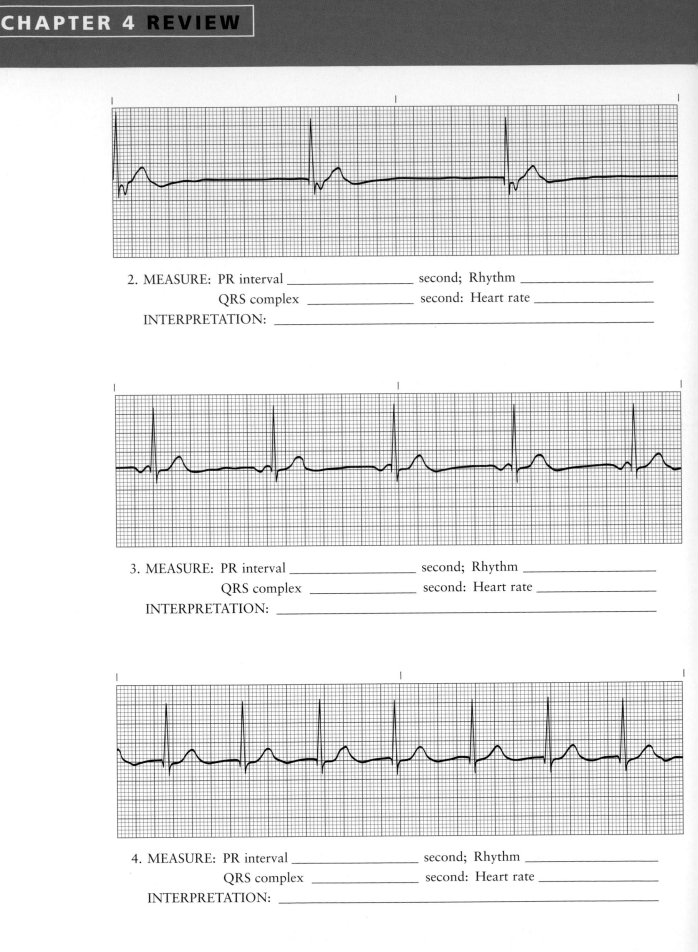

2. MEASURE: PR interval _____ second; Rhythm _____

QRS complex _____ second: Heart rate _____

INTERPRETATION: _____

3. MEASURE: PR interval _____ second; Rhythm _____

QRS complex _____ second: Heart rate _____

INTERPRETATION: _____

4. MEASURE: PR interval _____ second; Rhythm _____

QRS complex _____ second: Heart rate _____

INTERPRETATION: _____

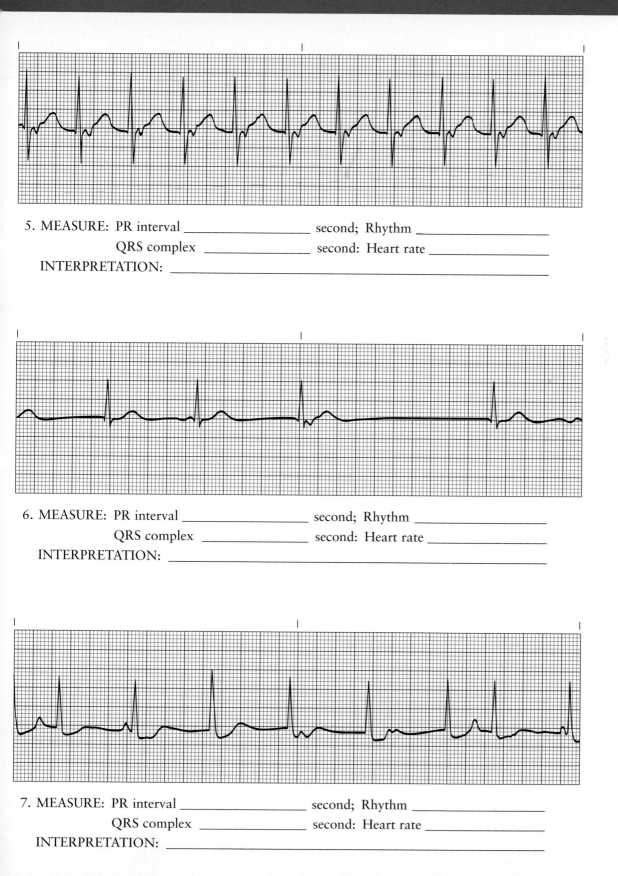

5. MEASURE: PR interval _____ second; Rhythm _____
         QRS complex _____ second: Heart rate _____
   INTERPRETATION: _____

6. MEASURE: PR interval _____ second; Rhythm _____
         QRS complex _____ second: Heart rate _____
   INTERPRETATION: _____

7. MEASURE: PR interval _____ second; Rhythm _____
         QRS complex _____ second: Heart rate _____
   INTERPRETATION: _____

Suggestion: You may find it helpful reviewing the Chapter 4 and 5 rhythm strips on the CD prior
to studying the next chapter.

CROSSWORD PUZZLE AND CLUES

Across

1 Junctional _____ occurs when all electrical impulses originate from a single site in the AV junction with a heart rate of less than 40 impulses per minute.

5 A dysrhythmia with both atrial and junctional complexes is called a wandering _____ pacemaker dysrhythmia.

7 Complex that originates in the AV junction, arrives early, and followed by a compensatory pause.

8 A wandering atrial pacemaker dysrhythmia originates from at least three different sites above the _____, including the SA node, the atria, the AV junction, or a combination of these sites.

15 A(n) _____ junctional pacemaker dysrhythmia originates from at least three sites within the junctional area and does not contain complexes that originate from any other area of the heart.

16 Secondary pacemaker of the heart. [2 words]

17 Patients with symptoms of poor cardiac output are medically _____.

Down

2 Upside down.

3 Hidden in another complex.

4 A junctional dysrhythmia with a heart rate of 101 or greater is known as junctional _____.

6 AV node and surrounding area.

9 The AV junction is located in right atria, near the _____.

10 The _____ _____ remains within 0.04 to 0.12 seconds in size.

12 Backwards; behind.

13 _____ is necessary to evaluate the patient's tolerance of the dysrhythmia.

14 The _____ heart rate of the AV junction is 40 to 60 impulses per minute.

The solution to this crossword puzzle is in the answer section.

WORD PUZZLE

This word puzzle is designed to help familiarize you with some of the new terminology found in this chapter. Have fun finding all the words on this list. The words can be spelled forward (normally), backward, up, down, or diagonally in any direction. The words will always be in upper case and found in a straight line. Good luck! Answers are found in the answer section.

```
R A P A T H W A Y K H H Z P A C E M A K E R M
T I D N K I P L C J F B Q Y W F M T I F N N M
O D L N L Q N Z P L R W Z M L T L Q M X H K B
R R L V R X X V Z Y Q C R R B V R N H F M G H
X A N R Q N A N E M T Q G Y X E M N T E C K R
E C F O N R J I L R K X T L T R B H Y S M M E
L Y W E I Q S Q D D T I G R L D Q E H U W K K
E H D T H T C C F R L E O R Y M D Z R A T H A
C C J U T K C T O I A G D S Z O M P S P R G M
T A B L V T Y A B M R C R M N L T W Y Y H W E
R T K O M T R A R A P H Y V L O K N D R N N C
I L H S Z Q T G D T Y L A D P W J H L O B J A
C A R B B I H E Q T N T E K A D X W A T U R P
A N R A R Q F H H B T O W X E R H V N A R R G
L O L R T G B M L K B W C T R V B T O S I M N
I I I H B B I K Q Q L H A D G L G K I N E V I
M T L P H A Q L W D M R P F K T K K T E D W R
P C T M P F Y F T X E N C T K N K N C P P K E
U N R V T L R B V L B P Q N T X D X N M W N D
L U D L B L N R E N H F J V M L T K U O A M N
S J A V J U N C T I O N M C Z X L N J C V W A
E R P C F C C M W Q K V K P N E D D I H E Z W
L K Q W Q A W W D T Q Q E R U T A M E R P X F
```

ABSOLUTE
ACCELERATED
AVJUNCTION
AVNODE
BRADYCARDIA
BURIED P WAVE
COMPENSATORY PAUSE
CONTRACTION

DYSRHYTHMIA
ELECTRICAL IMPULSE
HIDDEN
INVERTED
IRRITABILITY
JUNCTIONAL DYSRHYTHMIA
JUNCTIONAL TACHYCARDIA
PACEMAKER

PATHWAY
PJC
PREMATURE
P TOP
QRS COMPLEX
RETROGRADE
RTOR
WANDERING PACEMAKER

On completion of this chapter, the reader should be able to:

1 Describe first-degree heart block, including measurements of the components.

2 Explain the appearance of second-degree heart block, type I, including measurements of the components.

3 Describe the appearance of second-degree heart block, type II, including measurements of the components.

4 Describe third-degree heart block, including the appearance and measurements of the components.

5 Explain the appearance of a bundle branch block, including measurements of the components.

6 Define the terms *prolonged PR interval*, *progressive block*, *Wenckebach*, and *complete AV dissociation*.

Heart Blocks

DEFINITIONS

AV Dissociation—Dysrhythmia also known as third-degree heart block or complete heart block

Heart Block—Partial or complete interruption in the normal cardiac electrical conduction system

Intermittent Heart Block—Interruption of the conduction of an electrical impulse that occurs suddenly and without warning, completely blocking the conduction of the impulse to the ventricles

Lethal Dysrhythmia—A dysrhythmia that cannot sustain life; death producing

Mobitz I—Dysrhythmia also known as second-degree heart block, type I or Wenckebach

Mobitz II—Dysrhythmia also known as second-degree heart block, type II or classic

Progressive Heart Block—Interruption of the conduction of an electrical impulse that becomes longer with each impulse, until it is completely blocked and does not reach the ventricles

"Rabbit Ears"—An informal term used to describe the notched appearance of the widened QRS complexes in bundle branch blocks

HEART BLOCKS

Heart blocks occur when there is a *partial* or *complete interruption* in the cardiac electrical conduction system. This interruption occurs between the atria and the bundle of His, or in the ventricles between the AV junction and the Purkinje's fibers.

The appearance of the P wave and the QRS complex varies, depending on the type of heart block. The rate and the rhythm also may vary.

The location of the block and the resulting patient symptoms determine if the dysrhythmia is lethal.

First-Degree Heart Block

A *first-degree heart block* is caused by a delay in the conduction of an electrical impulse between the atria and the bundle of His. This delay occurs when there is a **partial interruption** or slowing in the conduction of an electrical impulse through the atrioventricular (AV) junctional area (Figure 5-1).

Although all electrical impulses are eventually conducted to the ventricles, the interruption causes the impulse to be delayed. Therefore, a first-degree heart block is **not** a true block, but simply a **delay** in the electrical conduction system. The delay is seen on the monitor screen or rhythm strip as a prolonged PR interval, greater than 0.20 second (Figure 5-2).

A P wave occurs before every QRS complex; however, the PR interval is always greater than 0.20 second. The size and shape of both the P wave and the QRS complex may vary, depending on the underlying rhythm. The P to P and the R to R intervals are usually regular, also depending on the underlying rhythm.

Because a first-degree heart block may be found in any rhythm that has a P wave before the QRS complex, the rate may be normal, bradycardic, or tachycardic. When describing a rhythm containing a first-degree heart block, identify the underlying rhythm first; for example, sinus bradycardia with a first-degree heart block (Figure 5-3).

Although a first-degree heart block is not usually a serious dysrhythmia, it is important to assess the patient carefully when the block indicates a recent change in the patient's electrical conduction system. This change may **indicate** damage to the myocardium, which can lead to a more serious dysrhythmia.

First-degree heart blocks may be caused by myocardial infarction or drugs.

Normal conduction   Abnormal conduction

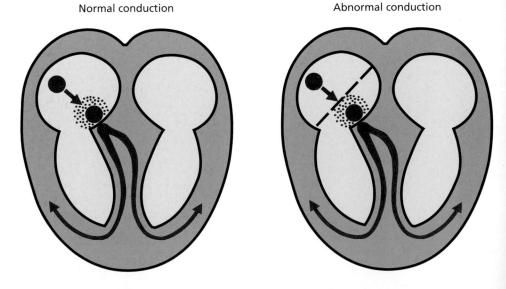

Figure 5-1 *Left heart* shows normal electrical conduction pathway. *Right heart* shows conduction pathway of a first-degree heart block with a delay between atria and AV junction.

Second-Degree Heart Blocks

There are two types of second-degree heart blocks, type I and type II. Both occur when there is an interruption in the conduction of an electrical impulse at or below the AV junctional area.

Second-Degree Heart Block, Type I

Second-degree heart block, type I (Mobitz I, Wenckebach), is a **progressive** heart block. This block occurs when the electrical impulse traveling from the atria is interrupted at the AV junction, slowing the conduction of the impulse to the ventricles.

The interruption becomes longer with each impulse, delaying the depolarization of the ventricles, until the interruption completely blocks the conduction of an electrical impulse to the ventricles. The cycle of **progressively delayed conduction** is then repeated (Figure 5-4, *A* through *E*).

The delay is seen on the rhythm strip as PR intervals become longer before each QRS complex, until a *dropped*, or *absent*, QRS complex occurs (P wave is seen without a QRS complex). This pattern is repeated throughout the dysrhythmia.

A P wave occurs before every QRS complex, and the P waves are the same size and shape. A QRS complex follows each P wave until a QRS is dropped. The QRS complex is usually less than 0.12 second.

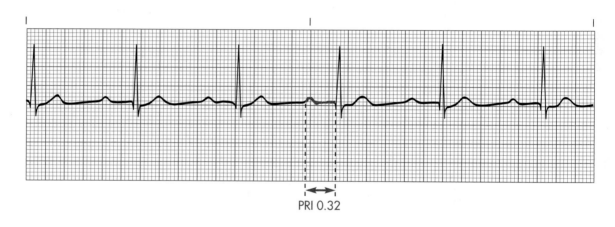

PRI 0.32

Figure 5-2 PR interval greater than 0.20 second: The delay is seen on the monitor screen or rhythm strip as a prolonged PR interval.

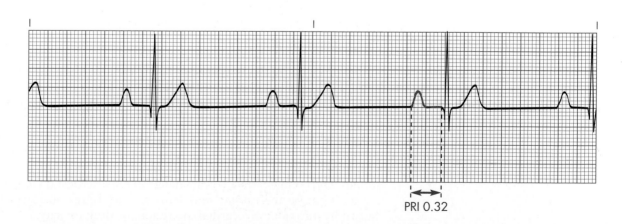

PRI 0.32

Figure 5-3 Sinus bradycardia with first-degree heart block: PR interval, 0.32 second; heart rate, 40 (notice peaked P waves).

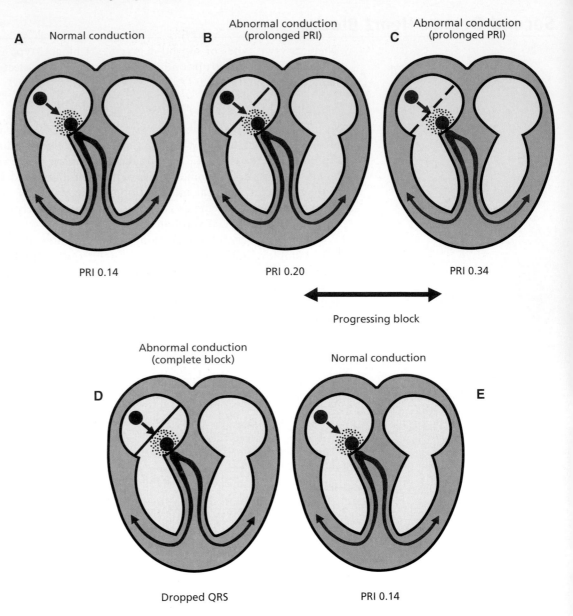

A Normal conduction

B Abnormal conduction (prolonged PRI)

C Abnormal conduction (prolonged PRI)

PRI 0.14

PRI 0.20

PRI 0.34

Progressing block

D Abnormal conduction (complete block)

E Normal conduction

Dropped QRS

PRI 0.14

Figure 5-4 A to E, Hearts show the cycle of progressive delay of second-degree heart block, type I (Mobitz I, Wenckebach).

Although the PR interval becomes progressively longer, the R to R intervals usually remain regular until the QRS complex is dropped. The pattern then repeats itself. The P to P interval remains regular; however, the overall rhythm is irregular. The rate may vary (Figure 5-5).

Although a second-degree heart block, type I, is not a lethal dysrhythmia, the patient may become medically unstable because of a bradycardic rate, recent injury to the cardiac muscle, or prior illness. A second-degree heart block, type I, may be serious when it indicates a recent change in the electrical conduction system following an injury to the cardiac muscle. A second-degree heart block, type I, may be caused by infection, myocardial infarction, or drug toxicity.

As with any rhythm, **patient assessment** is necessary to determine the patient's tolerance of the dysrhythmia.

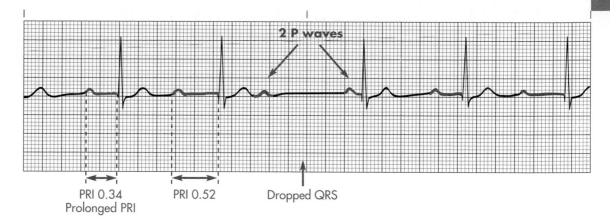

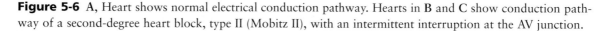

Figure 5-5 Second-degree heart block, type I (Mobitz I, Wenckebach): atrial heart rate, 60; ventricular heart rate, 50 (bradycardic rate).

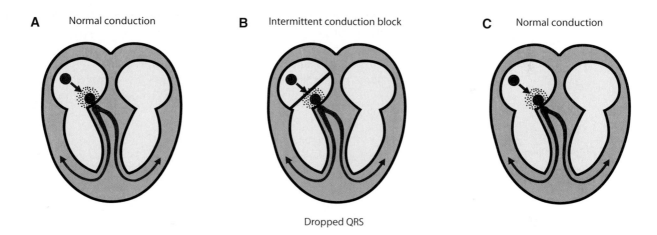

Figure 5-6 **A,** Heart shows normal electrical conduction pathway. Hearts in **B** and **C** show conduction pathway of a second-degree heart block, type II (Mobitz II), with an intermittent interruption at the AV junction.

Second-Degree Heart Block, Type II

Second-degree heart block, type II (Mobitz II, Classic), occurs when there is an **intermittent interruption** in the electrical conduction system near or below the AV junction. This interruption is **not** progressive but occurs **suddenly and without warning**, completely blocking the conduction of the impulse to the ventricles (Figure 5-6, *A* through *C*).

The rhythm strip shows a P wave before every QRS complex, and all P waves are the same size and shape. A QRS complex follows every P wave until an interruption occurs and a QRS complex is dropped (absent). The PR intervals of the underlying rhythm usually remain the same length and may be either normal or prolonged. Although the QRS complex usually measures less than 0.12 second, the complex will be wider if the block occurs low in the bundle branches.

A second-degree heart block, type II, can occur in any rhythm that has a P wave followed by a QRS complex. The P to P intervals are usually regular, and the R to R intervals are usually regular until a QRS complex is dropped. The overall rhythm is usually irregular, and the heart rate varies, depending on the underlying rhythm (Figure 5-7).

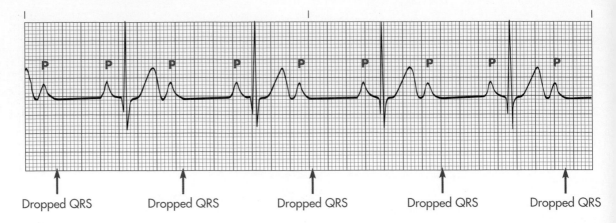

Dropped QRS   Dropped QRS   Dropped QRS   Dropped QRS   Dropped QRS

Figure 5-7 Sinus rhythm with a second-degree heart block, type II (Mobitz II), with a 2:1 block/ratio: atrial heart rate, 90; ventricular heart rate, 40 with bradycardic rate (notice peaked P waves).

When interpreting a dysrhythmia containing a second-degree heart block, type II, it is important to:

1. Identify the underlying rhythm, if possible.
2. Determine the ratio of P waves to each QRS complex. The number of P waves before each QRS complex helps to determine the severity of the block.

   Example: Two P waves before one QRS complex = 2:1 block/ratio
              Three P waves before one QRS complex = 3:1 block/ratio
              Four P waves before one QRS complex = 4:1 block/ratio

   This ratio may be constant or may vary. Second-degree heart block, type II, becomes more serious as the ratio of P waves to QRS complexes increases or if the ratio varies. A second-degree heart block, type II with a ratio greater than 3:1 may also be identified as an advanced AV heart block, due to an increase in the severity of the block/ratio.
3. Determine the frequency of occurrence. Second-degree heart block, type II, may occur in a pattern or at random. A second-degree heart block, type II, with no pattern (varying block/ratio) is more serious. The lack of a pattern indicates the block is irregular and may progress to a more dangerous dysrhythmia (Figure 5-8, *A* through *C*).

A second-degree heart block, type II, can be a **life threatening** dysrhythmia because of the increased irritability of the myocardium, if it leads to a more serious dysrhythmia such as third-degree heart block. If the block is severe enough, the ventricular rate may become bradycardic. A ventricular rate of 40 electrical impulses per minute or less is usually not sufficient to maintain adequate circulation to the vital organs of the body. Frequent assessment is very important to determine the patient's tolerance of the dysrhythmia.

A second-degree heart block, type II, may be caused by myocardial infarction, heart disease, or drug toxicity.

Third-Degree Heart Block

Third-degree heart block (complete heart block or complete AV dissociation) occurs when the electrical impulse is **completely blocked** between the atria and the ventricles. The interruption usually takes place between the AV junction and the bundle of His (Figure 5-9).

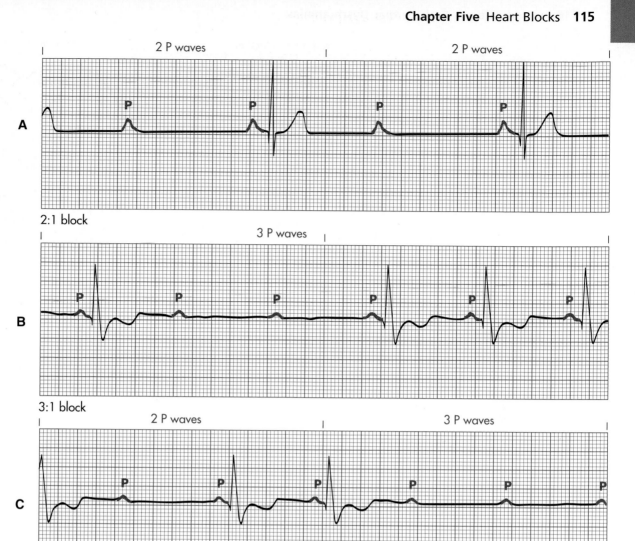

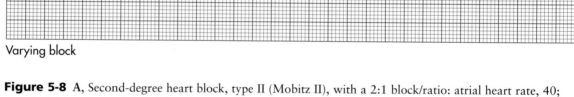

Figure 5-8 **A,** Second-degree heart block, type II (Mobitz II), with a 2:1 block/ratio: atrial heart rate, 40; ventricular heart rate, 20 with bradycardic rate (notice peaked P waves). **B,** Second-degree heart block, type II (Mobitz II), with a 3:1 block/ratio: atrial heart rate, 60; ventricular heart rate, 40 with bradycardic rate (notice diphasic T waves). **C,** Second-degree heart block, type II (Mobitz II), with a varying block/ratio: atrial heart rate, 60; ventricular heart rate, 30 with bradycardic rate (notice diphasic T waves).

Although the electrical impulse causes depolarization of the atria, the impulse is blocked before it can reach the ventricles. Because the electrical conduction system is completely interrupted, the ventricular muscle must initiate its own electrical impulses to cause cardiac muscle contraction. **Both** the atria and the ventricles **function independently,** as if they were two separate hearts (Figure 5-10).

The rhythm strip shows both P waves and QRS complexes, as well as what appear to be PR intervals that are constantly changing in length. However, the PR intervals do **not** become progressively longer as they do in second-degree heart block, type I.

On closer inspection of the rhythm strip, one can see that no relationship exists between the P waves and the QRS complexes. Because the atria and the ventricles are each functioning independently, no true PR interval occurs (Figure 5-11).

Normal conduction   Abnormal conduction

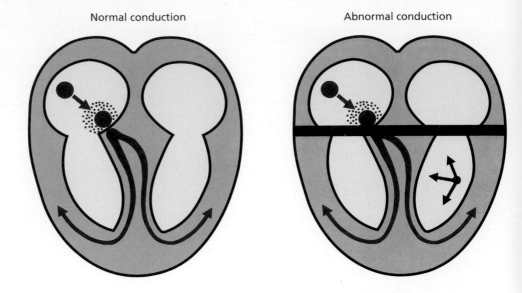

Figure 5-9 *Left heart* shows normal electrical conduction pathway. *Right heart* shows conduction pathway of a third-degree heart block with a complete interruption between the atria and the ventricles.

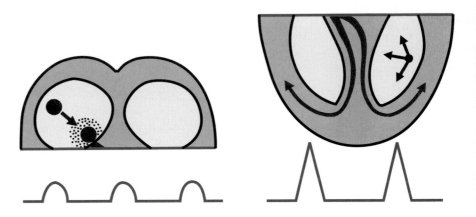

Figure 5-10 Third-degree heart block with separate atrial and ventricular responses.

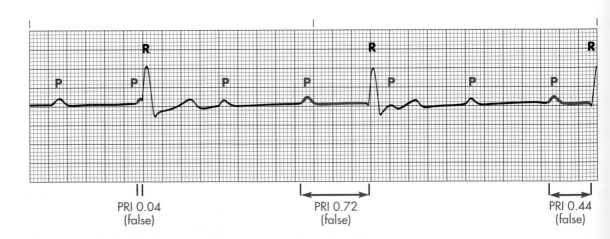

PRI 0.04
(false)

PRI 0.72
(false)

PRI 0.44
(false)

Figure 5-11 Separate P waves and QRS complexes of third-degree heart block: atrial heart rate, 70; ventricular heart rate, 20 to 30 with bradycardic rate (notice depressed ST segments).

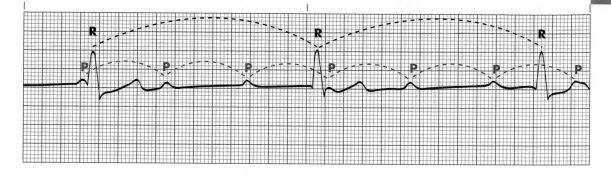

Figure 5-12 Third-degree heart block: atrial heart rate, 70; ventricular heart rate, 30 with bradycardic rate (notice depressed ST segments).

The P waves usually are the same size and shape, although some may be hidden in a QRS complex or in a T wave, changing their appearance. The QRS complexes are usually wide, longer than 0.12 second, and bizarre in appearance but are usually the same size and shape. Occasionally, the QRS complexes will measure less than 0.12 second, if the block occurs at the AV junction.

Because both the atria and the ventricles are generating their own electrical impulses, each will usually depolarize at its own inherent heart rate, causing the P to P intervals to be equal and the R to R intervals to be equal. However, the P to P intervals are usually not equal to the R to R intervals (Figure 5-12).

The atrial heart rate is usually 60 to 100 electrical impulses per minute; the ventricular heart rate is usually 20 to 40 electrical impulses, however, either rate may vary.

Third-degree heart block is considered a *life threatening dysrhythmia* because it may progress to asystole (no heart beat). It may be *lethal* if the ventricular rate is so slow and inefficient that the heart cannot maintain a cardiac output adequate to sustain life.

Third-degree heart block is often caused by a myocardial infarction or severe heart disease.

Bundle Branch Block

A *bundle branch block (BBB)* occurs when there is an **interruption** in the cardiac electrical conduction system of either the right or the left bundle branch. This interruption causes a **delay** in the conduction of the electrical impulse to the ventricle of the blocked bundle branch (Figure 5-13, *A* through *C*).

The atria are usually depolarized in a normal manner. The electrical impulse then follows the normal conduction pathway until it reaches the interruption in the bundle branch. The interruption in the electrical conduction system forces the impulse to "detour" and take an alternate route.

As with any detour, the alternate route takes more time to travel. This extra time causes the electrical impulse to reach the ventricle of the blocked bundle branch later than the ventricle of the normal bundle branch.

As a result, the blocked ventricle depolarizes slightly later than the normal ventricle, causing two separate depolarizations (Figure 5-14). The two depolarizations are shown on the rhythm strip as a single notched or widened QRS complex. The notched QRS is frequently referred to as "*rabbit ears.*" The QRS complex is wider than normal, measuring more than 0.12 second (Figure 5-15).

A bundle branch block can occur in any rhythm. The presence of P waves and PR intervals is determined by the underlying rhythm. The rate and rhythm also may vary, depending on the underlying rhythm.

Normal conduction

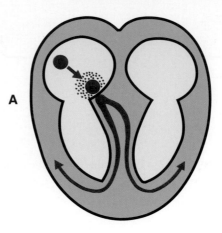

Abnormal conduction

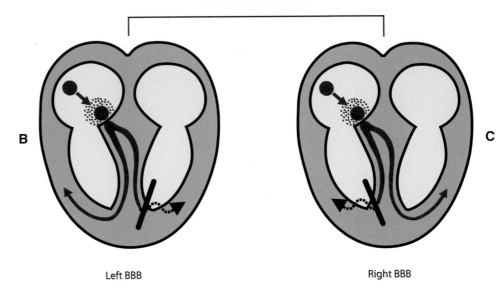

Left BBB   Right BBB

Figure 5-13 **A,** Heart shows normal electrical conduction pathway. Hearts in **B** and **C** show the delayed conduction pathway of a left and a right bundle branch block (BBB).

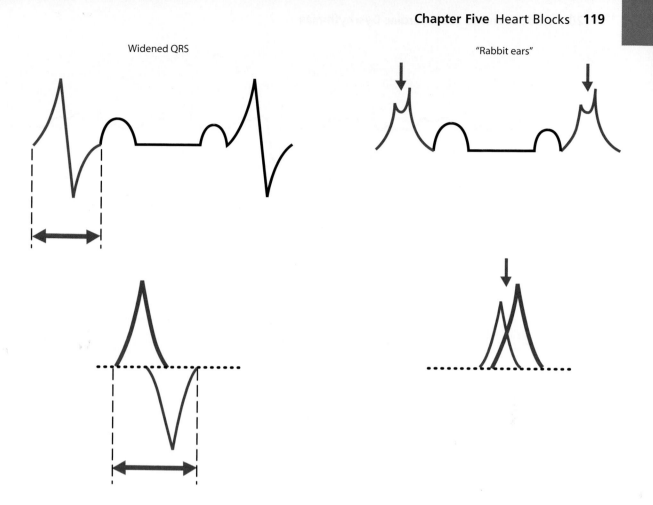

Widened QRS   "Rabbit ears"

Figure 5-14 Two types of ventricular depolarizations seen with a bundle branch block: either a widened QRS or "rabbit ears."

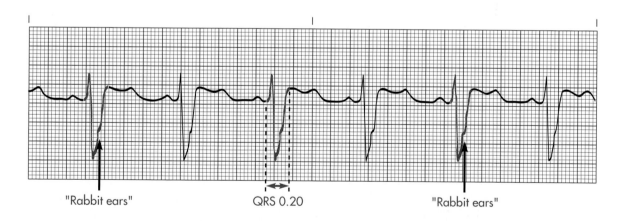

"Rabbit ears"   QRS 0.20   "Rabbit ears"

Figure 5-15 Typical "rabbit ears" and wide QRS seen with bundle branch block (notice elevated ST segments).

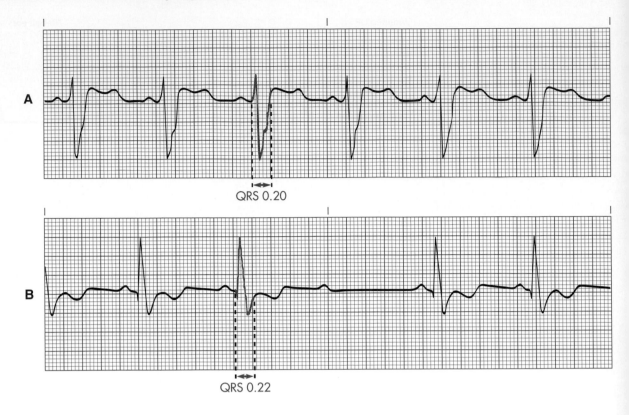

QRS 0.20

QRS 0.22

Figure 5-16 **A**, Sinus rhythm with a bundle branch block; heart rate, 60 (notice elevated ST segments and diphasic T waves). **B**, Second-degree heart block, type II (Mobitz II), with a bundle branch block; atrial heart rate, 50; ventricular heart rate, 40 to 50 with bradycardic rate (notice diphasic T wave).

When interpreting a rhythm strip containing a BBB, you must first identify the underlying rhythm; for example, sinus rhythm with a bundle branch block (Figure 5-16, *A* and *B*).

Although a BBB by itself is not usually a serious dysrhythmia, it **is** important to assess the patient carefully when the block indicates a recent change in the patient's electrical conduction pathway. This change may indicate damage to the myocardium, which can lead to a more serious dysrhythmia.

A 12-Lead electrocardiogram (ECG) is necessary to determine the seriousness of the block and if the block is in the right or left bundle branch.

Bundle branch blocks may be caused by heart disease or myocardial infarction.

REVIEW QUESTIONS

True   **False**   1. Heart blocks occur when there is a partial or complete interruption in the cardiac electrical conduction system.

True   **False**   2. A first-degree heart block occurs when there is a partial or complete interruption anywhere in the ventricles.

True   **False**   3. A third-degree heart block may progress to a Mobitz II heart block.

True   **False**   4. A third-degree heart block exists when the atria and ventricles function independently.

5. In a bundle branch block, the two depolarizations are seen on the rhythm strip as a notched or widened:

    a. T wave

    b. PR interval

    c. QRS complex

    d. ST segment

6. A third-degree heart block is a life threatening dysrhythmia because

    a. the additional force of the ventricular contraction can cause cardiac exhaustion

    b. it can progress to asystole

    c. the electrical impulse cannot be transmitted to the Purkinje's fibers

    d. the atria do not depolarize

7. Second-degree heart block, type I, is also known as:

    a. Mobitz II

    b. AV dissociation

    c. Mobitz I or Wenckebach

    d. bundle branch block

8. In a first-degree heart block, the PR interval is greater than _____ second.

9. Complete heart block, or AV dissociation, is also known as _____.

10. In a second-degree heart block, type I, the PR intervals become progressively _____, until a P wave is followed by a dropped or absent _____.

11. Explain why a second-degree heart block, type II, is considered a dangerous dysrhythmia.

_____

_____

12. When identifying a second-degree heart block, type II, which three aspects of a rhythm are important to evaluate?

    a. _____

    b. _____

    c. _____

RHYTHM STRIP REVIEW

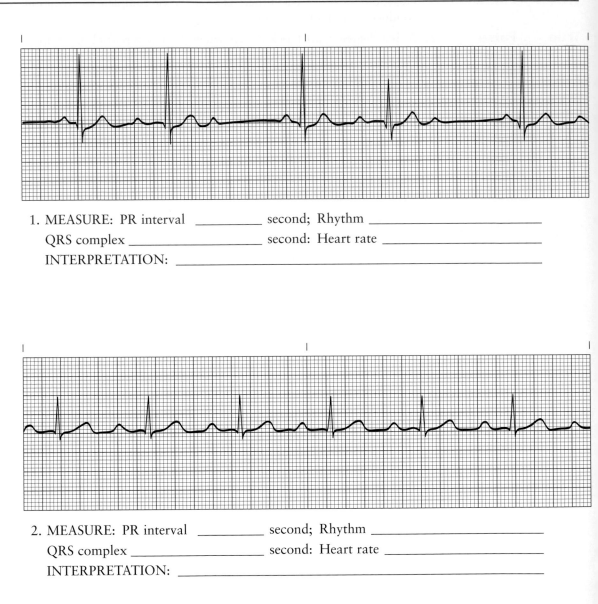

1. MEASURE: PR interval _____ second; Rhythm _____
   QRS complex _____ second: Heart rate _____
   INTERPRETATION: _____

2. MEASURE: PR interval _____ second; Rhythm _____
   QRS complex _____ second: Heart rate _____
   INTERPRETATION: _____

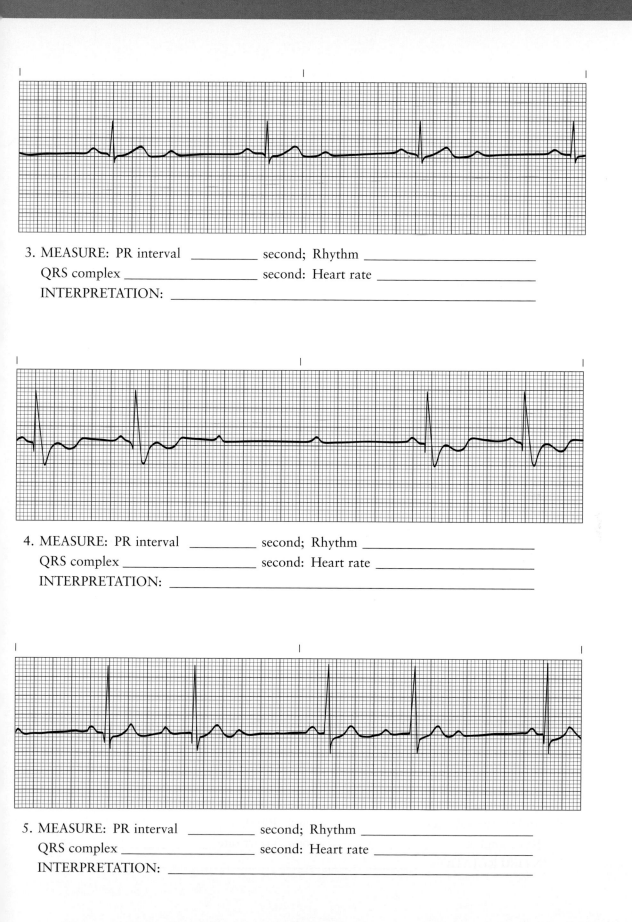

3. MEASURE: PR interval _____ second; Rhythm _____
   QRS complex _____ second: Heart rate _____
   INTERPRETATION: _____

4. MEASURE: PR interval _____ second; Rhythm _____
   QRS complex _____ second: Heart rate _____
   INTERPRETATION: _____

5. MEASURE: PR interval _____ second; Rhythm _____
   QRS complex _____ second: Heart rate _____
   INTERPRETATION: _____

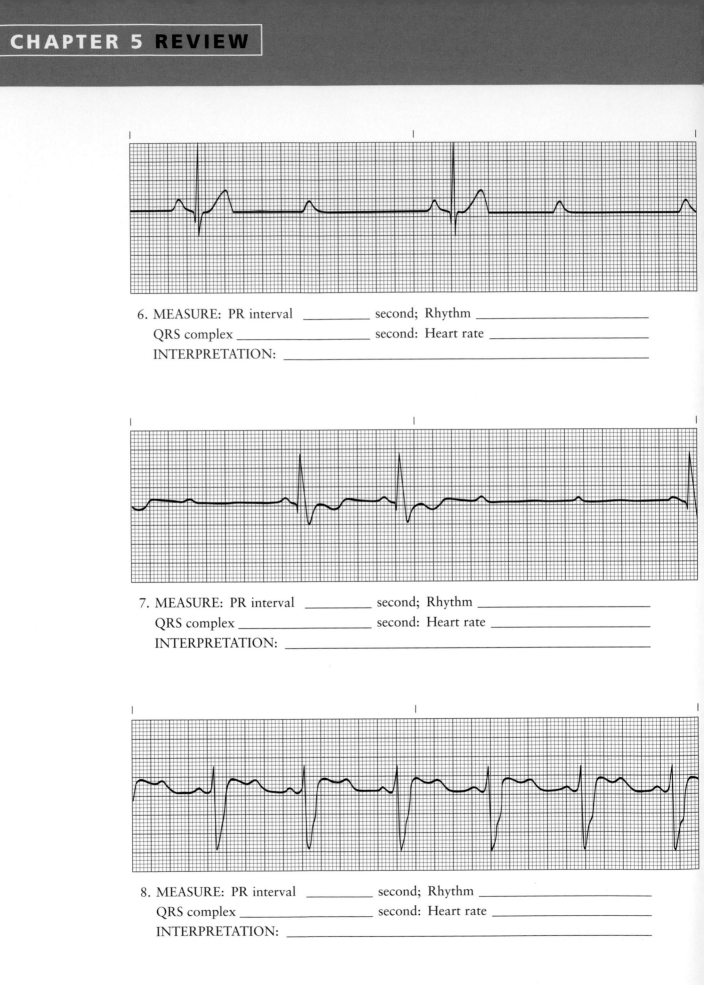

6. MEASURE: PR interval _____ second; Rhythm _____

   QRS complex _____ second: Heart rate _____

   INTERPRETATION: _____

7. MEASURE: PR interval _____ second; Rhythm _____

   QRS complex _____ second: Heart rate _____

   INTERPRETATION: _____

8. MEASURE: PR interval _____ second; Rhythm _____

   QRS complex _____ second: Heart rate _____

   INTERPRETATION: _____

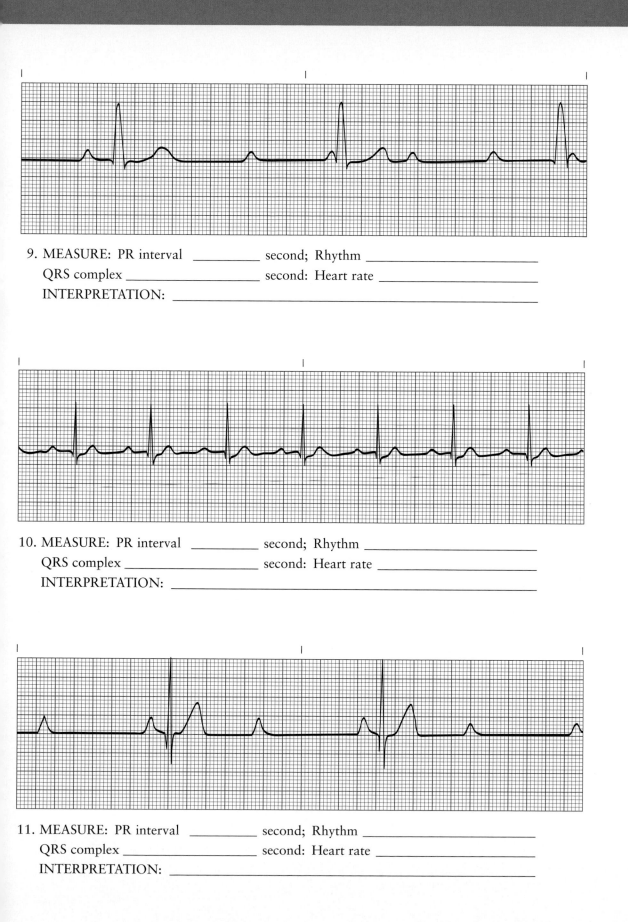

9. MEASURE: PR interval _____ second; Rhythm _____
   QRS complex _____ second: Heart rate _____
   INTERPRETATION: _____

10. MEASURE: PR interval _____ second; Rhythm _____
    QRS complex _____ second: Heart rate _____
    INTERPRETATION: _____

11. MEASURE: PR interval _____ second; Rhythm _____
    QRS complex _____ second: Heart rate _____
    INTERPRETATION: _____

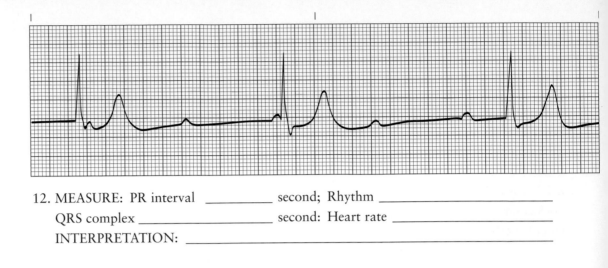

12. MEASURE: PR interval _____ second; Rhythm _____

QRS complex _____ second: Heart rate _____

INTERPRETATION: _____

Suggestion: You may find it helpful reviewing the Chapter 4 and 5 rhythm strips on the CD prior to studying the next chapter.

CROSSWORD PUZZLE AND CLUES

Across

1 Stops suddenly; intermittent conduction.

5 Complete block of the electrical conduction system between atria and ventricles; each functions separately.

7 Absent or _____ QRS complex.

9 Prolonged ___; first-degree block.

10 Upper heart chambers.

11 Second-degree heart block; type I or II.

12 Bundle of ____.

14 Number of P waves before each QRS complex in Mobitz II heart blocks.

15 Mobitz II is a(n) _____-degree heart block.

18 Second-degree heart block, type I.

21 Lower heart chambers.

22 Interruption of cardiac electrical conduction system.

24 _____ branch.

Down

2 Complete heart block.

3 Mobitz I is a(n) _____type of second-degree heart block.

4 ____-degree heart block is caused by a delay in conduction of electrical impulse through AV junctional area.

6 Pertaining to the heart.

8 Extended.

13 Identify the _____ rhythm when interpreting a Mobitz II heart block.

16 Life threatening.

17 _____node; primary cardiac pacemaker.

19 Heart blocks occur when there is a(n) _____ or complete interruption of the normal cardiac electrical conduction pathway.

20 Evaluate symptoms.

23 A "rabbit-ears" QRS is frequently seen in _____.

The solution to this crossword puzzle is in the answer section.

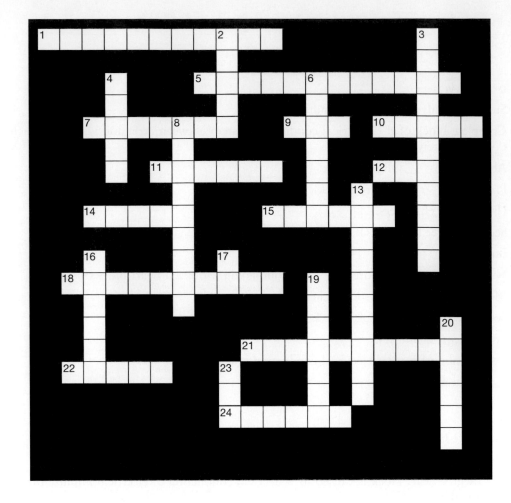

WORD PUZZLE

This word puzzle is designed to help familiarize you with some of the new terminology found in this chapter. Have fun finding all the words on this list. The words can be spelled forward (normally), backward, up, down, or diagonally in any direction. The words will always be in upper case and found in a straight line. Good luck. Answers are found in answer section.

```
Y  Z  S  T  U  N  D  E  R  L  Y  I  N  G  R  H  Y  T  H  M
N  W  C  U  K  R  L  T  N  T  N  E  S  B  A  N  J  W  N  W
E  Q  P  Z  D  M  A  O  Q  W  H  F  X  N  Y  M  N  T  Y  Z
V  N  H  R  F  D  I  B  G  X  I  H  C  R  M  V  M  K  L  C
I  J  Q  T  O  T  E  R  B  R  E  T  E  L  P  M  O  C  L  V
S  S  D  R  A  L  D  N  S  I  H  W  I  Y  Y  Z  K  J  I  E
S  H  R  R  X  J  O  T  M  W  T  I  N  V  B  N  C  D  N  E
E  C  M  Q  N  R  D  N  L  L  E  E  N  Y  T  O  O  F  T  R
R  N  W  L  D  E  N  L  G  P  A  F  A  M  R  T  L  T  E  G
G  A  X  W  G  E  M  O  Y  E  T  H  F  R  X  C  B  N  R  E
O  R  Y  R  H  W  P  T  I  M  D  Z  T  Y  S  H  T  E  M  D
R  B  E  W  I  L  V  P  O  T  D  P  L  E  M  E  R  M  I  D
P  E  D  D  D  B  Y  B  O  X  P  J  R  F  L  D  A  S  T  R
T  L  E  R  K  R  I  D  N  R  J  U  K  I  N  Q  E  S  T  I
C  D  L  M  K  T  Q  Z  T  N  D  W  R  R  N  R  H  E  E  H
N  N  A  Y  Z  K  Q  M  K  D  T  H  T  R  N  S  T  S  N  T
C  U  Y  I  F  M  K  M  D  R  C  M  X  L  E  G  V  S  T  B
X  B  E  K  H  F  B  B  B  Q  R  N  B  C  H  T  Z  A  W  W
Q  K  D  S  E  C  O  N  D  D  E  G  R  E  E  R  N  Q  K  J
C  A  V  D  I  S  S  O  C  I  A  T  I  O  N  G  W  I  H  T
```

ABSENT	HEART BLOCK	RATIO
ASSESSMENT	INTERMITTENT	SECOND DEGREE
AV DISSOCIATION	INTERRUPTION	SUDDEN
BBB	LETHAL	THIRD DEGREE
BUNDLE BRANCH	MOBITZ I	TYPE II
COMPLETE	NOTCHED QRS	UNDERLYING RHYTHM
DELAYED	PROGRESSIVE	WIDE
DROPPED QRS	PROLONGED PRI	
FIRST DEGREE	RABBIT EARS	

VENTRICULAR DYSRHYTHMIAS

When the sinoatrial (SA) node, other atrial pacemaker sites, and the atrioventricular (AV) junction all fail to initiate an electrical impulse, the ventricles may become the pacemaker of the heart. The electrical stimulus can be initiated from any pacemaker cell in the ventricles, including the bundle branches or the Purkinje's fibers.

Because the electrical impulse begins in the lower portion of the heart, the impulse must take an alternate conduction pathway. The electrical impulse must travel in a retrograde (backward) direction to depolarize the atria **and** also in a forward direction to depolarize the ventricles (Figure 6-1).

Since the atria depolarize at almost the same time as the ventricles, the P wave is usually hidden in the QRS complex and will not be seen (Figure 6-2). The QRS complex is wide and bizarre in appearance and measures greater than 0.12 second.

Because the ventricles are the least efficient pacemaker of the heart, they usually generate 20 to 40 electrical impulses per minute (inherent ventricular heart rate). However, many factors can affect the inherent heart rate. For example, poor cardiac output could cause a significant increase in the rate, as the heart beats faster in an attempt to improve the cardiac output.

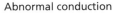

Abnormal conduction

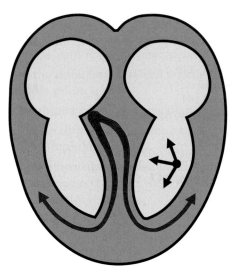

Figure 6-1 Ventricular electrical conduction pathway.

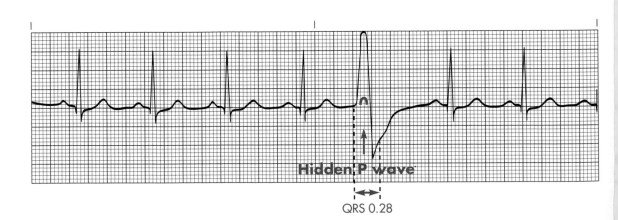

Figure 6-2 Ventricular response with hidden P wave within QRS complex.

Ventricular dysrhythmias are usually considered **life threatening**. However, as with any rhythm, **patient assessment** is essential to determine the patient's tolerance of the dysrhythmia.

Premature Ventricular Complex

A *premature ventricular complex* (PVC), formerly called a premature ventricular contraction, is an individual complex that originates from an area below the bundle of His, and also occurs earlier than the next expected complex of the underlying rhythm (Figure 6-3). PVCs are very common and can occur in any cardiac rhythm.

Although PVCs are *individual* complexes and not rhythms, they are included in this chapter because they originate from the ventricles.

When the ventricles initiate a PVC, the atria may or may not depolarize. If the atria do not depolarize, a P wave will not be formed. When atrial depolarization does occur, the P wave is usually hidden in the QRS complex because the ventricles depolarize at about the same time.

The QRS complex has a wide and bizarre appearance, is greater than 0.12 second, and may deflect in the opposite direction of the QRS complexes in the underlying rhythm.

The T wave immediately following the PVC is usually deflected in the opposite direction of the QRS complex of the premature ventricular complex. The ST segment of the PVC appears abnormal because of this opposite deflection.

A premature ventricular complex is usually followed by a complete compensatory pause. This pause allows the underlying rhythm to continue again at its normal rate, as if the PVC had never occurred (Figure 6-4).

You can check the complete compensatory pause by measuring the R to R intervals before and after the PVC. Measure from the R wave of the complex before the PVC to the R wave of the complex after the PVC. The distance will be equal to two times the R to R interval of the underlying rhythm (see Chapter 3).

The P to P and R to R intervals of the underlying rhythm will vary, depending on that rhythm. A PVC, in even the most regular rhythm, will cause the P to P and R to R intervals to be irregular.

The rate of the rhythm also varies, depending on the underlying rhythm and the number of PVCs within that rhythm. When determining the rate of a rhythm that

Normal conduction   Abnormal conduction

PVC

Figure 6-3 *Left heart* shows normal electrical conduction pathway. *Right heart* shows conduction pathway of a premature ventricular complex (PVC).

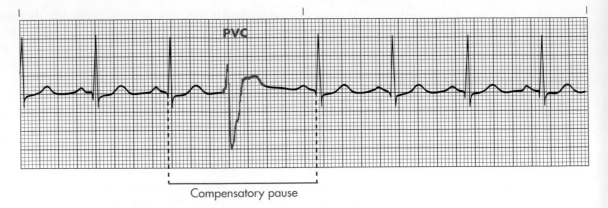

Figure 6-4 Premature ventricular complex with a complete compensatory pause.

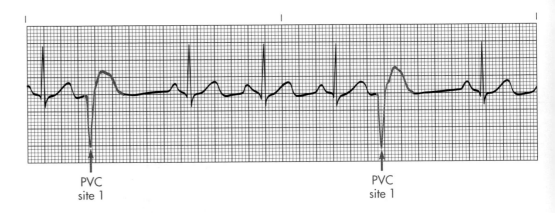

Figure 6-5 Sinus rhythm with unifocal premature ventricular complexes; heart rate, 70 (notice peaked P waves).

contains premature ventricular complexes, the PVCs **are** included in the total count of R waves.

Site of Origin

PVCs are further classified by the site of origin and the frequency of their occurrence.

1. *Unifocal* PVCs originate from a single site within the ventricles and therefore look alike. The term *unifocal* is also known as *monomorphic* (Figure 6-5).
2. *Multifocal* PVCs originate from different ventricular sites and have varying sizes and shapes. These PVCs are more dangerous because they are the result of increased irritability within the ventricles (Figure 6-6). The term *multifocal* is also known as *polymorphic*.

Frequency of Occurrence

When interpreting rhythm strips that contain premature ventricular complexes, it is important to look at how often the PVCs occur.

The frequency of occurrence is an indication of how irritable (excitable) the cardiac cells are. Less electrical stimulation is needed to cause depolarization when there is greater irritability. This can lead to a more serious, rapid rate dysrhythmia.

Also, when PVCs occur frequently, the ventricles have less time to refill with an adequate amount of blood. Either of these situations can cause poor cardiac output,

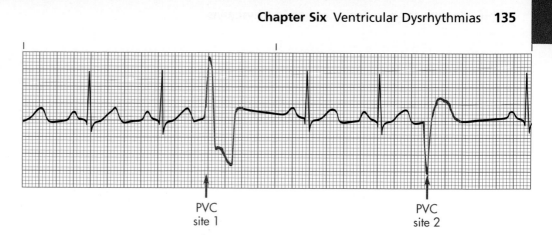

Figure 6-6 Sinus rhythm with multifocal premature ventricular complexes; heart rate, 70 (notice peaked P waves).

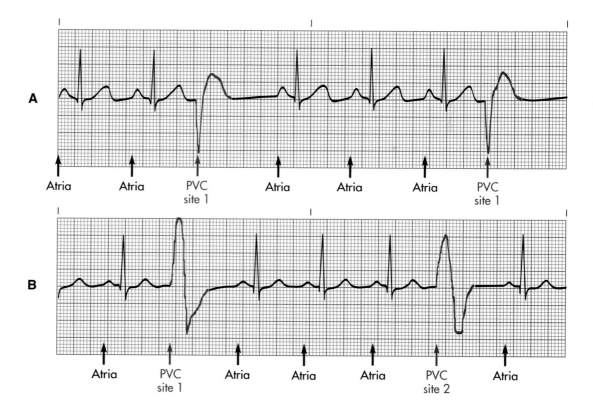

Figure 6-7 Quadrigeminy. **A,** Sinus rhythm with unifocal quadrigeminy of premature ventricular complexes; heart rate, 70. **B,** Sinus rhythm with multifocal quadrigeminy of premature ventricular complexes; heart rate, 70.

leading to serious symptoms. The following terms are used to describe the frequency of PVCs:

1. *Quadrigeminy* occurs when every fourth QRS complex is a PVC (Figure 6-7, *A* and *B*).
2. *Trigeminy* occurs when every third QRS complex is a PVC (Figure 6-8, *A* and *B*).
3. *Bigeminy* occurs when every other QRS complex is a PVC. This rate of occurrence is more serious than quadrigeminy or trigeminy because it usually indicates a higher degree of irritability in the ventricular muscle (Figure 6-9, *A* and *B*).

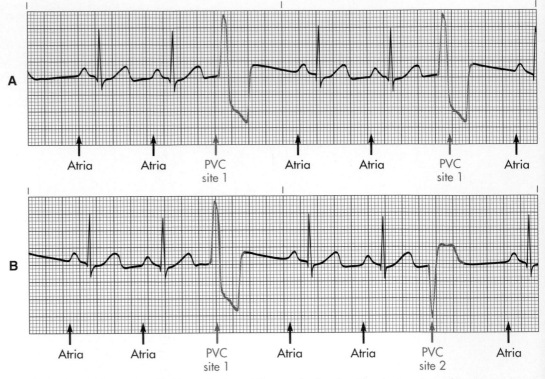

Figure 6-8 Trigeminy. **A,** Sinus rhythm with an episode of unifocal trigeminy of premature ventricular complexes; heart rate, 60 to 70. **B,** Sinus rhythm with an episode of multifocal trigeminy of premature ventricular complexes; heart rate, 70 (notice peaked P waves in **A** and **B**).

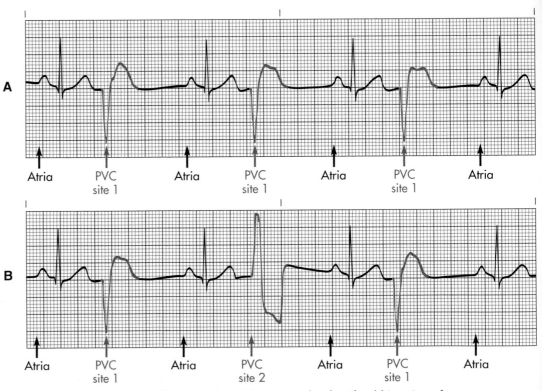

Figure 6-9 Bigeminy. **A,** Sinus rhythm with an episode of unifocal bigeminy of premature ventricular complexes; heart rate, 70. **B,** Sinus rhythm with multifocal bigeminy of premature ventricular complexes; heart rate, 70 (notice peaked P waves in **A** and **B**).

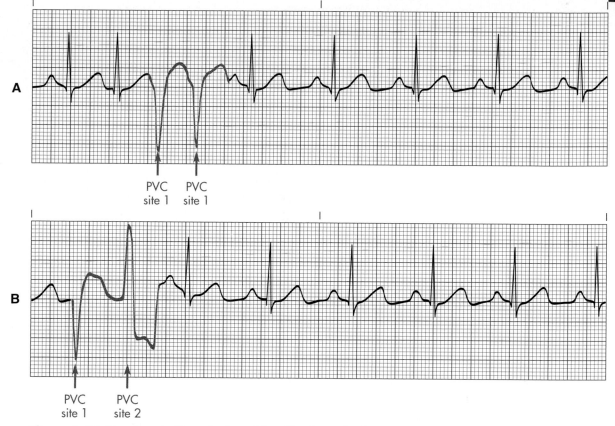

Figure 6-10 Couplets. **A**, Sinus rhythm with unifocal couplet; heart rate, 90. **B**, Sinus rhythm with multifocal couplet; heart rate, 80 (notice peaked P waves in **A** and **B**).

> **NOTE:** To identify bigeminy, trigeminy, and quadrigeminy in the clinical setting, there must be at least three episodes in a row on the monitor or rhythm strip.

4. *Couplet* (paired) describes two PVCs in a row that are not separated by a complex of the underlying rhythm (Figure 6-10, *A* and *B*).

5. *Run of ventricular tachycardia* (run of VT) occurs when three or more PVCs occur in a row, not separated by a QRS complex of the underlying rhythm. A run of VT is of short duration, and the PVCs are usually all unifocal, at a heart rate greater than 100. Both couplets and runs of VT indicate a high degree of irritability in the ventricles and may lead to a lethal dysrhythmia (Figure 6-11). A run of VT may be called a *salvo* or *burst* of PVCs.

R on T Phenomenon

R on T phenomenon (R on T) is an additional term used to describe PVCs. It occurs when the R wave of the PVC falls on the T wave of the previous complex. R on T phenomenon may lead to a lethal dysrhythmia, such as ventricular tachycardia (VT, V Tach), because the PVC occurs during the vulnerable period of ventricular repolarization (Figure 6-12, *A* and *B*). This vulnerable period, *(relative refractory period)* is the time during the cardiac cycle when cardiac cells have repolarized to the point that some cells can be stimulated to depolarize (contract) again, if the stimulus is strong enough (see Chapter 2).

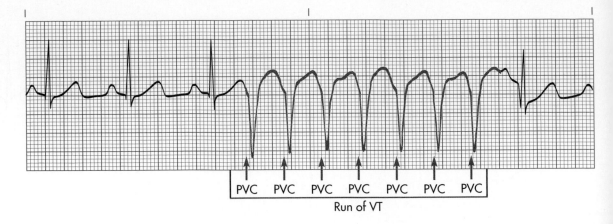

Figure 6-11 Sinus rhythm with a run of ventricular tachycardia; heart rate, 110 (notice peaked P waves).

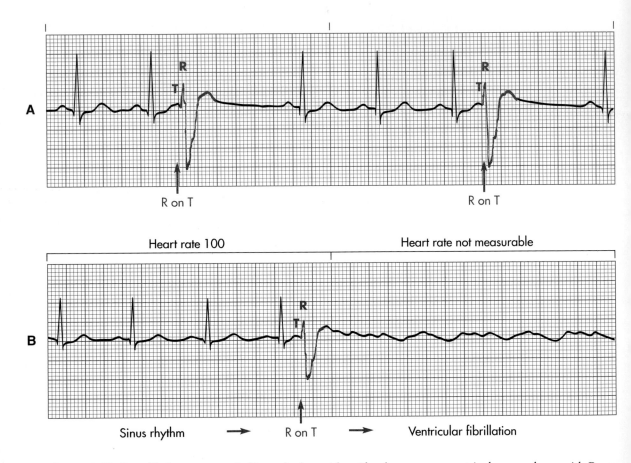

Figure 6-12 R on T phenomenon. **A,** Sinus rhythm with unifocal premature ventricular complexes with R on T; heart rate, 80. **B,** Sinus rhythm; heart rate, 100, with an R on T premature ventricular complex progressing to ventricular fibrillation (heart rate not measurable).

Other Aspects

Patients with PVCs do not always require treatment. PVCs may be the heart's attempt to increase the cardiac rate to maintain adequate circulation and cardiac output, when the rate of the underlying rhythm is bradycardic. However, PVCs are usually considered dangerous, and patients may require immediate treatment, if one or more of the following occur:

1. More than six PVCs in 1 minute
2. Multifocal PVCs
3. Couplets
4. Run of VT
5. R on T phenomenon
6. A patient who is medically unstable

When assessing the patient's condition, it is also important to remember that the patient's pulse may **not** match the heart rate seen on the monitor because of the following factors:

1. The ventricular muscle cells may not have repolarized enough to respond to the electrical impulse of the PVC and to contract effectively.
2. The PVC may not allow the ventricles to refill with enough blood to be felt as a pulse when the left ventricle contracts.

Because a PVC may not actually produce a pulse, it is **essential** to assess the patient and not rely on the monitor alone. This assessment will determine the patient's tolerance of the dysrhythmia and the possible need for immediate treatment.

PVCs can be caused by heart disease, myocardial infarction, or stimulants such as caffeine or nicotine. Stress and anxiety can also cause PVCs.

Ventricular Tachycardia

Ventricular tachycardia (VT, V Tach) is a dysrhythmia that usually originates from a single site in the ventricles at a rate of 101 to 250 electrical impulses per minute (Figure 6-13). A VT with a rate of 41 to 100 is considered an *accelerated idioventricular dysrhythmia*.

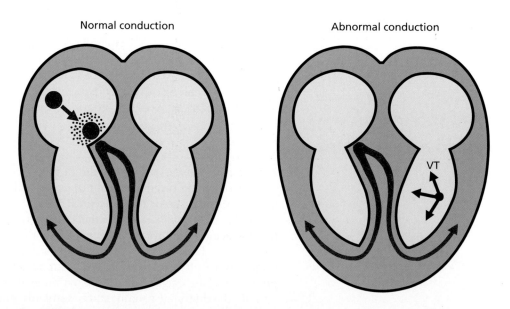

Normal conduction   Abnormal conduction

Figure 6-13 *Left heart* shows normal electrical conduction pathway. *Right heart* shows conduction pathway of ventricular tachycardia.

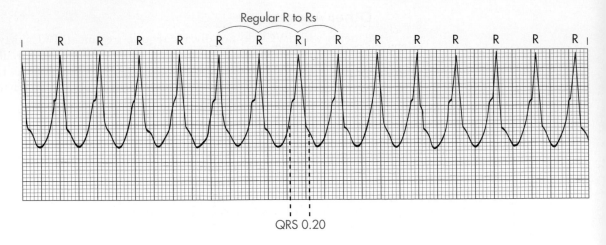

Figure 6-14 Ventricular tachycardia with regular R to R intervals and QRS greater than 0.12 second; heart rate, 140 to 150.

P waves, if present, are from the underlying rhythm, not the ventricular tachycardia. PR intervals and P to P intervals are not measurable.

The QRS complex is wide, bizarre, and measures greater than 0.12 second. The R to R interval is usually regular, although it may be slightly irregular (Figure 6-14).

This dysrhythmia starts suddenly and is frequently triggered by a PVC. Although the definition of ventricular tachycardia is more than three PVCs in a row, VT that lasts 30 seconds or less is usually called *unsustained VT* or a *run of VT*, while *sustained* (prolonged) *ventricular tachycardia* lasts longer than 30 seconds.

Ventricular tachycardia is a **life threatening** dysrhythmia. As the heart rate increases, the ventricles do not have time to completely empty and refill. Therefore, cardiac output is decreased, and adequate amounts of blood are not circulated to vital organs, such as the heart and brain.

Patient symptoms vary, depending on the duration of the ventricular tachycardia. For example, with a run of VT, the patient may feel slightly weak or complain of occasional "palpitations" or a "racing heart", (stable VT). However, in *sustained VT* the patient's condition usually becomes unstable, and may lead to unresponsiveness and **loss of pulse**, (pulseless VT) requiring immediate treatment. Again, the patient **must** be assessed frequently to determine the patient's tolerance of the dysrhythmia and the appropriate treatment.

Ventricular tachycardia may be the result of increased irritability within the ventricles, which can be caused by myocardial infarction, advanced heart disease, severe ischemia, electrical shock, or drugs such as epinephrine or digitalis.

Torsades de Pointes

Torsades de pointes is a dysrhythmia that looks similar to ventricular tachycardia. The dysrhythmia originates from the ventricular muscle, but it is unclear whether it is from a single site or multiple sites.

Unlike ventricular tachycardia, the wave amplitude (height) of torsades de pointes begins close to the baseline, gradually increasing and decreasing in a repeating pattern. The rhythm resembles a twisting and turning motion along the baseline (Figure 6-15). It is important to determine if the dysrhythmia is VT or torsades de pointes because each of these dysrhythmias is treated differently (see Chapter 9).

This dysrhythmia usually starts suddenly and is frequently preceded by a prolonged QT interval; more than one half the R to R interval of that complex and the R wave of the following complex (see Chapter 2). P waves, if seen, are from the underlying rhythm, not the torsades de pointes. PR intervals and P to P intervals are

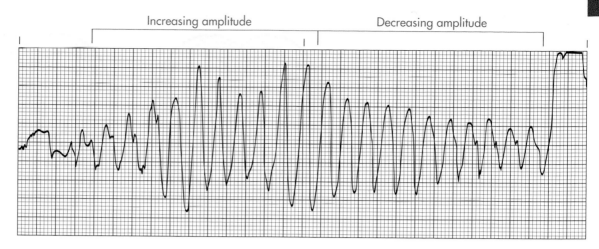

Figure 6-15 Torsades de pointes; heart rate, 240 to 250.

not measurable. The QRS complex is wide, bizarre, and greater than 0.12 second. The R to R interval is usually regular, although it may be slightly irregular. The ventricular rate is often greater than 150 electrical impulses per minute.

The duration of the torsades de pointes will affect the patient's tolerance of the dysrhythmia. If the torsades de pointes lasts only a few seconds, the patient may complain of symptoms such as slight weakness, occasional palpitations, or a "racing heart." However, a torsades de pointes with a longer duration usually leads to an unstable condition, with signs and symptoms of poor cardiac output such as hypotension or unresponsiveness, and may progress to a **loss of pulse.**

Torsades de pointes is a **life threatening** dysrhythmia. As the heart rate increases, the ventricles do not have enough time to completely empty and refill. Therefore, good cardiac output is not maintained, and adequate amounts of blood and oxygen are **not** circulated to the vital organs, such as the heart and brain.

Patient assessment **must** be performed frequently to determine the patient's tolerance of the dysrhythmia and the proper treatment protocol.

Some common causes of torsades de pointes include myocardial infarction, severe heart disease, low blood levels of magnesium, or drugs that prolong the QT interval, such as lidocaine or procainamide.

Ventricular Fibrillation

Ventricular fibrillation (VF, V Fib) is a **lethal** dysrhythmia that originates from many different sites within the ventricles (Figure 6-16). Because so many ventricular sites initiate electrical impulses, the cardiac cells do not have time to completely depolarize and repolarize. Therefore, electrical impulses are not transmitted through **any** conduction pathway of the heart.

Neither the atria nor the ventricles depolarize; therefore, P waves, QRS complexes, PR intervals, P to P intervals, and R to R intervals are **not** present. Only a chaotic, wavy line is seen on the monitor or rhythm strip. Because QRS complexes are not seen, it is impossible to measure a heart rate (Figure 6-17).

The ventricles make ineffective quivering movements, not actual contractions. Consequently, blood is not being pumped throughout the body, and the patient **does not** have a pulse. Death will occur if treatment is not begun immediately.

Ventricular fibrillation is described as either coarse or fine. *Coarse V Fib* waves have a higher amplitude (height) and are more irregular than fine V Fib waves. This difference indicates that a greater number of cardiac cells are able to respond to the electrical stimulation. Coarse V Fib may progress to fine V Fib, which responds less easily to treatment (Figure 6-18).

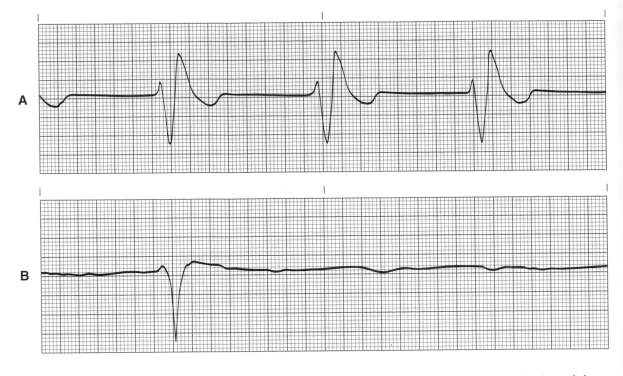

Figure 6-21 A, Idioventricular dysrhythmia; atrial heart rate, 0; ventricular heart rate, 30. B, Agonal dysrhythmia; atrial heart rate, 0; ventricular heart rate, 10.

complexes to be very wide and bizarre, measuring more than 0.12 second (Figure 6-21, A). The R to R intervals may be irregular.

The ventricular rate of an idioventricular dysrhythmia is usually less than 40 electrical impulses per minute. If the rate is 41 to 100 electrical impulses per minute, the dysrhythmia is known as *accelerated idioventricular dysrhythmia* or *accelerated idioventricular rhythm (AIVR)*. When the ventricular rate becomes less than 20 electrical impulses per minute, the rhythm is known as an *agonal (dying heart) dysrhythmia* (Figure 6-21, B). As the ventricles weaken and their electrical impulses become slower, the QRS complexes progressively show less amplitude and become wider, until **all** cardiac electrical activity stops.

The heart muscle is so damaged that cardiac contractions are ineffective, and cardiac output is so poor that oxygen is not reaching the body cells in sufficient amounts to maintain life. Both idioventricular and agonal dysrhythmias are **lethal** dysrhythmias, and treatment **must** be started immediately.

These dysrhythmias are usually seen in the end stage of advanced heart disease.

Ventricular Standstill

Ventricular standstill occurs when only atrial depolarization exists and there is **no** ventricular depolarization (Figure 6-22).

P waves are present, and the P to P intervals are regular. The ventricles do not depolarize; therefore QRS complexes, PR intervals, and R to R intervals are not present (Figure 6-23).

The atrial heart rate usually varies from 60 to 100 electrical impulses per minute; however, the ventricular rate is 0. Because the ventricles do not depolarize, there is **no** ventricular contraction. Blood **does not** circulate to any part of the body. The patient **does not** have a pulse. This dysrhythmia is **lethal** and requires **immediate** treatment.

Normal conduction   Abnormal conduction

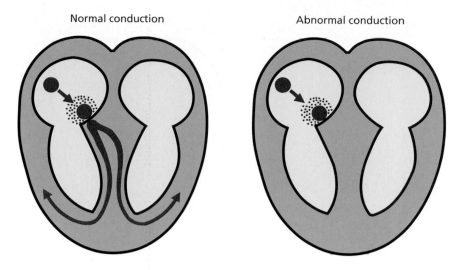

Figure 6-22 *Left heart* shows normal electrical conduction pathway. *Right heart* shows conduction pathway of ventricular standstill.

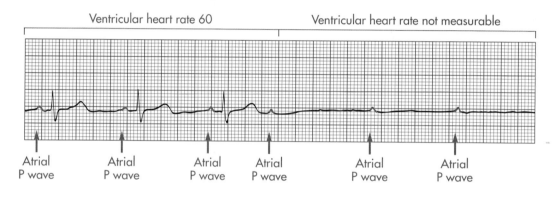

Ventricular heart rate 60   Ventricular heart rate not measurable

Atrial P wave   Atrial P wave   Atrial P wave   Atrial P wave   Atrial P wave   Atrial P wave

Figure 6-23 Sinus rhythm changing into ventricular standstill; atrial heart rate, 80; ventricular heart rate, 60; then changing to atrial heart rate, 40; ventricular heart rate, 0.

Ventricular standstill may be the result of third-degree heart block, massive myocardial infarction, or a ventricular rupture.

Asystole

Asystole occurs when there is a complete lack of electrical activity in both the atria and the ventricles. Therefore, the atria and ventricles do not depolarize (Figure 6-24).

No P waves, PR intervals, QRS complexes, P to P intervals, or R to R intervals exist. Asystole appears as a slightly wavy or straight line on the monitor screen or rhythm strip (Figure 6-25, *A* and *B*). Because it may be difficult to distinguish asystole from very fine V Fib, two different leads should be used to confirm asystole, for example, Lead II and MCL I (see Chapter 2).

This dysrhythmia is **lethal**. The patient will **not** have a pulse, and **immediate** assessment and treatment are required.

Asystole usually follows untreated VT or V Fib. It may also be caused by massive myocardial infarction, advanced cardiac disease, or electrical shock.

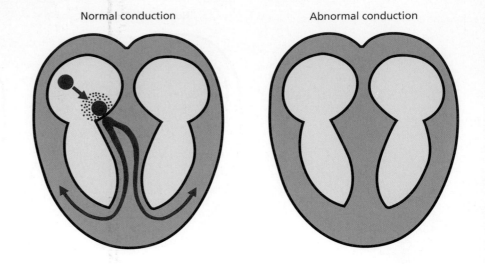

Normal conduction   Abnormal conduction

Figure 6-24 *Left heart* shows normal electrical conduction pathway. *Right heart* shows conduction pathway of asystole.

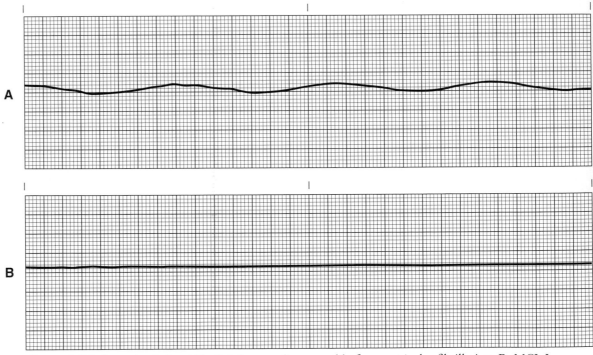

Figure 6-25 Asystole. A, Lead II, slightly wavy line, possibly fine ventricular fibrillation. B, MCL I, straight line. Rhythm is asystole. Atrial and ventricular heart rates of both strips are 0.

Tru
Tru
Tru
Tru
Tru

RHYTHM STRIP REVIEW

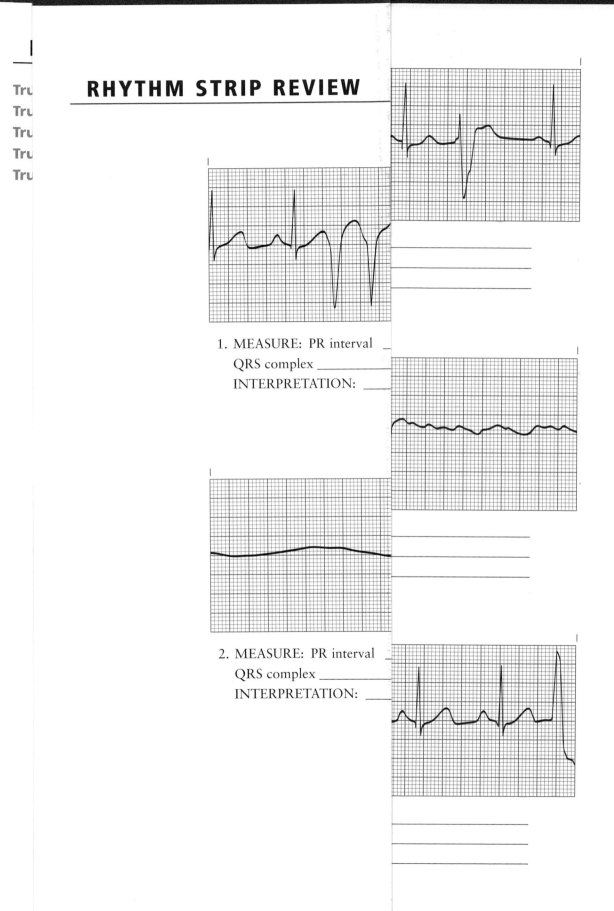

1. MEASURE: PR interval _____
   QRS complex _____
   INTERPRETATION: _____

2. MEASURE: PR interval _____
   QRS complex _____
   INTERPRETATION: _____

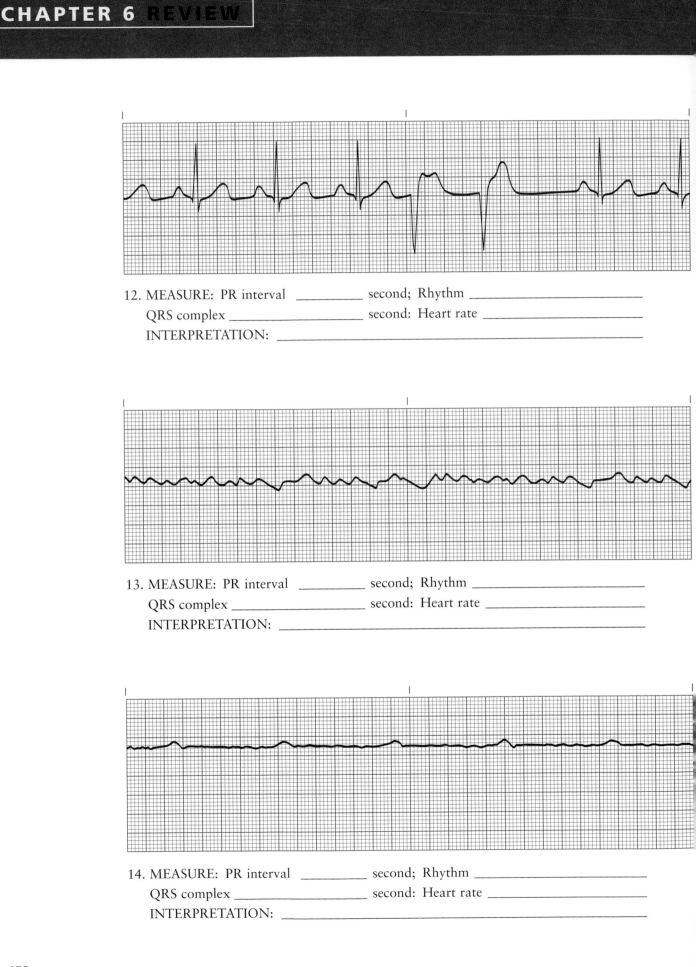

12. MEASURE: PR interval _____ second; Rhythm _____
    QRS complex _____ second: Heart rate _____
    INTERPRETATION: _____

13. MEASURE: PR interval _____ second; Rhythm _____
    QRS complex _____ second: Heart rate _____
    INTERPRETATION: _____

14. MEASURE: PR interval _____ second; Rhythm _____
    QRS complex _____ second: Heart rate _____
    INTERPRETATION: _____

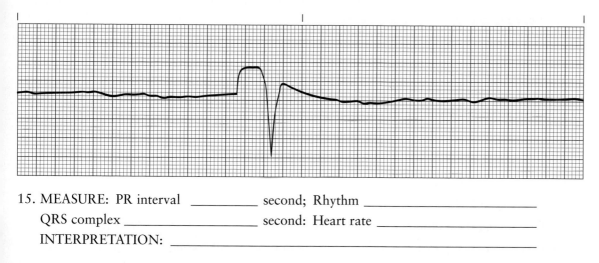

15. MEASURE: PR interval _____ second; Rhythm _____

    QRS complex _____ second: Heart rate _____

    INTERPRETATION: _____

Suggestion: You may find it helpful reviewing the Chapter 6 and 7 rhythm strips on the CD prior to studying the next chapter.

CROSSWORD PUZZLE AND CLUES

Across

1 Two PVCs in a row.

5 A PVC is usually followed by a(n) _____ compensatory pause.

9 Appears similar to ventricular tachycardia, but the amplitude begins close to baseline and gradually increases and decreases. (3 words)

10 Complete lack of electrical activity in the heart; no pulse.

13 Originates from one site in the ventricles.

17 A(n) ___ of V Tach consists of three or more PVCs in a row.

18 Originating from different sites in the ventricles.

20 Every other complex in a rhythm is a premature ventricular complex.

22 Patient _____ is essential to determine the patient's tolerance of and appropriate treatment for the dysrhythmia.

23 An idioventricular dysrhythmia with a rate of 41 to 100 electrical impulses per minute is known as a(n) _____ idioventricular dysrhythmia.

24 Ventricular _____ (VF).

25 In V Fib, the ventricular muscle makes ineffective _____ movements, not actual contractions.

Down

2 Complex that originates from any site below the bundle of His and occurs earlier than expected.

3 _____ ventricular tachycardia lasts longer than 30 seconds.

4 Idioventricular dysrhythmia; only the ventricular muscle can initiate an electrical impulse, but the heart muscle is too damaged to respond effectively. Heart rate: less than 20.

6 The R on T _____ is considered one of the danger signs that may indicate the need for treatment of PVCs.

7 _____ VF waves have a higher amplitude and are more irregular, indicating that a greater number of cardiac cells are able to respond to an electrical impulse.

8 Usually originates from a single site in the ventricles with a rate of 101 to 250 electrical impulses per minute.

11 Every 4th complex of a rhythm is premature.

12 _____ can mimic ventricular fibrillation.

14 Ventricular _____ occurs when only the atria depolarize and there is no ventricular depolarization.

15 The _____ ventricular heart rate is 20 to 40 impulses per minute.

16 The relative refractory period is also known as the _____ period.

19 The ___ complex is wide, bizarre looking, and measures greater than 0.12 second in ventricular dysrhythmias.

21 V Fib is a(n) _____ dysrhythmia. There is NO pulse.

The solution to this crossword puzzle is in the answer section.

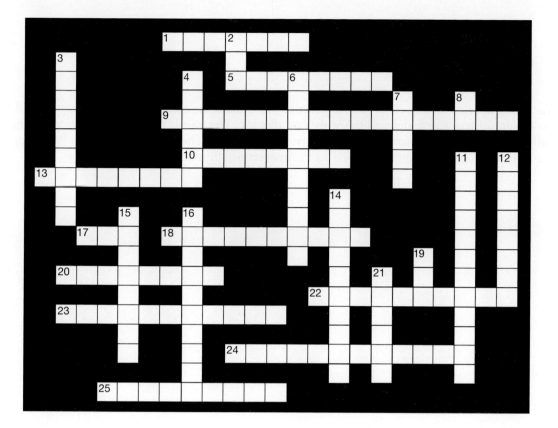

WORD PUZZLE

This word puzzle is designed to help familiarize you with some of the new terminology found in this chapter. Have fun finding all the words on this list. The words can be spelled forward (normally), backward, up, down, or diagonally in any direction. The words will always be in upper case and found in a straight line. Good luck. Answers are found in answer section.

```
T  N  O  R  I  D  I  O  V  E  N  T  R  I  C  U  L  A  R
L  X  M  D  O  I  R  E  P  E  L  B  A  R  E  N  L  U  V
M  Z  Q  C  Z  M  P  F  B  R  Y  V  G  B  K  X  M  X  Y
E  Z  T  C  O  K  K  B  Y  N  W  T  Q  N  K  W  D  Y  Y
R  N  L  Y  V  U  X  Q  I  T  R  I  G  E  M  I  N  Y  J
M  X  I  R  M  L  P  M  M  L  Z  W  G  G  K  K  T  Q  K
R  Q  X  F  S  Q  E  L  P  X  Q  R  R  P  T  L  V  H  H
Q  L  H  A  V  G  H  K  E  V  N  H  U  L  R  E  D  F  K
V  F  L  L  I  C  E  Y  Q  T  V  L  N  A  A  T  E  I  Z
Q  V  Z  B  A  A  H  L  J  K  L  L  O  C  E  H  N  B  Y
O  V  V  T  L  F  S  H  B  I  V  C  F  O  H  A  I  R  G
L  Y  V  F  B  A  Q  Y  T  A  O  R  V  F  G  L  A  I  G
A  V  T  R  I  B  C  S  S  C  T  M  T  I  N  K  T  L  C
N  W  C  V  P  B  D  O  O  T  R  S  N  T  I  K  S  L  X
O  V  G  K  J  N  F  A  F  G  O  K  N  L  Y  G  U  A  R
G  N  C  Y  A  T  R  L  L  I  K  L  Z  U  D  D  S  T  C
A  C  T  T  T  S  N  Y  B  B  N  K  E  M  H  Q  M  I  N
H  K  S  R  E  G  M  Q  X  J  V  U  W  T  X  V  M  O  G
T  O  R  S  A  D  E  S  D  E  P  O  I  N  T  E  S  N  K
```

AGONAL	IDIOVENTRICULAR	TORSADES DE POINTES
ASYSTOLE	LETHAL	TRIGEMINY
BIGEMINY	MULTIFOCAL	UNIFOCAL
CO	PVC	UNSTABLE
COARSE	R ON T	V FIB
COUPLET	RUN OF VT	V TACH
DYING HEART	SALVO	VULNERABLE PERIOD
FIBRILLATION	STANDSTILL	
FINE	SUSTAINED VT	

On completion of this chapter, the reader should be able to:

1 Describe an escape beat and an escape rhythm.

2 Define an *aberrantly conducted complex*.

3 Explain pulseless electrical activity (PEA).

4 Explain the difference between the two types of temporary pacemakers.

5 Explain the differences between atrial, ventricular, sequential, and biventricular pacemakers.

6 Define *capture* and *pacing* and give examples of 50% pacing and 75% capture.

7 Describe one function of an implantable cardioverter defibrillator.

8 Describe an automated external defibrillator and its use.

"Funny Looking" Beats (FLBs)

DEFINITIONS

AED—Automated external defibrillator; a temporary device that determines the patient's cardiac rhythm and defibrillates the heart, if necessary

Artificial Pacemaker—Small, battery-operated device that initiates electrical impulses in the heart; may be temporary or permanent

Capture—Ability of the cardiac muscle cells to conduct the electrical impulses generated by an artificial pacemaker

Cardiac Tamponade—Blood or extra fluid in the pericardial sac

Defibrillation—Procedure that uses measured electrical current to correct V Fib and pulseless V Tach

Escape Beat—An electrical impulse that "escapes" from a site other than the sinoatrial node and causes ventricular depolarization

"Funny Looking" Beats—Informal term for complexes that do not follow the usual patterns

ICD—Implantable cardioverter defibrillator; a surgically implanted device that both paces bradycardic rates and delivers programmed electrical impulses when the heart rate becomes too rapid; also known as AICD (automated implantable cardioverter defibrillator)

Pacing—Percentage of complexes generated by an artificial pacemaker, as seen on a monitor or rhythm strip

Pulseless Electrical Activity—Complex formations are seen on a monitor, but the heart muscle is not contracting

Shock—Informal term used to mean defibrillation

"FUNNY LOOKING" BEATS

Some complexes and wave formations do not fall into any of the specific patterns discussed in the previous chapters. In many parts of the United States, the slang expression for these complexes is *"funny looking beats"* or *FLBs*.

Escape Beats

When the cardiac electrical conduction system is interrupted for a brief period of time (sinus arrest) or when the heart rate is bradycardic, an impulse may "escape" from a site other than the sinoatrial (SA) node and cause depolarization of the myocardium. This electrical impulse is called an *escape beat* (Figure 7-1).

An escape beat is one way the heart attempts to maintain a normal rate or rhythm. For example, if the inherent heart rate of the SA node falls below 60, an electrical impulse may be initiated from outside the SA node. This escape beat is the heart's attempt to maintain normal cardiac output by increasing the heart rate. The escape beat will usually occur later than the next expected complex of the underlying rhythm, but it may be premature. The complex that ends a sinus arrest or sinus exit block is an example of an escape beat.

An escape beat may originate from the atria, the atrioventricular (AV) junction, or the ventricles and is named by the approximate point of origin. The rate of a rhythm containing an escape beat will vary, depending on the underlying rhythm and the number of escape beats.

Atrial escape beats can originate from anywhere in the atria, except the SA node, and usually meet the same criteria as other atrial complexes: an upright P wave before the QRS complex, a PR interval of 0.12 to 0.20 second, and a QRS complex of less than 0.12 second. An atrial complex that ends a sinus arrest or sinus exit block is usually the only atrial complex referred to as an escape beat (Figure 7-2, *A*).

If the SA node and atria fail to generate an electrical impulse or if the impulse is not conducted, the AV junctional area can initiate an electrical impulse that "escapes" to increase the heart rate. This impulse is a *junctional escape beat* and will

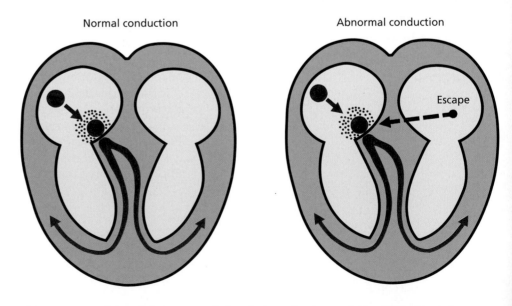

Normal conduction   Abnormal conduction

Escape

Figure 7-1 *Left heart* shows normal electrical conduction pathway. *Right heart* shows conduction pathway of an atrial escape beat.

have the same characteristics as all junctional complexes. The P wave is either inverted, hidden, or retrograde, and the QRS complex is usually less than 0.12 second (Figure 7-2, *B*).

If the SA node, the atria, and the AV junction fail to generate an electrical impulse or the heart rate falls below the junctional inherent rate of 40, a *ventricular escape beat* may be initiated from anywhere in the ventricles. As with all other ventricular complexes, the QRS complex of a ventricular escape beat is greater than 0.12 second and a P wave is usually not seen.

An escape beat can either remain a single complex or progress to an *escape rhythm,* if the atrial pacemaker cells do not initiate enough electrical impulses to maintain an adequate cardiac output. Junctional tachycardia and idioventricular dysrhythmias are examples of escape rhythms.

Aberrantly Conducted Complexes

An *aberrantly conducted complex* is formed when an electrical impulse is generated above the bundle of His and travels through the bundle branches in an abnormal manner. This causes one ventricle to depolarize at a slower rate than the other. One ventricle is then able to accept an electrical impulse causing depolarization earlier than the other ventricle, resulting in a QRS complex that resembles a bundle-branch block.

Aberrantly conducted complexes are individual complexes that appear different than the complexes of the underlying rhythm because they do not follow the same electrical conduction pathway as the underlying rhythm (Figure 7-3).

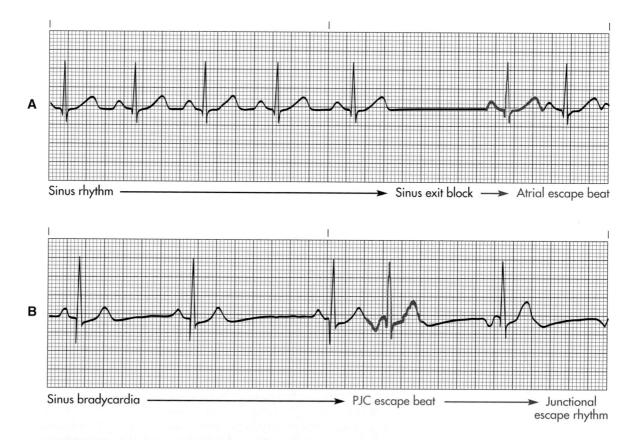

Figure 7-2 Escape beats and escape rhythm. **A,** Sinus rhythm with sinus exit block ended by an atrial escape beat; heart rate, 70. **B,** Sinus bradycardia with premature junctional complex (PJC) escape beat beginning a junctional escape rhythm; heart rate, 50.

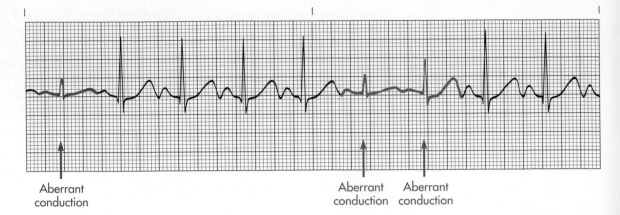

Figure 7-3 Aberrantly conducted complexes. Sinus rhythm with three aberrantly conducted complexes; heart rate, 90 (notice peaked P waves and prolonged QT intervals).

Examples of aberrantly conducted complexes include:

1. An aberrantly conducted complex that has a negative QRS complex when the underlying rhythm has a positive QRS complex.
2. The QRS of the aberrantly conducted complex may be wider, narrower, or shorter than the complexes of the underlying rhythm.

Aberrantly conducted complexes can originate from anywhere in the atria, the AV junction, or the ventricles. The origin of the aberrantly conducted complex will determine its size and shape. Because most aberrant complexes have a wide QRS complex, they may be hard to distinguish from a bundle branch block. However, aberrantly conducted complexes usually occur as individual complexes, not as entire rhythms.

The presence of P waves, PR intervals, and QRS complexes in the underlying rhythm varies. The rate and regularity of the rhythm containing the aberrantly conducted complex also vary, depending on the underlying rhythm.

Pulseless Electrical Activity

Pulseless electrical activity (PEA) is the current term used to describe any dysrhythmia that shows the conduction of electrical impulses, **without contraction** of the myocardium. Electrical depolarization of cardiac cells occurs throughout the heart, but the patient **does not** have a pulse or blood pressure. *Electromechanical dissociation* (EMD) is an older term for PEA dysrhythmia.

Almost any cardiac rhythm may be seen on the monitor screen or rhythm strip. The rhythm usually appears bradycardic and may have either wide or narrow QRS complexes (Figure 7-4).

Because the patient does not have a pulse and cardiac output has ceased, this dysrhythmia is **lethal,** and treatment **must** be started immediately. Patient assessment is the **only** means of determining the presence or absence of a pulse. The patient, **not** the monitor, must be treated.

Some types of pulseless electrical activity include idioventricular dysrhythmias, ventricular escape rhythms, and bradyasystolic (bradycardic rhythm without a pulse) dysrhythmias. These dysrhythmias all show complexes on the monitor screen indicating electrical activity. However, because there is **no mechanical** cardiac activity, blood is not being circulated and the patient does not have a pulse.

Pulseless electrical activity may be caused by hypovolemia (loss of blood volume), hypoxia (decrease in oxygen), cardiac tamponade (blood or excess fluid in pericar-

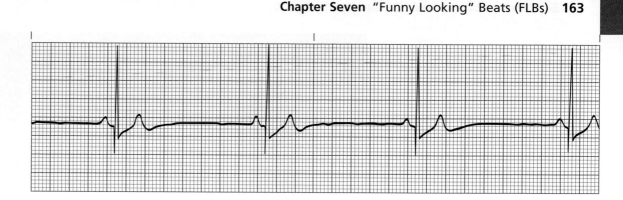

Figure 7-4 Pulseless electrical activity. Rhythm strip shows sinus bradycardia (heart rate, 40), but the patient does not have a pulse (notice depressed ST segments).

dial sac), or tension pneumothorax (air in the pleural cavity that prevents one lung from expanding). PEA may also occur when the cardiac muscle is too damaged to contract, although electrical impulses are still being conducted by the electrical conduction pathways.

> **NOTE:** Remember, although pulseless electrical activity mimics other rhythms that would ordinarily have a pulse, there is **NO pulse** with PEA! You **must** assess the patient to determine the presence of a PEA dysrhythmia.

PACEMAKER RHYTHMS

Many dysrhythmias have bradycardic rates that are too slow to maintain a normal cardiac output. Other dysrhythmias may be too rapid to allow complete filling of the ventricles before each contraction, resulting in poor cardiac output and decreased circulation to the vital organs of the body. These are **life threatening** dysrhythmias. Although many patients with these dysrhythmias respond to drug therapy, others will require assistance from an artificial pacemaker.

Pacemakers are small, battery-operated devices that initiate electrical impulses in the myocardium. The two main parts of a pacemaker are the generator and the lead wires (Figure 7-5). The *generator* is a small box that initiates and controls the rate and strength of each electrical impulse. The *lead wire* has an electrode at its tip that transmits the electrical impulse from the generator to the myocardium.

Temporary Pacemakers

Pacemakers may be either temporary or permanent. *Temporary pacemakers* are used to maintain a patient's heart rate in an emergency situation or until a permanent pacemaker can be surgically implanted.

There are two types of temporary pacemakers. Although the generator remains outside the patient's body with both types of pacemakers, the electrical impulse used to stimulate the cardiac muscle is delivered by two different means.

One method for delivery of the electrical impulse that has been used for many years is *transvenous* (through a vein). The lead wire is inserted through the skin and threaded through a large vein into the right atrium. The electrical impulse stimulates the atrium and is then conducted through the cardiac electrical conduction pathway, causing depolarization (Figure 7-6, *A*).

Transcutaneous (through the skin) pacemakers are the second method used for temporary pacing. This method delivers an electrical impulse through the skin and

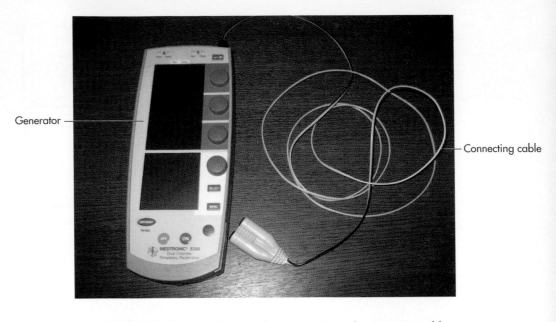

Generator

Connecting cable

Figure 7-5 External pacemaker generator and connecting cable.

body to the heart, stimulating the cardiac cells to depolarize in a normal manner, usually causing the cardiac muscle to contract.

Transcutaneous pacemakers have two lead wires connected to large adhesive pads, each containing an electrode. The pads have instructions describing where the pads should be placed, but if possible, the pads should not be placed over implanted functioning pacemakers.

The adhesive pads are placed on the body in one of two ways:

- One pad on the chest and the other pad on the back, (Figure 7-6, *B*).
- Both pads on the chest. Usually one on the right, upper chest and the other on the left side of the body, under the arm and slightly below the nipple line or on the upper left abdomen.

The generator for most pacemakers can be preset to initiate the rate of the electrical impulses by one of two methods:

Fixed: Set to generate electrical impulses at a constant rate, usually 70 to 80 impulses per minute.
Demand: Set to generate electrical impulses and maintain adequate cardiac output, only when the pacemaker senses the patient's own heart rate has fallen below a predetermined rate, usually less than 65 beats per minute. Transcutaneous pacemakers are the exception and can not be set for a demand rate because transcutaneous pacemakers can not sense the patient's heart rate.

NOTE: The terms *fire* and *pace* are often used in a clinical setting to mean the initiation of an electrical impulse from an artificial pacemaker.

Permanent Pacemakers

A *permanent pacemaker* is necessary when the patient's heart is unable to maintain a normal heart rate or a normal cardiac output, even with the aid of medications.

The generator of a permanent pacemaker is surgically implanted under the patient's skin, usually in the upper left chest, upper right chest or upper abdominal area. The lead wire is then inserted into the heart through a large vein (Figure 7-7).

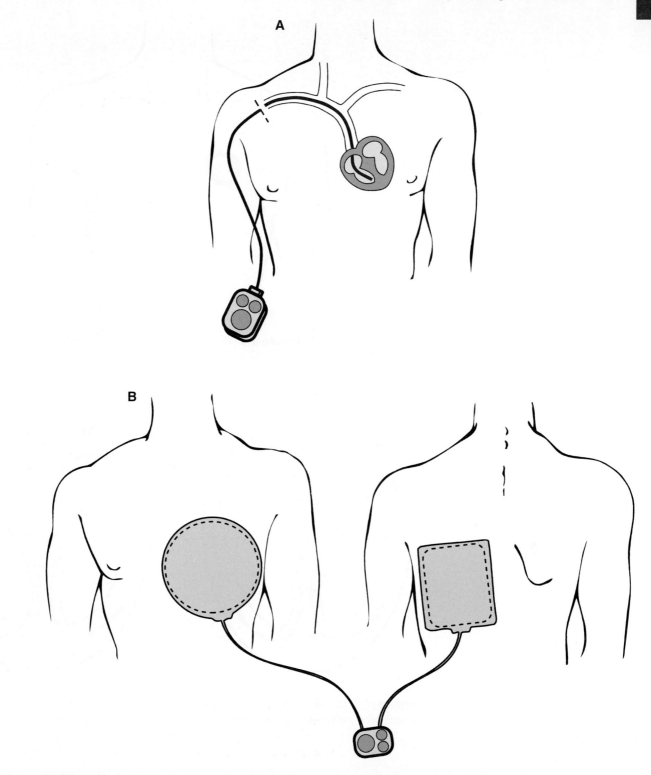

Figure 7-6 A, Temporary transvenous pacemaker placement. B, Temporary transcutaneous pacemaker placement.

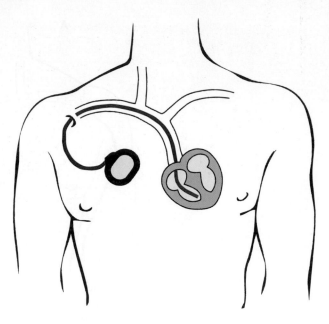

Figure 7-7 Permanent pacemaker placement.

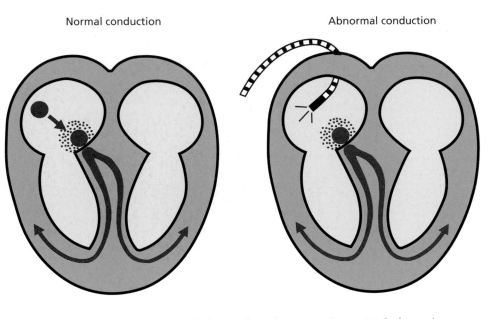

Figure 7-8 *Left heart* shows normal electrical conduction pathway. *Right heart* shows conduction pathway of atrial pacemaker.

There are four types of permanent pacemakers: atrial, ventricular, sequential, and biventricular.

Atrial Pacemakers

The lead wire and electrode of an *atrial pacemaker* are inserted into the right atrium. The electrical impulse that is generated by the pacemaker stimulates the atria, then follows the normal electrical conduction pathway through the heart to the ventricles (Figure 7-8).

The discharge of electrical energy from the pacemaker is represented on the rhythm strip by a vertical line, called a *pacer spike*, or *spike*. The pacer spike is usu-

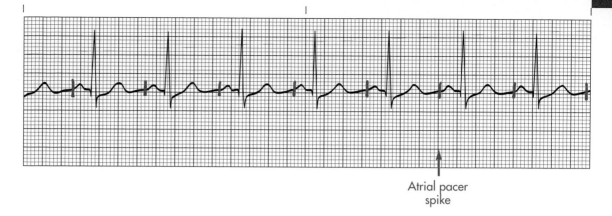

Figure 7-9 Atrial pacemaker rhythm showing pacer spikes; heart rate, 70; pacer rate, 70 (notice depressed ST segments).

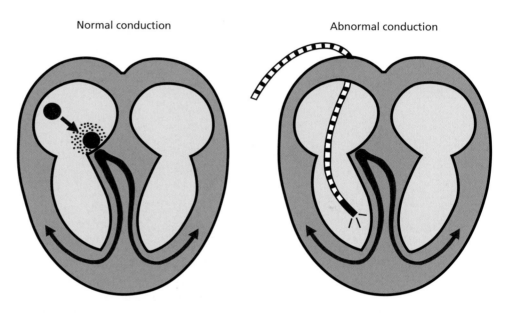

Normal conduction   Abnormal conduction

Figure 7-10 *Left heart* shows normal electrical conduction pathway. *Right heart* shows conduction pathway of ventricular pacemaker.

ally followed by a P wave and a QRS complex, although the P wave may not be seen unless the electrode is positioned high in the right atrium (Figure 7-9). P waves and QRS complexes that follow a pacer spike are usually not measured.

An atrial pacemaker can only be used if the AV junction and ventricular electrical conduction pathways are functioning. Atrial pacemakers are rarely used today because they are less efficient than ventricular or sequential pacemakers.

Ventricular Pacemakers

With *ventricular pacemakers*, the lead wire and electrode may be placed either in the right ventricle, or in the left ventricle (Figure 7-10). The pacemaker impulse causes depolarization of the ventricular muscle. The atria may not depolarize if they are extensively damaged.

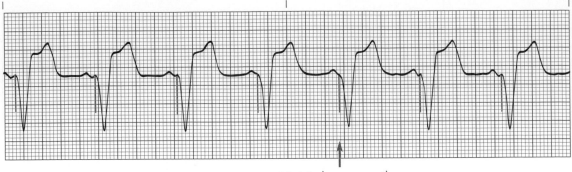

Ventricular pacer spike

Figure 7-11 Ventricular pacemaker rhythm with pacer spikes; heart rate, 70; pacer rate, 70 (notice elevated ST segments).

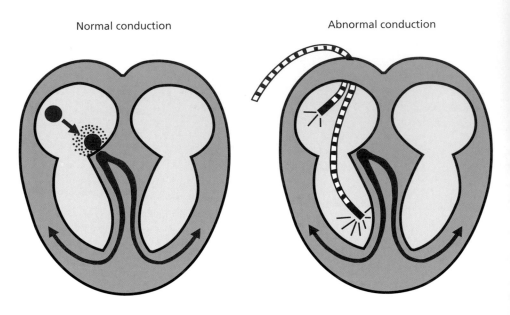

Normal conduction   Abnormal conduction

Figure 7-12 *Left heart* shows normal electrical conduction pathway. *Right heart* shows conduction pathway of sequential pacemaker.

A pacer spike, immediately followed by a QRS complex, will appear on the monitor screen or rhythm strip. Because the electrode is usually positioned low in the right ventricle, depolarization may not occur in a normal manner and the QRS is usually greater than 0.12 second (Figure 7-11). Both atrial and ventricular pacemakers are also known as single chamber pacemakers.

Sequential Pacemakers

The most commonly used type of pacemaker is the *sequential pacemaker*. The other two types of permanent pacemakers initiate depolarization of **either** the atria **or** the ventricles; however, the sequential pacemaker stimulates the depolarization of **both** the atria **and** the ventricles.

One type of sequential pacemaker has two lead wires, each with an electrode, one positioned in the right atrium and one positioned in the right ventricle. The use of two electrodes allows the atria and the ventricles to depolarize in a normal sequential manner (Figure 7-12). Another name for a sequential pacemaker is a dual chamber pacemaker.

Ventricular pacer spike

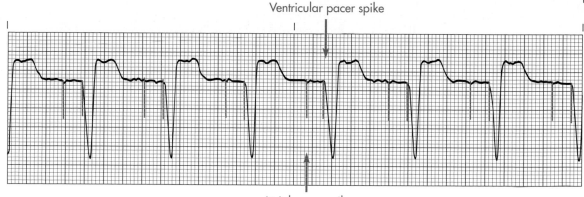

Atrial pacer spike

Figure 7-13 Sequential pacemaker or biventricular pacemaker rhythm with two pacer spikes before each QRS complex; heart rate, 70-80; pacer rate, 70 (notice elevated ST segment).

Biventricular Pacemakers

Normally, both the right and left ventricles depolarize and contract at the same time. However, diseases such as a myocardial infarction, congestive heart failure, or an enlarged heart (cardiomyopathy) can interrupt the normal electrical conduction system forcing the ventricles to depolarize and contract at different times. This decreases the cardiac output, producing symptoms.

Although ventricular and sequential pacemakers will increase cardiac output, *biventricular pacemakers* are used to greatly improve cardiac output, by causing both ventricles to contract at the same time. This allows adequate filling of the left ventricle with oxygenated blood and a more normal cardiac output.

Biventricular pacemakers usually have **three** lead wires, each with an electrode. One electrode is positioned in the right atrium, one in the right ventricle, and the third is in the left ventricle. The three electrodes cause the atria and both ventricles to depolarize in a more normal sequence.

The biventricular pacemaker controls depolarization using *overdrive pacing*. Overdrive pacing uses a stronger electrical impulse than the heart's own impulse. This causes the cardiac cells to depolarize in response to the artificial pacemaker, instead of to the weaker electrical impulse from the cardiac pacemaker cells. The biventricular pacemaker is also a sequential pacemaker, and is often called a sequential biventricular pacemaker.

The rhythm strip of either a sequential or a biventricular pacemaker may show two pacer spikes before each QRS complex (Figure 7-13). The spikes may occur so closely together that they appear as one long spike. The first spike represents the firing of the atrial electrode, and the second spike represents the firing of the ventricular electrode/electrodes. A P wave may not be seen, and the QRS is typically greater than 0.12 second.

Capture and Pacing

When interpreting a pacemaker rhythm, the percentage of capture and the percentage of pacing must be determined.

Capture, also known as *electrical capture,* refers to the cardiac cell's ability to depolarize in response to the electrical impulse generated by an artificial pacemaker. This depolarization is indicated by a P wave or QRS complex after **every** pacer spike. The presence of a QRS complex after a pacer spike **does not** always indicate the **contraction** of the myocardium, only the **conduction** of an electrical impulse through the cardiac muscle.

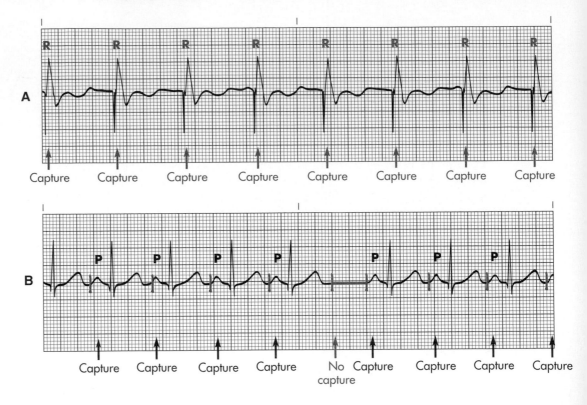

Figure 7-14 Pacemaker capture. **A,** Ventricular pacemaker with 100% capture (notice depressed ST segment and diphasic T waves); heart rate, 80; pacer rate, 80. **B,** Loss of capture; atrial pacemaker with 90% capture; heart rate, 80; pacer rate, 90.

A pulse indicates *mechanical capture* or the ability of the cardiac muscle to contract in response to the depolarization of the cardiac cells. The patient **must** be assessed to determine the presence of a pulse and adequate cardiac output.

The *percentage of capture* is determined by the number of pacer spikes that are followed by a complex in relationship to the total number of pacer spikes on the entire rhythm strip. For example, the rhythm strip will show 100% capture if every pacer spike is followed by a QRS complex (Figure 7-14, *A*). If only 9 of 10 pacer spikes are followed by a complex, the rhythm strip will show 90% capture.

Loss of capture occurs when a QRS complex does not follow a pacer spike (Figure 7-14, *B*). Loss of capture indicates that the electrical impulse generated by the artificial pacemaker has not been conducted and the cardiac cells have not depolarized. This situation may simply indicate that the voltage of the pacemaker electrical impulse needs to be increased. However, loss of capture may indicate that the myocardium is so damaged, it is unable to respond to every electrical impulse.

Pacing refers to the percentage of complexes generated by the artificial pacemaker. For example, if every QRS complex is preceded by a pacer spike, the rhythm is 100% paced (Figure 7-15, *A*). If a pacer spike occurs before only half of the QRS complexes, the strip is 50% paced (Figure 7-15, *B*). QRS complexes that do not have a pacer spike are initiated by the patient's heart, not the artificial pacemaker. These QRS complexes may appear normal or bizarre, depending on whether they follow the normal cardiac electrical conduction pathway.

The percentage of pacing depends on the pacemaking ability of the patient's own heart, as well as the type of pacemaker in use (demand or fixed-rate pacemaker).

The percentage of capture should **always** be 100%, regardless of the percent of pacing. For example, every pacer spike should be **followed** by a QRS complex.

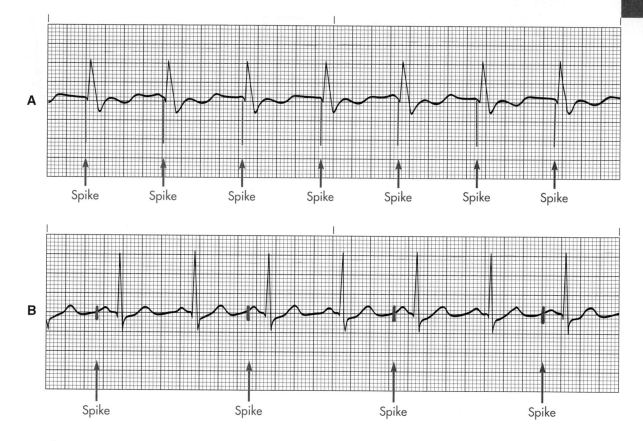

Figure 7-15 Pacemaker pacing. **A,** Ventricular pacemaker with 100% pacing; heart rate, 70; pacer rate 70 (notice depressed ST segment and diphasic T waves). **B,** Atrial pacemaker with 50% pacing; heart rate, 70; pacer rate, 40.

However, every QRS complex does **not** have to be **preceded** by a pacer spike. QRS complexes that appear without a pacer spike indicate that the patient's heart, not the artificial pacemaker, has initiated the electrical impulse.

IMPLANTABLE CARDIOVERTER DEFIBRILLATOR

Some potentially lethal dysrhythmias do not respond to artificial pacing alone but also require defibrillation for immediate treatment. An *implantable cardioverter defibrillator (ICD)*, also known as automatic implantable cardioverter defibrillator (AICD), is one type of pacemaker/defibrillator available for this use. Although some ICDs are not used to pace the heart, they all identify and treat the rapid heart rates of potentially lethal dysrhythmias, such as ventricular tachycardia.

The ICD generator is surgically implanted under the skin, similar to a pacemaker. Lead wires with electrodes and sensing units are then inserted into the atria and either one or both ventricles (Figure 7-16).

The implantable cardioverter defibrillator can be programmed to initiate low-voltage electrical impulses when the heart rate becomes rapid (usually more than 150 impulses per minute). The impulse from the ICD attempts to force the heart into a normal rate. If the first electrical impulse from the implantable cardioverter defibrillator is not strong enough, the ICD may be programmed to increase the voltage and initiate an additional one to two impulses, raising the voltage slightly each

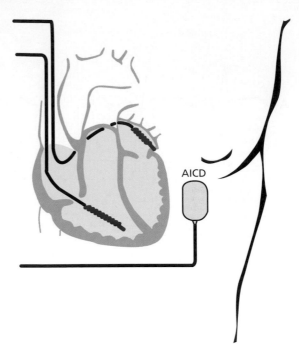

Figure 7-16 ICD (AICD) unit. Electrodes inserted into atrium and ventricle.

time. The patient may complain of a feeling of being "kicked" in the chest while defibrillation is occurring. Anyone touching the patient while the ICD is defibrillating may feel a mild tingling sensation. The patient may "jump" or "jerk" slightly as an effect of the defibrillation.

If the patient's heart rate remains rapid, the ICD will deliver an electrical impulse that is strong enough for cardiac defibrillation ("shock"). This defibrillation is an attempt to allow the SA node to again initiate electrical impulses at a normal rate.

The implantable cardioverter defibrillator will continue to defibrillate the patient until the heart has recovered its normal rate or until the ICD is turned off by medical personnel.

On the monitor screen or rhythm strip, the firing of the ICD appears similar to a pacing spike, but it may have a greater amplitude.

Some models of ICDs not only pace bradycardic dysrhythmias, but also function as biventricular pacemakers.

AUTOMATED EXTERNAL DEFIBRILLATOR

The *automated external defibrillator* (AED) is a device that can increase the survival rate of people who have a cardiac arrest in the community. The AED provides a method of immediate treatment by trained non-medical rescuers, before the arrival of the emergency medical personnel (9-1-1). The AED senses and evaluates the patient's heart rhythm and rate. Then the machine either delivers a defibrillation or instructs the rescuer on what steps to take (Figure 7-17).

Before attaching the AED, it is important to be sure that the patient is on a dry surface and not touching any metal objects. This is also an important precaution for the rescuer. If the patient is wearing a medication patch, such as nitroglycerin, remove the patch and wipe any moisture or medication from the chest. (Be careful not to touch the medication side of the patch with your bare fingers.) Do not place the AED pads directly over a pacemaker or ICD.

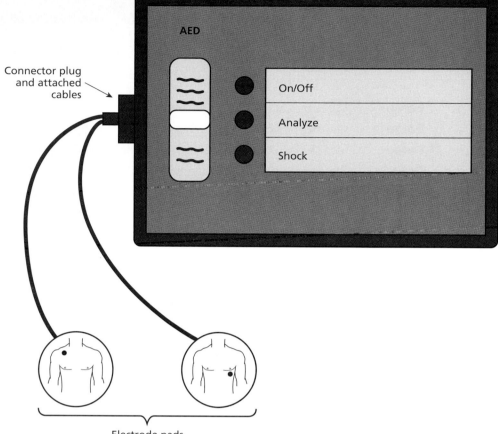

Connector plug and attached cables

AED

On/Off

Analyze

Shock

Electrode pads

Figure 7-17 AED unit.

The automated external defibrillator has two electrode pads and cables that are similar in appearance to telemetry electrodes and lead wires. The first electrode is attached to the skin, just below the collarbone on the patient's upper right chest. The second electrode is placed on the skin slightly beneath the left nipple. For a woman, the second electrode is placed beneath the left breast. Turn on the machine and ask everyone to stand back from the patient. The device will then analyze the patient's cardiac rhythm and provide defibrillation, if needed. **Do not** let anyone **touch** the patient while the machine analyzes or defibrillates the patient.

The machine will then analyze the cardiac rhythm again and instruct the rescuer when to begin cardiopulmonary resuscitation (CPR), if required.

When the emergency medical personnel arrive, tell them how long the AED has been in use, if defibrillation was given (and how many times), and/or the length of time that CPR has been performed.

The AED has been used successfully in identifying and defibrillating rapid lethal dysrhythmias, such as ventricular fibrillation and may recognize pulseless ventricular tachycardia.

REVIEW QUESTIONS

True	**False**	1. Sequential pacemakers are used to stimulate either the atria or the ventricles.
True	**False**	2. Escape beats are usually named for the approximate point of origin.
True	**False**	3. The AED can only be used by trained medical personnel.
True	**False**	4. PEA can only be identified on a 12-Lead electrocardiogram.
True	**False**	5. The two types of pacemakers are permanent and implanted.

6. List the main parts of an artificial pacemaker.

   a. _____

   b. _____

   c. _____

7. Explain the following terms

   a. 75% capture: _____

   _____

   _____

   b. 50% paced: _____

   _____

   _____

8. An escape beat

   a. occurs when a pacemaker fails and the next lower pacemaker "kicks in." It may occur later or earlier than expected.

   b. is an attempt by the heart to decrease the rate of a tachycardia.

   c. can only be initiated from the ventricles.

   d. is an attempt by the heart to increase the heart rate and maintain adequate cardiac output.

   (1) a, b, and c

   (2) b, c, and d

   (3) a and d

   (4) b and d

9. An ICD can automatically

   a. decrease PJCs.

   b. control quadrigeminy PVCs.

   c. identify and treat PEA.

   d. recognize and defibrillate ventricular tachycardia.

10. An AED

   a. is a device that can automatically sense the patient's rhythm and defibrillate, if necessary.

   b. should not be used if the patient is on wet ground or a rescuer is touching the patient.

   c. will instruct the rescuer when to begin CPR, if needed.

   d. all of the above.

11. An escape rhythm
    a. may be the heart's attempt to increase the heart rate and improve cardiac output.
    b. is never from the junctional area.
    c. may be generated by any part of the heart, except the SA node.
    d. is the heart's attempt to slow ventricular tachycardia.
        (1) a and b
        (2) b and c
        (3) a and c
        (4) b and d

12. Define an aberrantly conducted complex.

    _____

    _____

13. List the four types of permanent artificial pacemakers and the area of the heart stimulated by each.
    a. _____
    b. _____
    c. _____
    d. _____

14. List two ways temporary pacemakers can be applied to a patient.
    a. _____
    b. _____

15. List two ways the heart rate can be set on pacemaker generators.
    a. _____
    b. _____

RHYTHM STRIP REVIEW

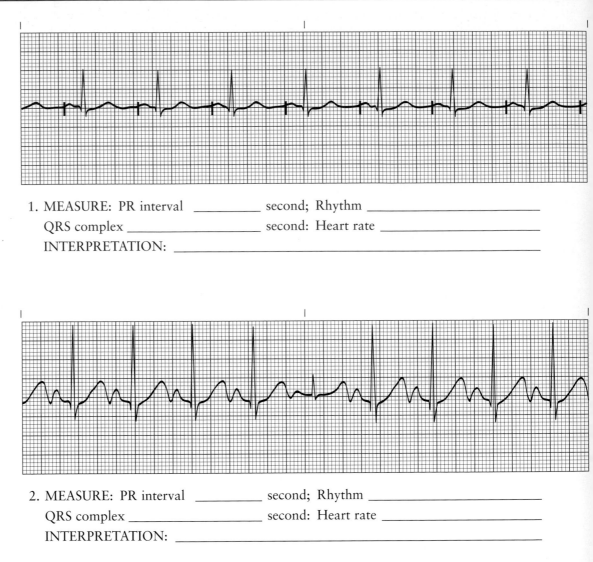

1. MEASURE: PR interval _____ second; Rhythm _____

   QRS complex _____ second: Heart rate _____

   INTERPRETATION: _____

2. MEASURE: PR interval _____ second; Rhythm _____

   QRS complex _____ second: Heart rate _____

   INTERPRETATION: _____

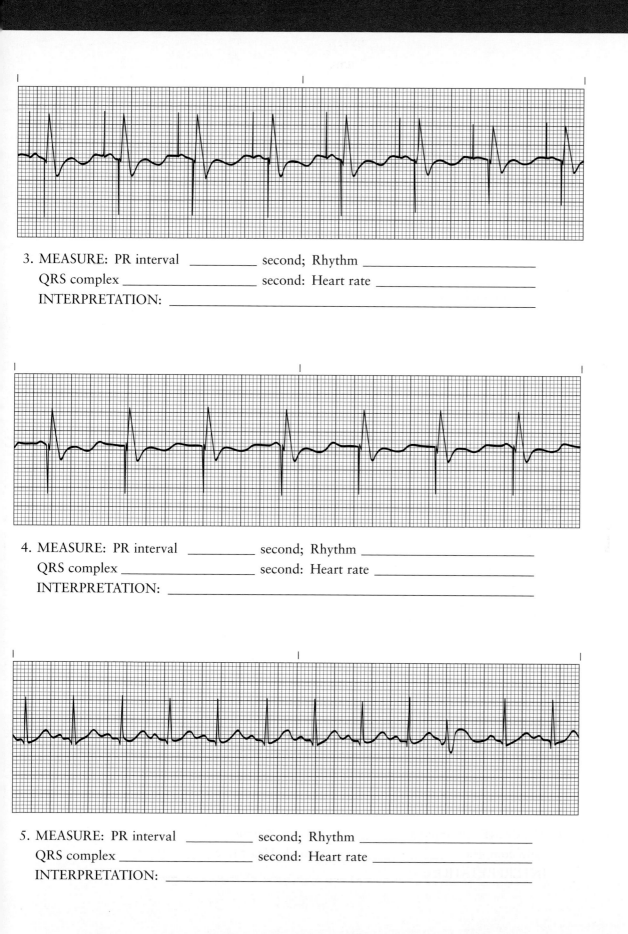

3. MEASURE: PR interval _____ second; Rhythm _____
   QRS complex _____ second: Heart rate _____
   INTERPRETATION: _____

4. MEASURE: PR interval _____ second; Rhythm _____
   QRS complex _____ second: Heart rate _____
   INTERPRETATION: _____

5. MEASURE: PR interval _____ second; Rhythm _____
   QRS complex _____ second: Heart rate _____
   INTERPRETATION: _____

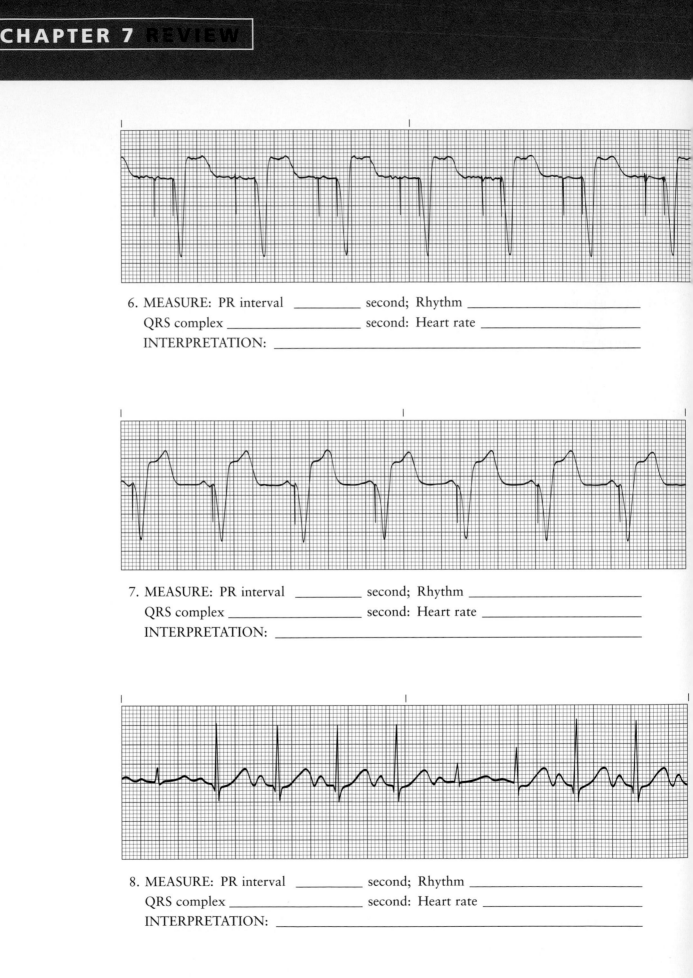

6. MEASURE: PR interval _____ second; Rhythm _____

    QRS complex _____ second: Heart rate _____

    INTERPRETATION: _____

7. MEASURE: PR interval _____ second; Rhythm _____

    QRS complex _____ second: Heart rate _____

    INTERPRETATION: _____

8. MEASURE: PR interval _____ second; Rhythm _____

    QRS complex _____ second: Heart rate _____

    INTERPRETATION: _____

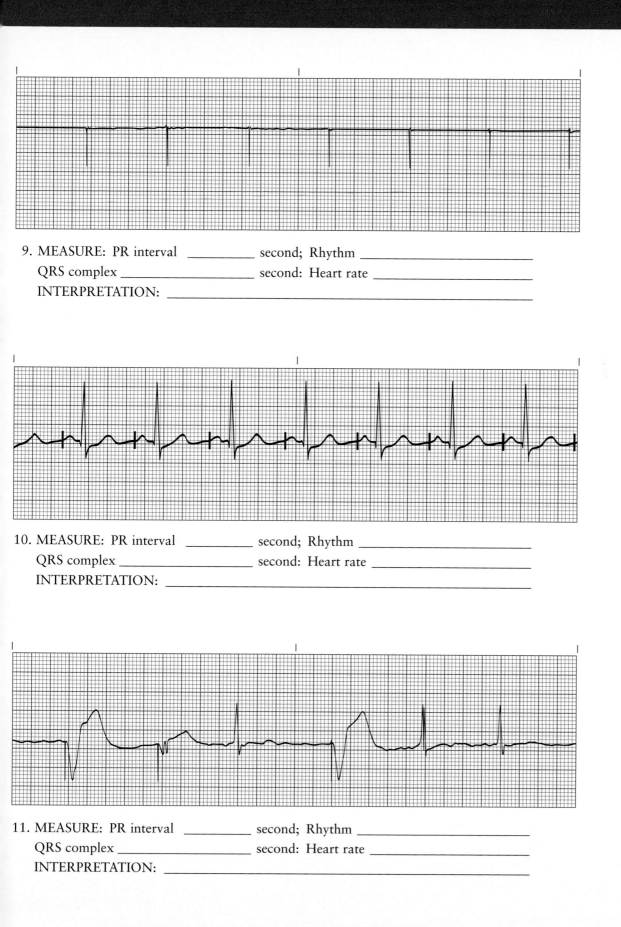

9. MEASURE: PR interval _____ second; Rhythm _____

   QRS complex _____ second: Heart rate _____

   INTERPRETATION: _____

10. MEASURE: PR interval _____ second; Rhythm _____

   QRS complex _____ second: Heart rate _____

   INTERPRETATION: _____

11. MEASURE: PR interval _____ second; Rhythm _____

   QRS complex _____ second: Heart rate _____

   INTERPRETATION: _____

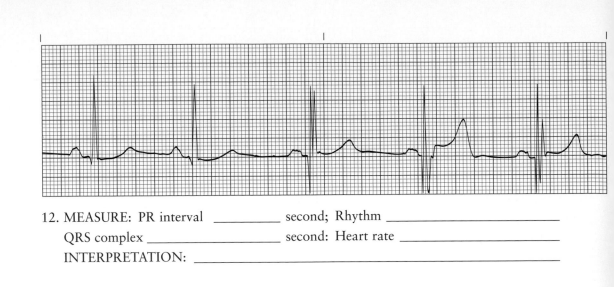

12. MEASURE: PR interval _____ second; Rhythm _____

    QRS complex _____ second: Heart rate _____

    INTERPRETATION: _____

Suggestion: You may find it helpful reviewing the Chapter 6 and 7 rhythm strips on the CD prior to studying the next chapter.

CROSSWORD PUZZLE AND CLUES

Across

1 A(n) _____ pacemaker is necessary when the patient's heart is unable to maintain a normal heart rate for adequate cardiac output.

3 Describes complexes that do not follow the normal cardiac electrical conduction pathways.

7 Ability of cardiac cells to conduct an electrical impulse generated by an artificial pacemaker.

8 Pacemaker set to initiate an electrical impulse only when the patient's heart rate falls below a predetermined rate, usually less than 65 beats per minute.

9 Small box that initiates and controls the rate and strength of electrical impulses.

11 Death producing.

13 An electrical impulse that "escapes" from a site outside the SA node to end the pause of a sinus exit block (Two words).

15 Surgically implanted pacemaker; also capable of delivering measured electrical current to treat potentially lethal dysrhythmias such as V Tach.

17 Loss of blood volume.

18 A QRS complex should _____ every pacer spike.

19 Type of an artificial pacemaker used to stimulate depolarization of both the atria and the ventricles.

20 Electrical impulse is transmitted through the skin by means of electrodes placed on the patient's chest and back.

22 Abbreviation for any dysrhythmia that shows complexes on a monitor; however, the cardiac muscle is not contracting and the patient does not have a pulse.

23 Artificial _____ capable of generating electrical impulses in the heart.

24 Lack of oxygen in the cells of body tissue or organs.

25 The generator remains outside the body with a(n) _____ pacemaker.

26 Pacemaker set to initiate an electrical impulse at a constant rate, between 70 to 80 impulses per minute.

Down

1 The percentage of complexes generated by an artificial pacemaker.

2 Blood or extra fluid in the pericardial sac occurs in cardiac _____.

3 A(n) _____ pacemaker can only be used if the AV junctional and ventricular electrical conduction pathways are functioning.

4 Lead wire inserted through the skin and threaded through a large vein into the right atrium.

5 Device able to monitor and interpret a patient's cardiac rhythm and if necessary, defibrillate automatically.

6 An AED can be used by trained _____ rescuers.

10 Transmits the electrical impulses to the cardiac muscle; located on the lead wire from the generator.

12 Procedure that uses measured electrical current to correct VF and pulseless VT.

14 Type of an artificial pacemaker that stimulates depolarization of the ventricles.

16 _____ of the patient is essential to determine the presence of a PEA dysrhythmia.

18 _____ and paced are terms meaning the initiation of an electrical impulse from an artificial pacemaker.

19 Slang term meaning "to defibrillate."

21 Vertical line on monitor or rhythm strip that indicates the electrical impulse generated by an artificial pacemaker.

The solution to this crossword puzzle is in the answer section.

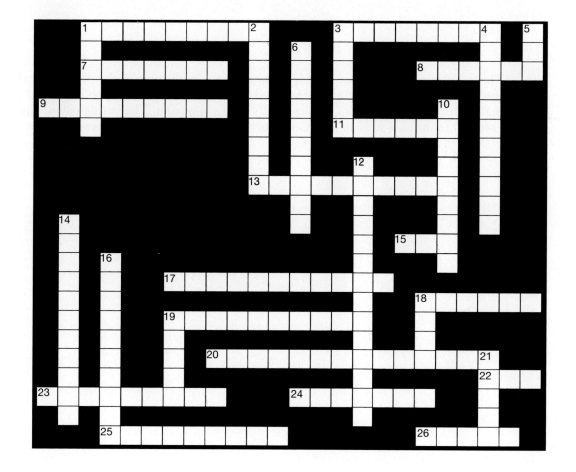

WORD PUZZLE

This word puzzle is designed to help familiarize you with some of the new terminology found in this chapter. Have fun finding all the words on this list. The words can be spelled forward (normally), backward, up, down, or diagonally in any direction. The words will always be in upper case and found in a straight line. Good luck! Answers are found in answer section.

```
Z E S C A P E B E A T R M F V K L D M H
F I X E D R A T E Y A V K Y Q V A G K T
E D O R T C E L E L L Z H P Z P I N B R
R N D L T E P Y U B Y R S T A A T I J A
H E N K R F K C S P C U P C B B N C R N
A K K I K D I G E S O Q E K H E E A N S
E L F D P R X R P N E M R Y F R U P N C
K R H Y T X M L E E A L P B H R Q B D U
C L U N K A V V G K A O E V T A E K J T
W L E T N F S X E E V S R S J N S T P A
H V E P N K R J O N T E Z L T N W E N
Y L N T A A V T L L B E N R Y U R F R E
P T F R H J C E R J G L R X I T P Y C O
O R T Z T A M T K D L M N A K W R X E U
X C N T C I L D T C R Q V L T V D M N S
I L V C A X H F K I M L L P R O K A T G
A T X D E F I B R I L L A T O R R V E F
L W E T A R D N A M E D K R N N Q Z T L
M N Z D F M W P A C E R S P I K E T R Z
R C K N J Z Y R A R O P M E T W N G Z O
```

ABERRANT
AED
CAPTURE
DEFIBRILLATOR
DEMAND RATE
ELECTRODE
ESCAPE BEAT
FIRE
FIXED RATE

GENERATOR
HYPOVOLEMIA
HYPOXIA
ICD
LEAD WIRES
LETHAL
PACEMAKER
PACER SPIKE
PACING

PEA
PERCENT
PERMANENT
PULSELESS
SEQUENTIAL
TEMPORARY
TRANSCUTANEOUS
TRANSVENOUS
VENTRICULAR

Dysrhythmia Review

This chapter is designed as a review of all the dysrhythmias discussed in Chapters 3 through 7. Each dysrhythmia is presented with a rhythm strip followed by the criteria for that dysrhythmia.

SINUS DYSRHYTHMIAS (Chapter 3)

Normal Sinus Rhythm, p 59

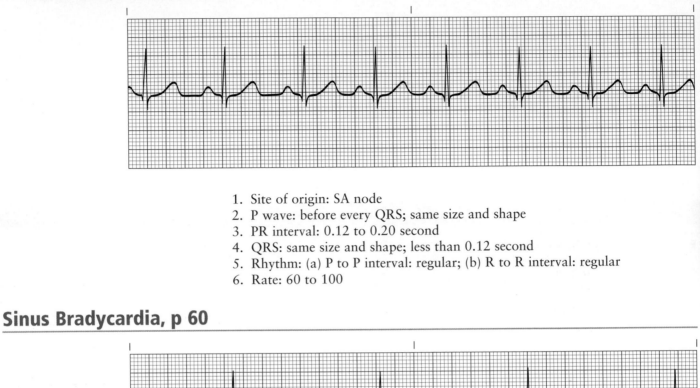

1. Site of origin: SA node
2. P wave: before every QRS; same size and shape
3. PR interval: 0.12 to 0.20 second
4. QRS: same size and shape; less than 0.12 second
5. Rhythm: (a) P to P interval: regular; (b) R to R interval: regular
6. Rate: 60 to 100

Sinus Bradycardia, p 60

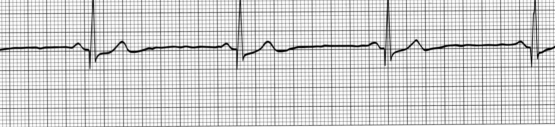

1. Site of origin: SA node
2. P wave: before every QRS; same size and shape
3. PR interval: 0.12 to 0.20 second
4. QRS: same size and shape; less than 0.12 second
5. Rhythm: (a) P to P interval: regular; (b) R to R interval: regular
6. Rate: less than 60

Sinus Tachycardia, p 60

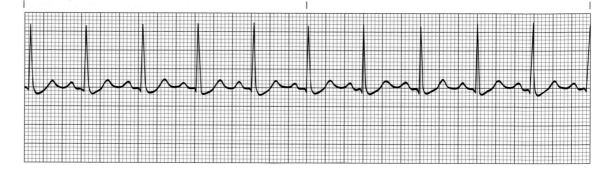

1. Site of origin: SA node
2. P wave: before every QRS; same size and shape
3. PR interval: 0.12 to 0.20 second
4. QRS: same size and shape; less than 0.12 second
5. Rhythm: (a) P to P interval: regular; (b) R to R interval: regular
6. Rate: 101 to 150

Sinus Arrhythmia, p 61

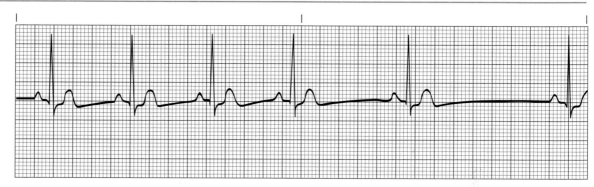

1. Site of origin: SA node
2. P wave: before every QRS; same size and shape
3. PR interval: 0.12 to 0.20 second
4. QRS: same size and shape; less than 0.12 second
5. Rhythm: (a) P to P interval: irregular; (b) R to R interval: irregular; (c) the longest R to R interval will be less than twice the length of remaining R to R intervals
6. Rate: overall rate varies with respirations; usually 60 to 100
   a. Increases as patient inhales
   b. Decreases as patient exhales

Sinus Exit Block; Sinus Arrest, p. 62

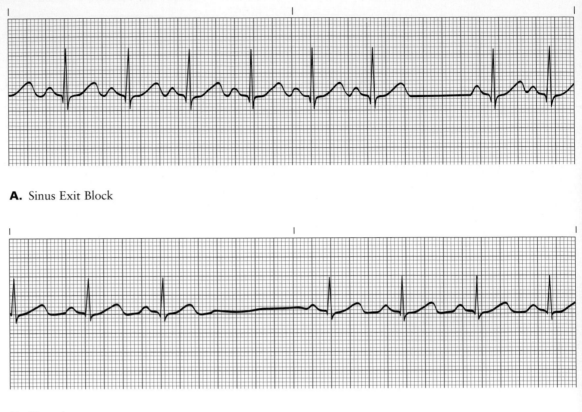

A. Sinus Exit Block

B. Sinus Arrest

1. Site of origin:
   a. Sinus Exit Block: SA node fires, but impulse is blocked to the atria
   b. Sinus Arrest: SA node fails to fire for at least two cardiac cycles
2. P wave: before every QRS; same size and shape
3. PR interval: varies slightly within normal limits of 0.12 to 0.20 second
4. QRS: same size and shape; less than 0.12 second
5. Rhythm: (a) P to P interval: regular, except during pause; (b) R to R interval: regular, except during pause
6. Rate: varies according to underlying rhythm
7. Pause: (a) **Sinus exit block**: the distance from the last normal beat to the next beat is equal to exactly two or more previous cardiac cycles; able to divide pause equally; (b) **Sinus arrest**: equal to more than two previous cardiac cycles; not able to divide pause equally

ATRIAL DYSRHYTHMIAS (Chapter 3)

Premature Atrial Complex, p 64

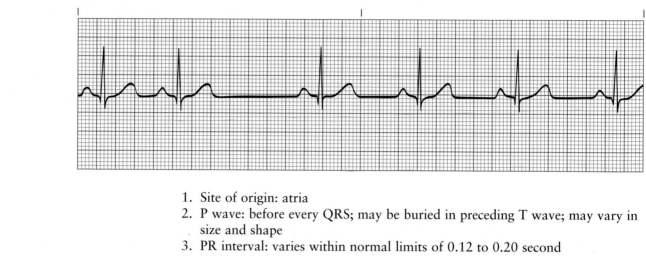

1. Site of origin: atria
2. P wave: before every QRS; may be buried in preceding T wave; may vary in size and shape
3. PR interval: varies within normal limits of 0.12 to 0.20 second
4. QRS: same size and shape; less than 0.12 second
5. Rhythm: (a) P to P interval: varies according to the underlying rhythm and the number of PACs; (b) R to R interval: varies according to the underlying rhythm and the number of PACs
6. Rate: varies according to the underlying rhythm and the number of PACs
7. Occurs: premature; usually followed by a noncompensatory pause

Paroxysmal Atrial Tachycardia/Paroxysmal Supraventricular Tachycardia, p 66

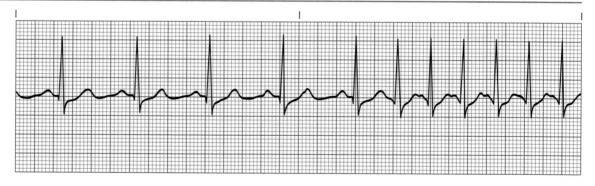

1. Site of origin: atria
2. P wave: before every QRS; may be buried in preceding T wave; same size and shape
3. PR interval: 0.12 to 0.20 second
4. QRS: same size and shape; less than 0.12 second
5. Rhythm: (a) P to P interval: regular; (b) R to R interval: regular
6. Rate: 151 to 250
7. Onset: starts suddenly; onset must be observed

Supraventricular Tachycardia, p 66

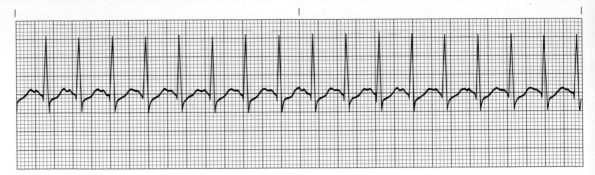

1. Site of origin: above bundle of His
2. P wave: (a) atrial: before every QRS or buried in preceding T wave; same size and shape; (b) junctional: inverted, hidden, or retrograde; same size and shape
3. PR interval: normal to not measurable
4. QRS: same size and shape; less than 0.12 second
5. Rhythm: (a) P to P interval: regular, if present; (b) R to R interval: regular
6. Rate: 151 to 250
7. Onset: starts suddenly; onset is not observed

Atrial Flutter, p 68

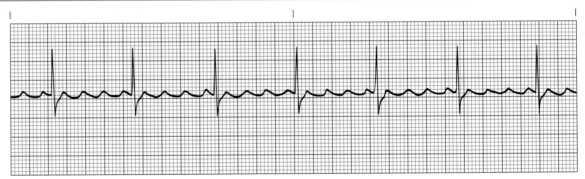

1. Site of origin: one atrial site
2. P wave: not present; T waves may be hidden in the flutter waves
3. Flutter waves: "saw-toothed" in shape; size may vary
4. PR interval: cannot be measured
5. QRS: same size and shape; less than 0.12 second
6. Rhythm: (a) P to P interval: not present; (b) F to F interval: regular; (c) R to R interval: regular, except in varying block/ratio
7. Rate:
   a. Atrial: 250 to 350
   b. Ventricular: usually 60 to 100 but may vary
      (1) Less than 60; slow ventricular response
      (2) 101 to 150; rapid ventricular response
8. Ratio of block:
   a. Two F waves to 1 QRS = 2:1 block/ratio
   b. Three F waves to 1 QRS = 3:1 block/ratio
   c. Four F waves to 1 QRS = 4:1 block/ratio
   d. Varying number of F waves to 1 QRS = varying block/ratio
      This strip shows a 4:1 block/ratio.

Atrial Fibrillation, p 70

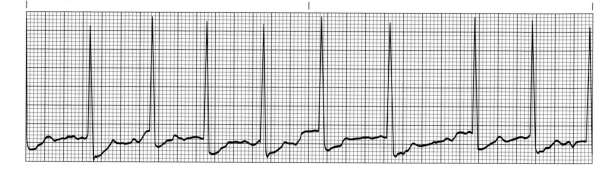

1. Site of origin: multiple sites in the atria
2. P wave: no distinctive P wave
3. PR interval: cannot be measured
4. QRS: same size and shape; less than 0.12 second
5. Rhythm: (a) P to P interval: cannot be measured; (b) R to R interval: irregular
6. Rate:
   a. Atrial: 350 to 500 or more
   b. Ventricular:
      (1) Less than 60; slow ventricular response
      (2) 60 to 100; controlled A Fib
      (3) 101 to 150; rapid ventricular response
      (4) Greater than 150; uncontrolled A Fib

Wolff-Parkinson-White Syndrome, p 73

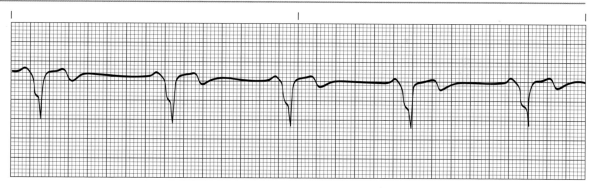

1. Site of origin: accessory pathway (bundle of Kent)
   a. Atria to ventricle (antegrade)
   b. Ventricle to atria (retrograde)
   c. Both a and b in a continuous cycle
2. P wave: present, unless rhythm is an SVT, atrial flutter or atrial fibrillation
3. PR interval: less than 0.12 second, if P waves are present
4. QRS: (a) can be greater than 0.12 second; (b) slurring (curving of QRS complex); (c) may contain a delta wave
5. Rhythm: (a) P to P interval: varies according to the underlying rhythm; (b) R to R interval: varies according to the underlying rhythm
6. Rate:
   a. Varies according to the underlying rhythm
   b. Associated with SVT, including atrial flutter and atrial fibrillation, with uncontrolled ventricular response
   c. Ventricular rates of 200 to 300 can occur and become life threatening

JUNCTIONAL DYSRHYTHMIAS (Chapter 4)

Junctional Dysrhythmia, p 90

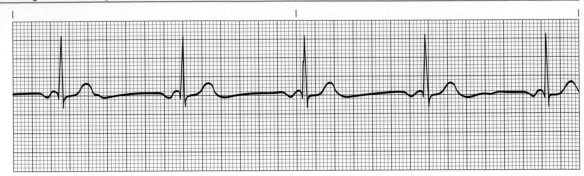

1. Site of origin: AV junction
2. P wave: inverted, buried, or retrograde; same size and shape, if present
3. PR interval: usually less than 0.12 second, if inverted P wave is present before the QRS
4. QRS: same size and shape; less than 0.12 second
5. Rhythm: (a) P to P interval: regular if present; (b) R to R interval: regular
6. Rate: 40 to 60

Junctional Bradycardia Dysrhythmia, p 94

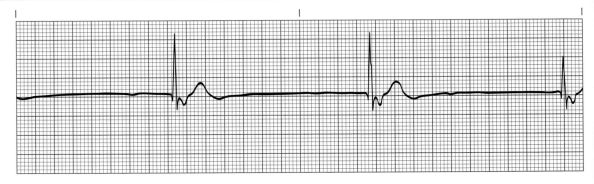

1. Site of origin: AV junction
2. P wave: inverted, buried, or retrograde; same size and shape, if present
3. PR interval: usually less than 0.12 second, if inverted P wave is present before the QRS
4. QRS: same size and shape, less than 0.12 second
5. Rhythm: (a) P to P interval: regular, if present; (b) R to R interval: regular
6. Rate: less than 40

Accelerated Junctional Dysrhythmia/Junctional Tachycardia Dysrhythmia, p 95

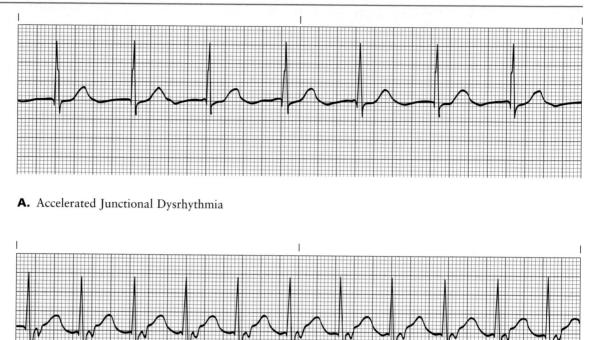

A. Accelerated Junctional Dysrhythmia

B. Junctional Tachycardia Dysrhythmia

1. Site of origin: AV junction
2. P wave: inverted, buried, or retrograde; same size and shape, if present
3. PR interval: usually less than 0.12 second, if inverted P wave is present before the QRS
4. QRS: same size and shape, less than 0.12 second
5. Rhythm: (a) P to P interval: regular, if present; (b) R to R interval: regular
6. Rate:
   a. Accelerated junctional dysrhythmia 61 to 100
   b. Junctional tachycardia dysrhythmia 101 to 150

Premature Junctional Complex, p 96

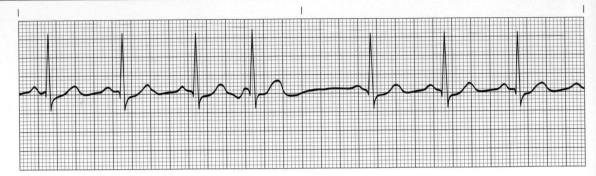

1. Site of origin: AV junction
2. P wave: inverted, buried, or retrograde
3. PR interval: usually less than 0.12 second, if inverted P wave is present before the QRS
4. QRS: less than 0.12 second
5. Rhythm: (a) P to P interval: varies according to the underlying rhythm and number of PJCs; (b) R to R interval: varies according to the underlying rhythm and number of PJCs
6. Rate: varies according to underlying rhythm and number of PJCs
7. Occurs: prematurely; usually followed by a compensatory pause

Wandering Junctional Pacemaker Dysrhythmia, p 97

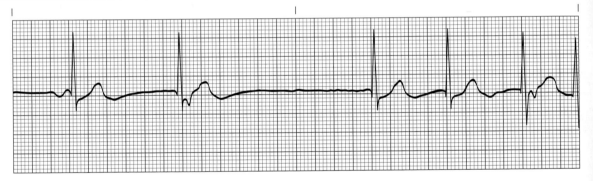

1. Site of origin: at least three junctional sites
2. P wave: inverted, buried, or retrograde; varies in size and shape, if present
3. PR interval: usually less than 0.12 second, if inverted P wave is present before the QRS
4. QRS: less than 0.12 second; size and shape may vary
5. Rhythm: (a) P to P interval: irregular, if present; (b) R to R interval: irregular
6. Rate: varies, usually 40 to 60

Wandering Atrial Pacemaker Dysrhythmia, p 98

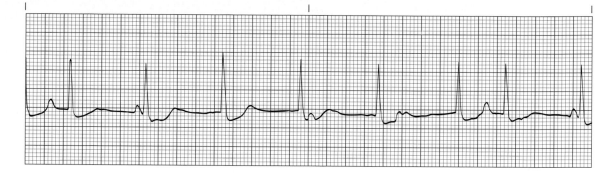

1. Site of origin: must be combination of three or more sites from above bundle of His
2. P wave: varies according to site of origin
3. PR interval: varies, if present
4. QRS: varies according to site of origin; may be greater than 0.12 second
5. Rhythm: (a) P to P interval: irregular; (b) R to R interval: irregular
6. Rate: varies, usually 60-100

HEART BLOCKS (Chapter 5)

First-Degree Heart Block, p 110

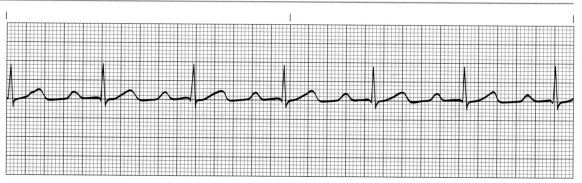

1. Site of origin: underlying rhythm usually atrial
2. Site of delay: between atria and bundle of His
3. P wave: before every QRS; same size and shape
4. PR interval: greater than 0.20 second
5. QRS: same size and shape; usually less than 0.12 second
6. Rhythm: (a) P to P interval: varies according to underlying rhythm; (b) R to R interval: varies according to underlying rhythm
7. Rate: varies according to underlying rhythm

Second-Degree Heart Block, Type I (Mobitz I, Wenckebach), p 111

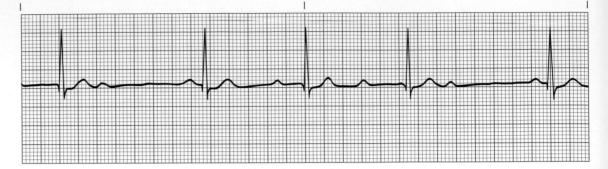

1. Site of origin: atria
2. Site of block: AV junction; progressive
3. P wave: at least one for every QRS; same size and shape
4. PR interval: becomes progressively longer, until QRS is dropped
5. QRS: same size and shape; less than 0.12 second
6. Rhythm: (a) P to P interval: regular; (b) R to R interval: irregular
7. Rate: Atrial and ventricular rates vary

Second-Degree Heart Block, Type II (Mobitz II, Classic), p 113

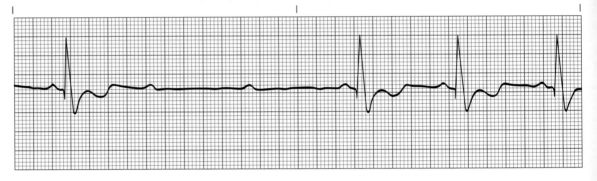

1. Site of origin: atria
2. Site of block: AV junction; intermittent block
3. P wave: at least one for every QRS; same size and shape
4. PR interval: equal throughout; may be normal or prolonged
5. QRS: same size and shape; usually less than 0.12 second
6. Rhythm: (a) P to P interval: varies according to underlying rhythm; (b) R to R interval: irregular
7. Rate: Atrial and ventricular rates vary; can be life threatening
8. Ratio of block:
   a. 2 P waves to 1 QRS = 2:1 block/ratio
   b. 3 P waves to 1 QRS = 3:1 block/ratio
   c. 4 P waves to 1 QRS = 4:1 block/ratio
   d. Varying number of P waves to 1 QRS = varying block/ratio
      This strip shows a 3:1 block/ratio.

Third-Degree Heart Block (Complete Heart Block, Complete AV Dissociation), p 114

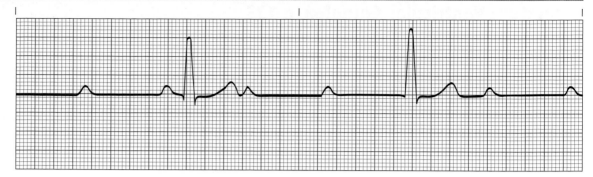

1. Site of origin: atria and ventricles
2. Site of block: between atria and ventricles
3. P wave: no relationship to QRS; same size and shape
4. PR interval: appears to vary; no true PR interval
5. QRS: same size and shape; usually wide, bizarre, and greater than 0.12 second
6. Rhythm: (a) P to P interval: regular; (b) R to R interval: regular
7. Rate:
   a. Atrial: usually 60 to 100
   b. Ventricular: usually 20 to 40
   c. Life threatening; can progress to a **lethal** dysrhythmia

Bundle Branch Block, p 117

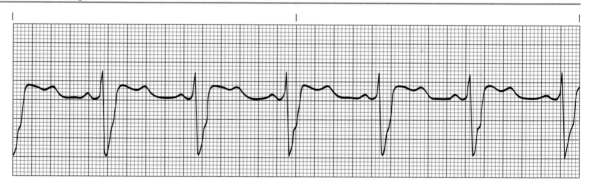

1. Site of origin: usually atria
2. Site of block: bundle branch (right or left)
3. P wave: varies according to underlying rhythm
4. PR interval: varies according to underlying rhythm
5. QRS: usually same size and shape; notched appearance; usually greater than 0.12 second
6. Rhythm: (a) P to P interval: varies according to the underlying rhythm; (b) R to R interval: varies according to the underlying rhythm
7. Rate: varies according to the underlying rhythm

VENTRICULAR DYSRHYTHMIAS (Chapter 6)

Premature Ventricular Complex, p 133

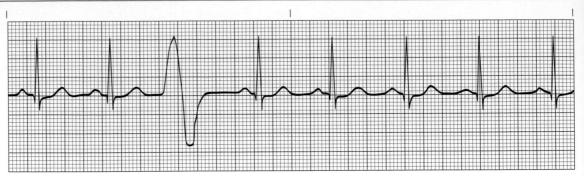

1. Site of origin: ventricles
2. P waves: not present, or hidden in PVC
3. PR interval: not measurable
4. QRS: may vary in size and shape; wide, bizarre, greater than 0.12 second
5. Rhythm: (a) P to P interval: not measurable in PVC; varies according to underlying rhythm and number of PVCs; (b) R to R interval: varies according to the underlying rhythm and number of PVCs
6. Rate: varies according to the underlying rhythm and number of PVCs
7. Occurs: premature; followed by a compensatory pause
8. T wave: deflected in the opposite direction of the QRS

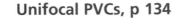

NOTE: The following are classifications of PVCs

Unifocal PVCs, p 134

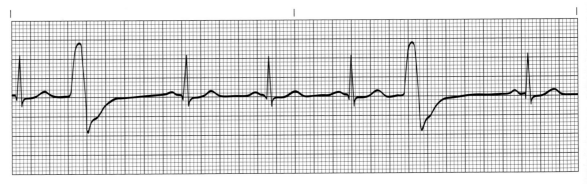

1. Site of origin: one ventricular site
2. QRS: same size and shape
3. Other characteristics: same as PVC

Multifocal PVCs, p 134

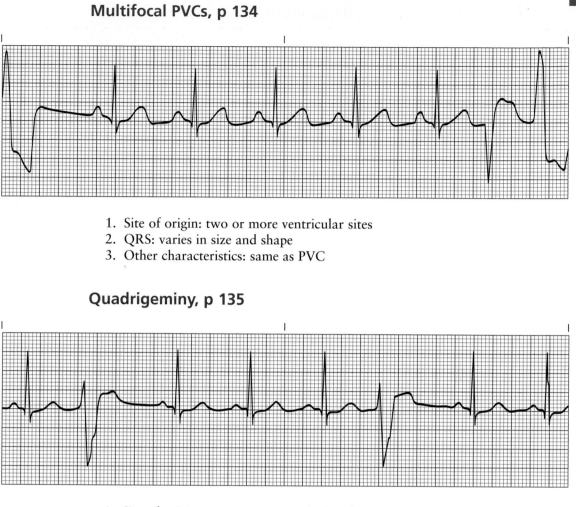

1. Site of origin: two or more ventricular sites
2. QRS: varies in size and shape
3. Other characteristics: same as PVC

Quadrigeminy, p 135

1. Site of origin: one or more ventricular sites
2. QRS: unifocal or multifocal
3. Occurs: every fourth complex is a PVC
4. Other characteristics: same as PVC

Trigeminy, p 136

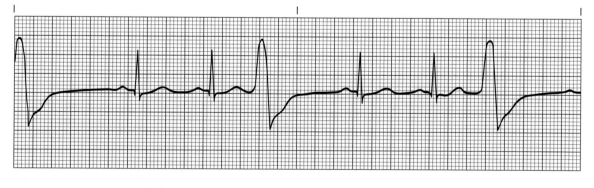

1. Site of origin: one or more ventricular sites
2. QRS: unifocal or multifocal
3. Occurs: every third complex is a PVC
4. Other characteristics: same as PVC

Bigeminy, p 136

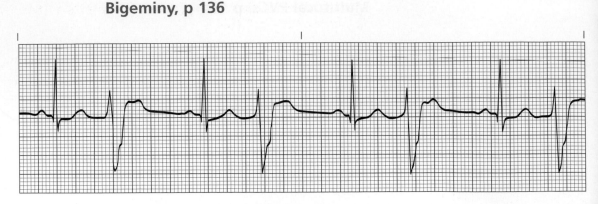

1. Site of origin: one or more ventricular sites
2. QRS: unifocal or multifocal
3. Occurs: every other complex is a PVC
4. Other characteristics: same as PVC

Couplet, p 137

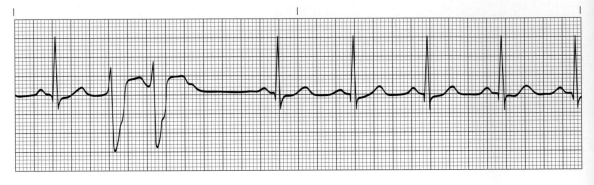

1. Site of origin: one or more ventricular sites
2. QRS: unifocal or multifocal
3. Occurs: two PVCs in a row
4. Other characteristics: same as PVC

R on T Phenomenon, p 137

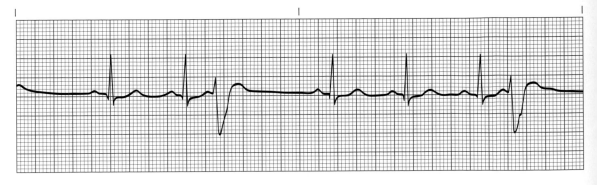

1. Site of origin: one or more ventricular sites
2. QRS: unifocal or multifocal
3. Occurs: R wave of PVC falls on the T wave of the preceding QRS
4. Other characteristics: same as PVC

Run of Ventricular Tachycardia (Unsustained Ventricular Tachycardia), p 138

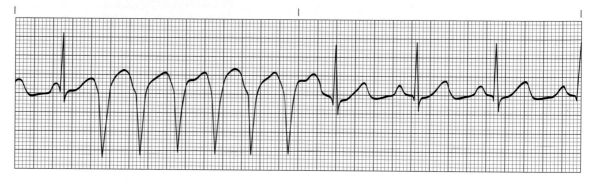

1. Site of origin: one or more ventricular sites
2. QRS: usually unifocal
3. Occurs: three or more PVCs in a row, at a heart rate greater than 100
4. Duration: less than 30 seconds; can be life threatening
5. Other characteristics: same as PVC

Ventricular Tachycardia (Sustained Ventricular Tachycardia), p 139

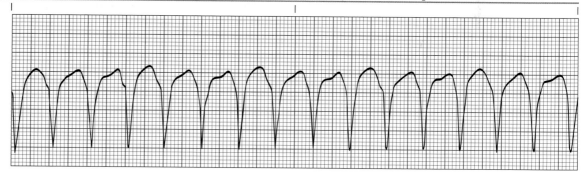

1. Site of origin: one or more ventricular sites
2. P wave: usually not present
3. PR interval: not measurable
4. QRS: usually same size and shape; wide, bizarre, greater than 0.12 second
5. Rhythm: (a) P to P interval: not measurable; (b) R to R interval: usually regular
6. Rate: 101 to 250 or more
7. Occurs: more than three PVCs in a row; sudden onset
8. Duration: usually greater than 30 seconds; life threatening; can progress to a **lethal** dysrhythmia

Torsades de Pointes, p 140

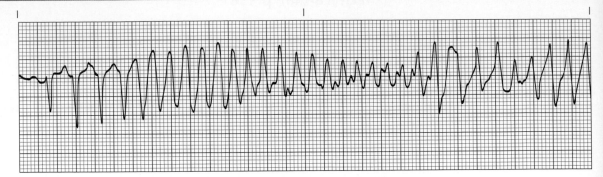

1. Site of origin: unclear if one or more ventricular sites
2. P wave: usually not present
3. PR interval: not measurable
4. QRS: usually same shape; varies in size, going from low to high and back to low amplitude
5. Rhythm: (a) P to P interval: not measurable; (b) R to R interval: usually regular
6. Rate: usually greater than 150
7. Occurs: sudden onset; frequently seen in a rhythm with prolonged QT intervals
8. Duration: varies; life threatening; can progress to a **lethal** dysrhythmia

Ventricular Fibrillation, p 141

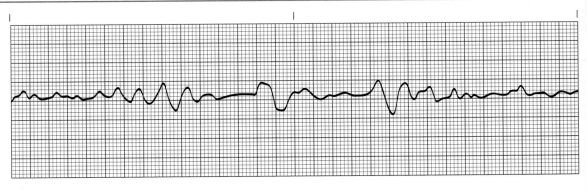

1. Site of origin: many ventricular sites
2. P wave: not present
3. PR interval: not measurable
4. QRS: not present; only a chaotic, wavy line
5. Rhythm: (a) P to P interval: not present; (b) R to R interval: not present
6. Rate: not measurable; patient does **not** have a pulse; this is a **lethal** dysrhythmia
7. Wave amplitude: coarse or fine

Idioventricular Dysrhythmia/Agonal Dysrhythmia (Dying Heart), p 143

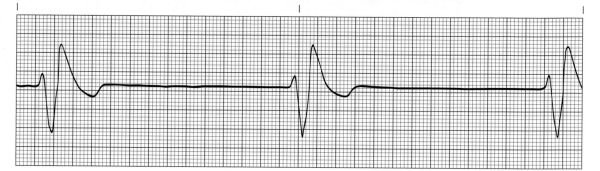

A. Idioventricular Dysrhythmia

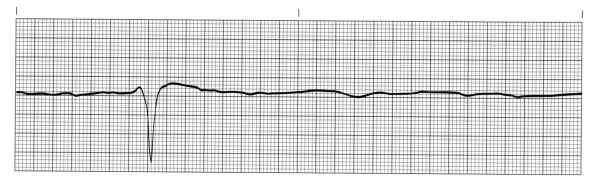

B. Agonal Dysrhythmia (dying heart)

1. Site of origin: usually one ventricular site
2. P wave: not present
3. PR interval: not measurable
4. QRS: gradually decreases in amplitude and increases in width; wide, bizarre, greater than 0.12 second
5. Rhythm: (a) P to P interval: not present; (b) R to R interval: usually irregular
6. Rate:
   a. Idioventricular dysrhythmia: 20 to 40; life threatening; can progress to a **lethal** dysrhythmia
   b. Agonal dysrhythmia: less than 20; becomes slower until it completely stops; a **lethal** dysrhythmia

NOTE: If the ventricular rate is 41 to 100, it is known as accelerated idioventricular dysrhythmia or accelerated idioventricular rhythm (AIVR).

Ventricular Standstill, p 144

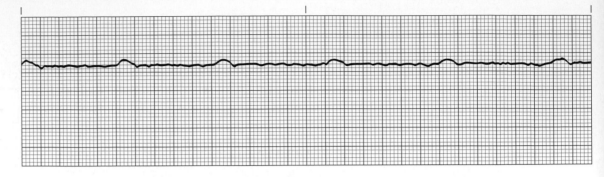

1. Site of origin: atria
2. P wave: seen without QRS; usually same size and shape
3. PR interval: not measurable
4. QRS: not present
5. Rhythm: (a) P to P interval: usually regular; (b) R to R interval: not present
6. Rate:
   a. Atrial: usually 60 to 100
   b. Ventricular: 0; a **lethal** dysrhythmia

Asystole, p 145

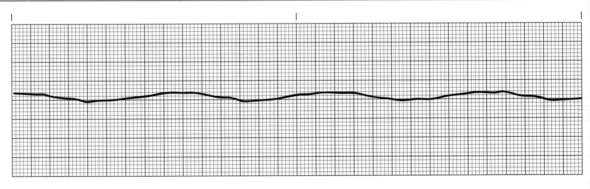

1. Site of origin: no electrical activity in heart muscle
2. P wave: not present
3. PR interval: not present
4. QRS: not present; only a straight or slightly wavy line
5. Rhythm: (a) P to P interval: not present; (b) R to R interval: not present
6. Rate: atrial and ventricular heart rates are 0; a **lethal** dysrhythmia

"FUNNY LOOKING" BEATS (Chapter 7)

Escape Beats, p 160

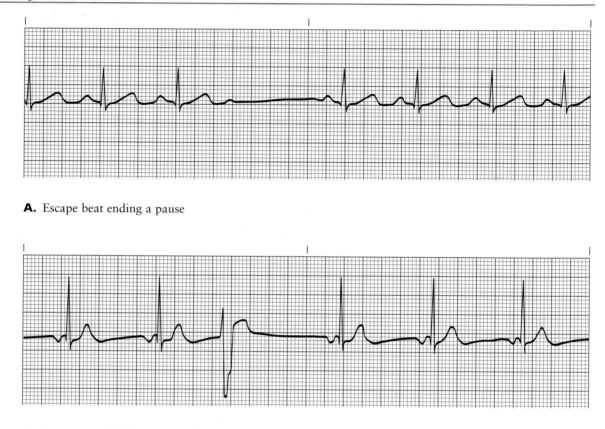

A. Escape beat ending a pause

B. Escape beat (PVC) increasing heart rate

1. Site of origin: single atrial, junctional, or ventricular site; other than the SA node
2. P wave: varies according to site of origin
3. PR interval: varies according to site of origin
4. QRS: varies according to site of origin
5. Rhythm: (a) P to P interval: irregular, if present; (b) R to R interval: irregular
6. Rate: varies according to site of origin and underlying rhythm
7. Occurs:
   a. Complex that ends the pause of a sinus exit block or sinus arrest
   b. Premature complexes that increase the rate of a bradycardic rhythm

Aberrantly Conducted Complex, p 161

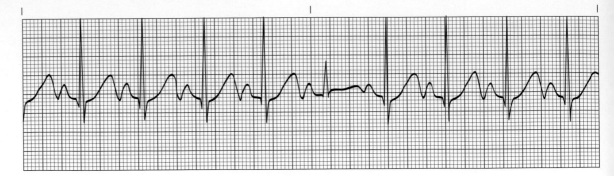

1. Site of origin: varies
2. P wave: varies according to site of origin
3. PR interval: varies according to site of origin
4. QRS: varies according to site of origin
5. Rhythm: (a) P to P interval: varies according to underlying rhythm; (b) R to R interval: varies according to underlying rhythm
6. Rate: varies according to underlying rhythm
7. Occurs:
   a. Single complex that follows different electrical conduction pathway than the underlying rhythm
   b. Complex usually does not occur prematurely

Pulseless Electrical Activity, p 162

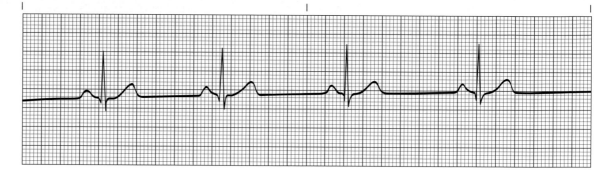

1. Site of origin: **mimics any rhythm with a pulse**
2. P wave: mimics any rhythm
3. PR interval: mimics any rhythm
4. QRS: mimics any rhythm
5. Rhythm: (a) P to P interval: mimics any rhythm; (b) R to R interval: mimics any rhythm
6. Rate: mimics any rhythm; patient **does not** have a pulse; this is a **lethal** dysrhythmia
7. Includes: idioventricular dysrhythmias, bradyasystole dysrhythmias

Pacemaker Rhythms, p 163

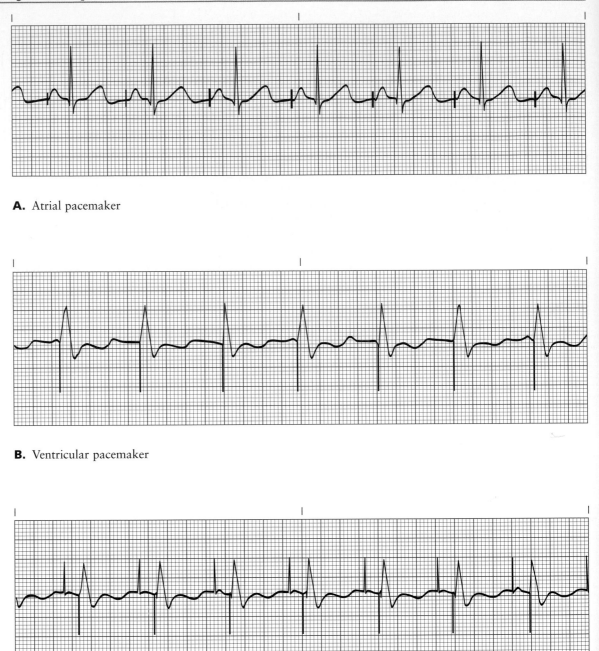

A. Atrial pacemaker

B. Ventricular pacemaker

C. Sequential or biventricular pacemaker

1. Site of origin:
   a. Atrial pacemaker: right atrium (strip **A**)
   b. Ventricular pacemaker: either right or left ventricle (strip **B**)
   c. Sequential pacemaker: right atrium and right ventricle (strip **C**)
   d. Biventricular pacemaker: right atrium, right and left ventricles (strip **C**)
2. P wave: may be replaced by pacer spike
3. PR interval: not measured in paced rhythm
4. QRS: usually greater than 0.12 second; occurs after ventricular pacer spike
5. Rhythm:
   a. P to P interval: varies if present
   b. R to R interval:
      (1) Fixed rate pacemaker: regular
      (2) Demand pacemaker: varies
   c. Pacer spike to pacer spike
      (1) Fixed rate: regular
      (2) Demand rate: varies with the rate of the underlying rhythm
6. Rate: varies according to pacemaker; fixed rate or demand rate
7. Pacing: varies
8. Capture: 100%
9. Types:
   a. Temporary
      (1) Transvenous
      (2) Transcutaneous
   b. Permanent

CHAPTER 9

Medication Review and Adult Treatment Guidelines

DEFINITIONS

ACE inhibitors—Medications that increase cardiac output, lower blood pressure, reduce sodium and water retention (edema)

Antiarrhythmics—Medications that act on the electrical conduction pathway of the heart to prevent or reverse dysrhythmias by slowing the conduction of the electrical impulse, stopping or slowing the reentry pathways, and/or by blocking electrolytes such as potassium or calcium

Anticoagulants—Medications that help prevent the formation of blood clots

Beta-Adrenergic Blockers (β-Blockers)—Medications that decrease the rate and force of heart contractions; reduce cardiac ischemia by reducing the heart muscle's need for oxygen; also lower blood pressure, reduce occurrence of dysrhythmias and pain of angina

Calcium Channel Blockers—Drugs that decrease the heart rate by slowing conduction of the AV node and by lengthening the refractory periods; drugs that prevent spasms of the coronary arteries by relaxing the smooth muscle of the blood vessels

Fibrinolytic Agents—Drugs that dissolve clots in the coronary arteries that cause ischemia and infarction; may reduce the number of deaths from MI. May also be called thrombolytic agents or reperfusers ("clot busters")

Glycoprotein IIb/IIIa Inhibitors—Medications that stop or slow the ability of platelets to form clots

Reperfusion—Process of opening blocked arteries in order to reestablish the flow of blood; can be done with medications or surgical procedures

MEDICATION REVIEW AND ADULT TREATMENT GUIDELINES

This chapter is divided into two sections. The first section is a brief and simplified summary of the most common medications used to treat cardiac dysrhythmias, myocardial infarctions (MIs), and poor cardiac output. This review does **not** include all medications that might be used in the treatment of any dysrhythmia or cardiac disease and is **not** meant to take the place of a pharmacology course. Anyone administering medications should do so only after competency/certification by his or her institution and as governed by the laws and regulations of his or her state. All medications should be administered under the direction of a physician.

The treatments outlined in the second section of this chapter are only general guidelines. They should be used in conjunction with, **not** instead of, your institution's policies and procedures. All treatments should be performed under the guidance of a physician.

The medication and adult treatment guidelines are based on the American Heart Association advanced cardiac life support (ACLS) protocols of 2005 and the most recent updates from the 2005 *Handbook of Emergency Cardiac Care for Healthcare Providers.* Anyone wanting more information regarding medications and treatments used in treating dysrhythmias and cardiac disease is encouraged to attend an ACLS course.

MEDICATION REVIEW

Medications Used to Treat Dysrhythmias

Adenosine

Action: Decreases HR by depressing the SA node and AV node activity.

Indications: To treat narrow complex tachycardias such as PAT/PSVT or SVT.

Dosage: 6 mg IV push rapidly over 1 to 3 seconds, followed immediately by a 20 ml IV saline solution flush, and elevation of the extremity. If no response in 1 to 2 minutes, repeat adenosine at 12 mg IV push rapidly, followed by 20 ml IV saline solution flush; may repeat once more at 12 mg IV push, if there is no response in 1 to 2 minutes.

Precautions: Side effects usually last only 1 to 2 minutes and include flushing, difficulty breathing, and mild chest pain; may also have short-lasting episodes of bradycardia, asystole, or ventricular ectopy (abnormal beats); PAT/PSVT and SVT may recur because the effects of this medication last only a short time; may interact with theophylline (aminophylline), dipyridamole, or carbamazepine. Use with caution in the elderly. Safe and effective in pregnancy. Contraindicated in hypersensitivity to adenosine. May be harmful if used in atrial flutter, A Fib or WPW syndrome.

Amiodarone

Action: Decreases HR by altering impulses through conduction pathways; slows conduction; prolongs effective refractory period.

Indications: To treat V Fib, VT, and pulseless VT.

Dosage: **V Fib/pulseless VT:** 300 mg IV/IO push; if no response within 3 to 5 minutes, repeat once. If dysrhythmia is controlled, begin a continuous infusion at 1 mg/min for 6 hours, followed by 0.5 mg/min for 18 hours; up to a total of 2.2 g in 24 hours. **VT with a pulse:** an infusion of 150 mg IV over 10 minutes can be delivered; if no response, repeat 150 mg IV once. If dysrhythmia is controlled, begin a continuous infusion at 1 mg/min for 6 hours, followed by 0.5 mg/min for 18 hours; up to a total dose of 2.2 g in 24 hours. A slow infusion is 360 mg IV over 6 hours; a maintenance infusion is 540 mg IV over 18 hours.

Precautions: May cause bradycardia, vasodilation, hypotension, and prolonged QT intervals. Use with caution in patients with congestive heart failure (CHF), kidney, liver, or lung disease. Contraindicated in hypersensitivity to amiodarone, pregnancy, second- and third-degree heart block. Amiodarone is incompatible with saline solution and should be administered only in D5W solution, with the use of an inline filter. Always put in a glass bottle. Has a tendency to foam when shaken. May cause hypotension for several months; may also cause scarring of lung tissue or thyroid problems.

Atropine Sulfate

Action: Increases HR and sinus node automaticity; improves AV conduction.

Indications: To correct symptomatic bradycardias; asystole; PEA; to increase HR in a bradycardic rhythm with PVCs, to at least 60 beats/minute.

Dosage: **Symptomatic bradycardia:** 0.5 mg IV, repeated at 3 to 5 minute intervals to a total dose of 3 mg; **Asystole/PEA:** 1 mg IV/IO, repeated every 3 to 5 minutes for a total dose of 3 mg.

Precautions: May cause tachycardia; may increase ischemia due to increased need for oxygen by the myocardium. Use with caution in pregnancy, in the elderly, in MI, and in ACS. Contraindicated in hypersensitivity to atropine sulfate. Not effective in second-degree heart block, type II, or third-degree heart block.

NOTE: Any single dose less than 0.5 mg may cause bradycardia.

Beta-Adrenergic Blockers (Atenolol, Esmolol Hydrochloride, Labetalol, Metoprolol Tartrate, and Propranolol Hydrochloride)	Action:	May reduce cardiac ischemia in patients receiving fibrinolytic agents; may reduce occurrence of V Fib after MI.
	Indications:	Recurrent VT and V Fib; after emergency treatment of MI; severe hypertension, and to decrease ventricular response in patients with narrow complex tachycardias.
	Dosage:	**Atenolol:** 5 mg IV over 5 minutes; wait 10 minutes, repeat dose of 5 mg IV over 5 minutes. **Esmolol:** initial dose: 0.5 mg/kg IV over 1 minute, followed by a four minute infusion at 0.05 mg/kg per minute. Titrate to a maximum dose of 0.3 mg/kg per minute, to a total of 200 mcg/kg. **Labetalol:** 10 to 20 mg IV push over 1 to 2 minutes. May either repeat or double the dose every 10 minutes to a maximum dose of 150 mg, or follow initial bolus dose with an IV infusion of 2 to 8 mg/min. **Metoprolol:** 5 mg slow IV push, over 2 to 5 minutes, repeated at 5-minute intervals to a total dose of 15 mg. **Propranolol:** give 1 to 3 mg divided into 3 equal doses, slow IV push. Give no more than 1 mg/min at 2 to 3 minute intervals.
	Precautions:	May cause bradycardia, AV conduction delays, and hypotension. Use with caution in pregnancy and kidney disease. Contraindicated in hypersensitivity to these beta-adrenergic blockers, second- or third-degree heart blocks, congestive heart failure, cocaine-induced ACS, WPW syndrome, bronchospasm, bradycardia, or hypotension. Do not mix with furosemide or sodium bicarbonate, or use with calcium channel blockers.
Calcium Channel Blockers (Diltiazem Hydrochloride; Verapamil Hydrochloride)	Action:	Decrease the HR by slowing conduction of the AV node and by lengthening the refractory periods. Decreases hypertension by dilating coronary arteries.
	Indications:	To treat narrow complex tachycardias, and rapid ventricular response in atrial flutter and A Fib; to treat hypertension.
	Dosage:	**Diltiazem:** initial bolus: 0.25 mg/kg (average 15 to 20 mg) IV over 2 minutes; repeat dose: 0.35 mg/kg (average 20 to 25 mg) IV over 2 minutes, 15 minutes after the first dose; maintenance dose: continuous IV infusion of 5 to 15 mg/hr, titrated to heart rate. **Verapamil:** give 1 to 3 mg divided into 3 equal doses, slow IV push. Give no more than 1 mg/min, at 2 to 3 minute intervals.
	Precautions:	May cause a short period of hypotension and/or bradycardia. Older patients should be given lower doses (2.5 mg) verapamil at slower rates of infusion (over 3 minutes). Use with caution in pregnancy. Contraindicated if systolic blood pressure is less than 90 mm Hg, in hypersensitivity to these calcium channel blockers, sick sinus syndrome, and acute MI. Do not use in the following: patients with WPW syndrome; in wide QRS tachycardias (VT); with beta blockers. Do not use in patients with an AV block, unless a temporary pacemaker is available.
Epinephrine Hydrochloride (Adrenalin)	Action:	Increases rate and force of cardiac contractions; increases coronary and cerebral blood flow; increases automaticity.
	Indications:	During CPR for cardiac arrest: V Fib, pulseless VT, asystole, PEA, or anaphylaxis (severe allergic reaction). Use in severe bradycardia or hypotension that has not responded to other therapies.
	Dosage:	**IV/IO bolus:** 1 mg of a 1:10,000 dilution; may be repeated at 3 to 5 minute intervals. **Continuous IV infusion:** 1 mg (1 ml) of a 1:1000 dilution in 500 ml D5W or NS, starting at a rate of 1 mcg/min and titrated as needed.
	Precautions:	May increase ischemia due to increased rate and force of contractions; may cause or increase ventricular ectopy (abnormal beat). Use with caution in patients with hypertension, in pregnancy, and in the elderly. Contraindicated in hypersensitivity to epinephrine. Do not mix with sodium bicarbonate; continuous infusion is only used in patients with a pulse.

Ibutilide	Action:	Decreases the HR by slowing conduction through the AV junction and by lengthening the refractory periods.
	Indications:	To treat rapid ventricular response in atrial flutter and A Fib, of less than 48 hours duration.
	Dosage:	**Adults weighing more than 60 kg:** 1 mg (10 ml) IV over 10 minutes. May repeat the second dose after 10 minutes, at the same rate, if needed. **Adults weighing less than 60 kg:** 0.01 mg/kg IV. May repeat the second dose after 10 minutes, at the same rate, if needed.
	Precautions:	May cause VT or torsades de pointes; should be monitored during use and up to 6 hours after infusion, with a defibrillator readily available; use with caution in liver or kidney disease, second- or third-degree heart block, bradycardia, in pregnancy, and in the elderly. Contraindicated in hypersensitivity to ibutilide.
Intravenous Fluids (IV Fluids); Intraosseous Fluids (IO Fluids)	Action:	Replaces lost body fluids; provides IV/IO access for administration of medications; used to dilute and deliver medications.
	Indications:	Hypovolemia; IV or IO access for medication administration.
	Dosage:	1000 ml of 0.9% normal saline (NS) solution or lactated Ringer's (LR) solution. **Intravenous fluids (IV):** access in vein via needle or specialized catheter. **Intraosseous fluids (IO):** access into the bone marrow of specific areas of the arms, legs, sternum or pelvic bones via an adult IO device. **Hypovolemia:** bolus (rapid infusion) of 300 ml/hr or greater. **Medication access:** usually 60 ml/hr or less. **Continuous infusion:** varies because the rate is titrated (adjusted) to the patient's needs.
	Precautions:	Must be used with caution in elderly patients or patients with chronic lung problems to prevent complications such as congestive heart failure. Must be used with caution in patients with brain injury. Monitor IV site to prevent infiltration (IV catheter slips out of vein and solution infuses into tissue).

NOTE: If unable to obtain IV or IO access, consider endotracheal route for lidocaine, epinephrine, atropine and naloxone.

Lidocaine Hydrochloride (Xylocaine)	Action:	Decreases automaticity, helping to decrease ventricular dysrhythmias.
	Indications:	To control ventricular dysrhythmias such as PVCs or VT. Alternative treatment for pulseless VT or V Fib.
	Dosage:	1 to 1.5 mg/kg IV/IO, repeated at 5 to 10 minute intervals in doses of 0.5 to 0.75 mg/kg IV, until a total of 3 mg/kg has been given; if the ventricular ectopy has been suppressed and the patient has a pulse, begin a continuous infusion at 1 to 4 mg/min.

NOTE: If underlying rhythm is bradycardic, consider giving atropine first.

	Precautions:	Signs of toxicity include numbness in hands or feet, drowsiness, slurred speech, decreased hearing, confusion, muscle twitching or tremors, and/or agitation. In severe cases of toxicity, seizures may occur; large doses of lidocaine may cause bradycardia, heart block, or AV conduction dysrhythmias. Use with caution in pregnancy and in the elderly. Contraindicated in hypersensitivity to lidocaine and in patients with WPW syndrome, or severe heart block.
Magnesium Sulfate	Action:	Reduces ventricular dysrhythmias that may follow an MI (decreased magnesium levels may cause V Fib and may also prevent VT from responding to treatment).
	Indications:	Treatment of choice in torsades de pointes; may be used in V Fib or pulseless VT, or digoxin toxicity; magnesium sulfate should be used whenever magnesium levels are decreased.

Magnesium Sulfate, cont'd	Dosage:	**Torsades de pointes without a pulse or hypomagnesemia:** 1 to 2 g diluted in 10 ml IV fluid over 5 to 20 minutes IV/IO. **Torsades de pointes with a pulse:** loading dose of 1 to 2 g in 50 to 100 ml IV fluid, over 5 to 60 minutes. Follow with 0.5 to 1 g/hr IV, titrating dosage to control torsades de pointes.
	Precautions:	May cause flushing, sweating, slight bradycardia, and hypotension. Use with caution in patients with kidney failure and in pregnancy. Contraindicated in hypersensitivity to magnesium sulfate. Should be diluted in IV fluid.
Oxygen (O₂)	Action:	Increases oxygen available to all tissue cells; helps to reduce shortness of breath; may help to decrease ischemia.
	Indications:	For all patients with respiratory distress, SOB, chest pain, dysrhythmias, decreased cardiac output, and in all cardiopulmonary arrests; part of "MONA" protocol for acute MI (acute coronary syndrome [ACS]).
	Dosage:	**For alert patients with mild distress:** 1 to 6 L/min (liters per minute) delivered by nasal cannula. **For patients with moderate respiratory distress:** 4 to 12 L/min by Venturi mask, at 24% to 50%. **For patients with severe respiratory distress:** 6 to 10 L/min of 100% oxygen, delivered by a partial rebreather mask at 35% to 60% or non-rebreather mask with reservoir at 6 to 15 L/min for 60% to 100%. **During CPR:** give by bag-mask device or endotracheal tube at 15 L/min at 100%. Pulse oximetry may be helpful in oxygen titration.
	Precautions:	Flammable; do not use in presence of flames, sparks, or during cardioversion or defibrillation. Use with caution in alert patients with chronic lung disease. Should be used at 100% in all resuscitation attempts. Pulse oximetry may be inaccurate with low cardiac output or anemia.
Procainamide Hydrochloride	Action:	Suppresses ventricular and atrial ectopy; decreases excitability and automaticity.
	Indications:	To control a variety of dysrhythmias.
	Dosage:	20 mg/min IV until any of the following occur: (1) The dysrhythmia is suppressed. (2) The patient becomes hypotensive. (3) The QRS complex widens by 50% of its original width. (4) A total of 17 mg/kg has been given. If necessary, 50 mg/min IV up to 17 mg/kg IV can be given, until any of the above symptoms occur. A continuous IV infusion of procainamide at a rate of 1 to 4 mg/min should be started if the ventricular dysrhythmia has been suppressed and the patient has a pulse.
	Precautions:	May cause hypotension if administered too quickly; decrease maintenance dose if patient has kidney failure. Use with caution in bradycardia and in pregnancy. Contraindicated in hypersensitivity to procainamide hydrochloride, second- and third-degree heart blocks, myasthenia gravis, or systemic lupus. Avoid using in patients with prolonged QT intervals or in torsades de pointes; monitor BP closely.
Vasopressin	Action:	Constricts smooth muscle in blood vessels.
	Indications:	Alternative to epinephrine in the treatment of refractory V Fib, pulseless VT, asystole, and PEA.
	Dosage:	40 units IV/IO push, **once only,** to replace the <u>first</u> or <u>second</u> dose of epinephrine in pulseless VT, VF, asystole, and PEA.
	Precautions:	Potent peripheral vasoconstrictor, which may lead to severe hypertension, increased cardiac ischemia, and chest pain. Use with caution in pregnancy, in the elderly, and in coronary artery disease. Not recommended for patients with chronic kidney disease or hypersensitivity to vasopressin.

Medications Used to Treat Myocardial Infarctions

Aspirin (Acetylsalicylic Acid)

Action: Decreases platelet formation of clots against the inside of arterial walls.

Indications: Part of "MONA" protocol for acute MI (ACS); consider using as a preventive measure for MI, stroke, and angina.

Dosage: 160 to 325 mg PO immediately in acute MI; recommend chewing over swallowing whole tablet. Do not use enteric coated tablets.

Precautions: May cause gastrointestinal bleeding, tinnitus (ringing in the ears), dizziness, wheezing, confusion, and convulsions. Giving increased doses (1000 mg) may limit the positive effects that are needed. Use with caution in liver or kidney disease, asthma, Hodgkin's disease, ulcer disease, pregnancy, or in patients taking warfarin (Coumadin). Contraindicated in hypersensitivity to salicylates or bleeding disorders.

Clopidogrel Bisulfate

Action: Anticoagulant.

Indications: Antiplatelet therapy when aspirin cannot be tolerated; give as soon as possible to patients with UA/NSTEMI if contraindications are not present; give after cardiac catheterization and before (PCI) percutaneous coronary intervention, (i.e., angioplasty, stent) when risk of bleeding is low.

Dosage: Initial dose of 300 mg PO, followed by 75 mg PO daily for 1 to 9 months (it will take several days for full effects to develop).

Precautions: May cause nausea, vomiting, heartburn, or gastrointestinal (GI) bleeding. Use with caution in kidney or liver disease, or in pregnancy. Contraindicated in patients with ulcer disease, hypersensitivity to this drug, or active bleeding. Do **not** give in ACS if coronary artery bypass graft (CABG) is planned within 5 to 7 days.

Glycoprotein IIb/IIIa Inhibitors (Abciximab, Eptifbatide, Tirofiban)

Action: Platelet inhibitor.

Indications: Acute coronary syndrome (ACS) with NSTEMI or UA/NSTEMI.

Dosage: **Abciximab:** ACS with planned PCI within 24 hours: 0.25 mg/kg bolus (10 to 60 minutes before procedure), then 0.125 mcg/kg per min. IV infusion for 12 hours; PCI only: 0.25 mg/kg IV bolus, then 10 mcg/min IV infusion. **Eptifibatide:** ACS: 180 mcg/kg IV bolus over 1 to 2 min, then 2 mcg/kg per min IV infusion for 72 to 96 hours; undergoing PCI: 180 mcg/kg IV bolus over 1 to 2 min, then 2 mcg/kg per min IV infusion, then repeat bolus in 10 min.; adjust dose if creatinine clearance less than 50 ml/min. **Tirofiban:** ACS or undergoing PCI: 0.4 mcg/kg per min IV for 30 minutes, then 0.1 mcg/kg per min IV infusion for 48 to 96 hours; adjust dose if creatinine clearance less than 30 ml/min.

> **NOTE:** Check package insert for current indications, dosage, and duration of therapy, since optimal duration of therapy has not been established.

Precautions: Use with caution in patients over age 65 and in pregnancy. Contraindications: bleeding, bleeding disorders, surgery, or trauma within 30 days; platelet count below 150,000/mm^3, hypersensitivity to glycoproteins; **Abciximab:** must use with heparin; platelet function recovery takes 48 hours; readministration may cause hypersensitivity; **Eptifibatide:** platelet function recovers within 4 to 8 hours; **Tirofiban:** platelet function recovers within 4 to 8 hours.

Fibrinolytic/ Thrombolytic Agents ("Clot Busters") Alteplase (Activase, tissue plasminogen activator, t-PA); Reteplase (Retavase); Streptokinase (Streptase); Tenecteplase (TNKase)	Action:	Dissolves clots in the coronary arteries that cause ischemia and infarction; may reduce number of deaths from MI.
	Indications:	All patients with symptoms and electrocardiographic findings of STEMI, when PCI (percutaneous coronary intervention) is not available within a reasonable period of time. Fibrinolytics must be given within 12 hours of onset of symptoms; patients must meet specific criteria determined by the manufacturer and your institution.
	Dosage:	Varies with specific thrombolytic agent; follow manufacturer's instructions or the policy of your institution and specific instructions of the physician.
	Precautions:	May lead to increased bleeding, decreased clot formation, and intracranial bleeding. Use with caution in pregnancy. Should not be used in patients with bleeding disorders, recent surgery, recent CVAs (hemorrhagic strokes), or with hypersensitivity to these agents. All patients receiving fibrinolytic therapy should receive 160 to 325 mg of chewable aspirin as soon as possible; patients may require heparinization to help keep blood vessels open after fibrinolytic therapy.

Heparin Unfractionated (UFH)	Action:	Anticoagulant; prevents or delays the formation of clots.
	Indications:	Acute MI (STEMI, NSTEMI).
	Dosage:	**Initial bolus:** 60 to 70 units/kg, with a maximum dose of 4000 units. **Continuous infusion:** 12 units/kg per hour with maximum dose of 1000 units/hr for patients weighing more than 70 kg. Follow heparin protocol of your institution.
	Precautions:	May cause active bleeding, severe hypertension, bleeding disorders, and gastrointestinal bleeding. Use with caution in pregnancy and in the elderly. Contraindicated in recent surgery, severe hypertension, liver or kidney disease, known thrombocytopenia (low platelet count), or hypersensitivity to heparin.

Heparin Low Molecular Weight (LMWH); Enoxaparin (Lovenox)	Action:	Anticoagulant; inhibits formation of clots.
	Indications:	ACS, STEMI, NSTEMI.
	Dosage:	**NSTEMI Enoxaparin Protocol:** 1 mg/kg subcutaneous twice daily (BID); the first dose may be preceded by 30 mg IV bolus; **STEMI Enoxaparin Protocol:** used with fibrinolytic treatment: 30 mg IV bolus; then 1 mg/kg subcutaneous twice daily (BID) until hospital discharge.
	Precautions:	May cause active bleeding or hypertension. Use with caution: pregnancy, in the elderly, kidney or liver disease, severe hypertension, or blood disorders. Contraindicated if given with **tenecteplase** in men with creatinine blood level greater than 2.5mg/dl or in women greater than 2 mg/dl; contraindicated in hypersensitivity to pork products or heparin; with platelet count less than 100,000/mm^3; recent surgeries. Not to be used in conjunction with epidural therapy.

Morphine Sulfate	Action:	Narcotic analgesic that provides relief for severe chest pain; reduces need for oxygen in the myocardium.
	Indications:	Pain relief of choice for MIs. Part of "MONA" protocol for acute MI (ACS); cardiogenic pulmonary edema (fluid in the lung caused by heart disease) with stable BP.
	Dosage:	1 to 5 mg IV titrated over 1 to 5 minutes; may repeat in 5 to 30 minutes until pain is relieved.
	Precautions:	May cause hypotension. Monitor respirations frequently because morphine may depress respiratory function. Use with caution in pregnancy, in the elderly, or with liver or kidney disease. Contraindicated in hypersensitivity to morphine or in patients with asthma. Follow your institution's guidelines for use of a narcotic.

Nitroglycerin

Action: Relieves cardiac chest pain and hypertension by relaxing and dilating smooth muscle in blood vessels, including coronary arteries.

Indications: To treat acute angina, unstable angina, and congestive heart failure associated with MIs; reduce pain and hypertension associated with MIs; part of "MONA" protocol for acute MI (ACS).

Dosage: **Sublingual** (under the tongue): one tablet (0.3 or 0.4 mg); repeat at 5-minute intervals; maximum dose is three tablets. **Spray: (Caution: Do Not Shake)** 0.4 mg under or on the tongue by metered-dose canister (patient should wait 10 seconds before swallowing); maximum dose, three sprays in 15 minutes. **IV:** an initial dose of 10 to 20 mcg titrated to pain and hypertension relief. May increase by 5 to 10 mcg per minute, every 5 to 10 minutes as needed.

Precautions: Do not use if systolic BP is less than 90 mm Hg. May cause severe hypotension soon after administration of medication (monitor vital signs frequently). Headache, nausea, and vomiting may also occur. Use with caution in pregnancy, liver or kidney disease, or IV use in the elderly. Contraindicated in hypersensitivity to nitroglycerin or nitrites. Administer with an infusion pump. Incompatible with dobutamine; be aware of other drug incompatibilities. Absorbed by plastic (must be administered in glass bottles with polyethylene tubing). Should also avoid use in patients who have taken medications for erectile dysfunction and impotency.

Medications Used to Treat Poor Cardiac Output/ Serious Respiratory Conditions

ACE Inhibitors (Captopril, Enalapril, Enalaprilat, Lisinopril, Ramipril)

Action: Increases cardiac output; lowers blood pressure; reduces sodium and water retention (edema).

Indications: To improve left ventricular function; reduce death rate after acute MI; to treat high blood pressure or heart failure.

Dosage: **Captopril:** initial single dose of 6.25 mg PO; advance to 25 mg three times daily (TID), then 50 mg three times daily, as tolerated. **Enalapril:** initial dose 2.5 mg PO; titrate to 20 mg PO, twice daily (BID). **Enalaprilat:** initial dose 0.625 mg IV over 5 min, then 1.25 to 5 mg IV every 6 hours. **Lisinopril:** 5 mg PO within 24 hours of onset of symptoms, then 5 mg PO given after 24 hours, then 10 mg PO given after 48 hours, then 10 mg PO once daily. **Ramipril:** begin with single dose of 2.5 mg PO; titrate to 5 mg PO twice daily (BID), as tolerated.

Precautions: Use with caution in dialysis, diabetes, and kidney disease. Contraindicated in pregnancy or edema; do not give if patient is hypotensive, has serum potassium greater than 5 mEq/L, or has hypersensitivity to ACE inhibitors; Enalaprilat IV is contraindicated in STEMI, due to risk of hypotension. Generally not started in emergency department. Begin within 24 hours of onset of symptoms, after reperfusion therapy has been completed and blood pressure (BP) has been stabilized.

Calcium Chloride

Action: Increases myocardial contractility.

Indications: Replace and maintain calcium levels; hyperkalemia (increased potassium level); calcium channel blocker toxicity.

Dosage: 500 to 1000 mg slowly IV; may repeat if necessary.

Precautions: Give slowly; rapid administration may cause slowing of the HR. May cause spasms of the coronary and cerebral (brain) arteries. Use with caution in patients receiving digitalis, in pregnancy, and in kidney disease. Contraindicated in hypercalcemia and V Fib; incompatible with sodium bicarbonate. Not routinely used in cardiac arrest.

Digitalis Glycoside (Digoxin [Lanoxin])

Action: Increases myocardial contractility, resulting in increased cardiac output; helps control ventricular response to atrial dysrhythmias.

Indications: Used with atrial flutter or A Fib; is an alternate treatment for atrial tachycardias, including PAT/PSVT and SVT. Used in treatment of chronic congestive heart failure.

Dosage: Initial dose of 10 to 15 mcg/kg administered IV in three divided doses.

Precautions: Use with caution in patients with acute MI because the drug may cause AV block, sinus bradycardia, or VT; use with caution in pregnancy and in the elderly. Contraindicated for patients with WPW syndrome, second- or third-degree heart block, digitalis toxicity, torsades de pointes, VT, V Fib, or hypersensitivity to digitalis glycoside. When given with amiodarone, decrease dose by 50%; do not administer if HR is less than 60 beats/min; usually not used outside hospital setting because of slow onset of action. Avoid use of cardioversion if patient is taking digoxin, unless condition is life threatening. If necessary, use low settings of 10 to 20 Joules.

Digoxin Immune FAB (ovine) (Digibind, DigiFab)

Action: Corrects digoxin toxicity.

Indications: Used in digoxin toxicity that causes life-threatening dysrhythmias, shock, CHF; hyperkalemia (potassium level greater than 5.5 mEq/L); elevated digitalis blood levels, if patient is symptomatic.

Dosage: **Chronic toxicity:** 3 to 5 vials (120 to 200 mg); each vial binds 0.6 mg digoxin. **Acute toxicity:** 10 vials (400 mg), may require up to 20 vials (800 mg). Dosage varies with the amount of digoxin taken.

Precautions: May cause congestive heart failure (CHF), ventricular rate increase, atrial fibrillation, or hypokalemia. Serum digoxin level should not be used to calculate additional dosage of Digibind because serum levels usually rise after treatment. Use with caution in pregnancy, in the elderly, cardiac or kidney disease, or sheep protein allergy. Contraindicated in hypersensitivity to Digibind/DigiFab or mild digoxin toxicity. Do not mix with any other medication.

Dobutamine Hydrochloride

Action: Increases force and rate of contraction of heart muscle, increasing cardiac output and increasing coronary artery blood flow.

Indications: Short-term treatment of heart failure.

Dosage: 2 to 20 mcg/kg per minute IV infusion. Titrate so HR does not increase by more than 10% of the HR before treatment.

Precautions: May cause rapid-rate dysrhythmias, changes in BP, headache, nausea, and vomiting; monitor vital signs and patient's rhythm continuously. Administer with infusion pump. Use with caution in patients who have the following:
1. Atrial fibrillation: increases AV conduction and rapid ventricular response.
2. MI: high doses may increase myocardium's need for oxygen and increase ischemia.
3. PVCs: may increase incidence of PVCs.
Use with caution in patients with hypertension and in pregnancy. Contraindicated in hypersensitivity to dobutamine hydrochloride and sulfites. Do not use in patients with systolic BP less than 100 mm Hg who are in shock, or in shock caused by known poison or drugs. Incompatible with aminophylline, verapamil, digoxin, and heparin. Do not mix with sodium bicarbonate.

Dopamine Hydrochloride

Action: Increases cardiac output by improving myocardial contractility; increases BP by constricting peripheral arteries and veins.

Indications: To treat hypotension accompanied by other symptoms, when there is no hypovolemia; for symptomatic bradycardia.

Dosage: 2 to 20 mcg/kg per minute continuous IV infusion. Titrate all doses to patient's blood pressure and heart rate.

	Precautions:	May cause nausea and vomiting. Increased HR may produce supraventricular or ventricular dysrhythmias. May increase need for oxygen by the myocardium, which can lead to ischemia. Use with caution in pregnancy and in the elderly. Contraindicated in V Fib, tachycardic dysrhythmias, or hypersensitivity to dopamine. Use with an infusion pump; check IV site frequently for infiltration; monitor vital signs and cardiac rhythm frequently. Do not mix with sodium bicarbonate. Discontinue drug administration slowly.
Flumazenil	Action:	Complete or partial reversal of sedative effects of benzodiazepines.
	Indications:	Benzodiazepine overdose; benzodiazepines are used to treat cocaine overdose or cocaine-induced ACS.
	Dosage:	Initial dose: 0.2 mg IV over 15 seconds; second dose: 0.3 mg IV over 30 seconds, if consciousness does not occur. Repeat every minute until patient regains consciousness or a total of 1 mg in 5 minutes or 3 mg in one hour is given. Most patients respond after 0.6 to 1 mg of drug.
	Precautions:	May cause nausea, vomiting, dizziness, blurred vision, hypertension, seizures, or chest pain. Use with caution in pregnancy, in the elderly, liver or kidney disease, or seizure disorders. Contraindicated in hypersensitivity to drug, long-term benzodiazepine use, tricyclic antidepressant overdose, or patients being given benzodiazepines for a life-threatening condition. Monitor respirations for recurrent depression.
Furosemide (Lasix)	Action:	Removes excess fluid from tissues; increases formation of urine.
	Indications:	Acute pulmonary edema; congestive heart failure; cerebral edema after MI; hypertensive emergencies.
	Dosage:	20 to 40 mg IV, over 1 to 2 minutes; if there is no response, double the dose to 40 to 80 mg IV over 1 to 2 minutes. Start at 40 mg IV for patients with new onset of pulmonary edema without hypovolemia.
	Precautions:	May cause severe dehydration, hypotension, hypovolemia, electrolyte imbalances, high blood glucose levels, or damage to hearing. Use with caution in pregnancy, diabetes, severe liver or kidney disease, or dehydration. Contraindicated in hypersensitivity to sulfonamides, hypovolemia, or severely decreased electrolyte levels.
Glucagon	Action:	Relaxes smooth muscle; raises glucose level.
	Indications:	Treatment of toxic effects of calcium channel blockers or beta-blockers.
	Dosage:	Initial dose: 3 mg IV slowly, followed by IV infusion at 3 mg/hour, as needed.
	Precautions:	May cause nausea, vomiting and high blood glucose levels; contraindicated in hypersensitivity.
Inamrinone (Amrinone)	Action:	Improves cardiac output by increasing strength of cardiac contractions; decreases BP by relaxing and dilating blood vessel walls.
	Indications:	Consider using in congestive heart failure (CHF) that has not responded to other drug therapy.
	Dosage:	**Initial dose:** 0.75 mg/kg slow IV push; repeat 0.75 mg/kg after 30 minutes, if needed. **Maintenance dose:** 5 to 10 mcg/kg per minute, titrated to desired BP. Reduce dose by 50% to 75% when creatinine clearance is less than 10 ml/min.
	Precautions:	May cause stomach upset, fever, liver problems, kidney failure, and decreased platelet count. Increases myocardial demand for oxygen, which can cause ischemia or cardiac dysrhythmias; may also increase ventricular irritability. Use with caution in pregnancy and in the elderly. Contraindicated in hypersensitivity to this drug, sulfites, or patients with an acute MI. Incompatible with furosemide, sodium bicarbonate, or dextrose. Use an infusion pump to administer.

Isoproterenol Hydrochloride (Isuprel)	Action:	Increases force and rate of myocardial contractions, improving cardiac output and systolic BP.
	Indications:	Torsades de pointes that does not respond to magnesium sulfate; used for symptomatic bradycardia unresponsive to atropine, until temporary pacing can be established.
	Dosage:	**Continuous infusion:** 2 to 10 mcg/min, titrated to patient's BP and pulse. **Torsades de pointes:** titrate to increase the HR of the underlying rhythm (causing the QT intervals to shorten), until the torsades de pointes is resolved.
	Precautions:	**Use with extreme caution.** Do not use with other tachycardic dysrhythmias or cardiac arrest; must be used with infusion pump; incompatible with aminophylline and sodium bicarbonate; use lower doses in the elderly; use with caution in pregnancy. Contraindicated in hypersensitivity to this drug or sulfite allergy (may contain sulfite preservative); do not use with epinephrine (can cause V Fib or VT).
Milrinone	Actions:	Improves cardiac output by increasing strength of cardiac contractions; decreases BP by relaxing and dilating blood vessel walls.
	Indications:	Consider using in congestive heart failure that has not responded to other drug therapy.
	Dosage:	**Initial bolus:** 50 mcg/kg IV over 10 minutes. **Maintenance dose:** 0.375 to 0.750 mcg/kg per minute for 2 to 3 days; reduce dose with kidney problems.
	Precautions:	May cause stomach upset, fever, liver problems, kidney failure, or reduction of platelets. Increases myocardial demand for oxygen, which can increase cardiac ischemia; may also increase ventricular irritability, therefore cardiac monitoring and patient assessment are required. Use with caution in patients with atrial flutter, A Fib, liver or kidney disease; use with caution in pregnancy and in the elderly. Should not be used in acute MI patients, cardiac valve disease, and patients who are allergic to this drug or to sulfites. Incompatible with furosemide or procainamide. Use an infusion pump to administer.
Naloxone Hydrochloride (Narcan)	Action:	Unknown; may replace narcotics at narcotic receptor sites.
	Indications:	Respiratory depression or unconsciousness due to known or suspected narcotic overdose.
	Dosage:	Give 0.4 to 2 mg IV, titrate until respirations are adequate; may repeat dose every 2 to 3 min, as needed; can give up to 6 to 10 mg over less than 10 minutes; respiratory rate increases within 1 to 2 minutes.
	Precautions:	May cause narcotic withdrawal (example: nausea, vomiting, anxiety, abdominal cramping, hypertension). May need to repeat dosing, since narcotic effect lasts longer than Narcan. Monitor for recurrent respiratory depression; use with caution in patients with increased cardiac irritability, pregnancy, or seizure disorder. Contraindications include hypersensitivity to drug or to sulfite allergies. Do not mix with other medications.
Nitroprusside Sodium (Sodium Nitroprusside)	Action:	Dilates and relaxes the smooth muscle of blood vessels; increases cardiac output; reduces myocardium's need for oxygen (may reduce ischemia); relieves chest pain.
	Indications:	Hypertensive emergencies (when high BP will not respond to other drugs), and acute congestive heart failure.
	Dosage:	50 mg diluted in 250 ml D_5W solution; **initial IV dose:** 0.25 to 0.3 mcg/kg per minute; titrate every 3 to 5 minutes until desired BP or maximum dose of 10 mcg/kg per minute. Action occurs within 1 to 2 minutes. Use D_5W solution to reconstitute medication; do not add any other drugs or preservatives to nitroprusside solution.

	Precautions:	May cause headache, nausea and vomiting, abdominal cramps, and severe hypotension. Monitor vital signs every 2 to 3 minutes because medication may decrease BP rapidly. Use with caution in patients with liver or kidney disease, in pregnancy, and the elderly. Contraindicated in hypersensitivity to sodium nitroprusside. Solution must be protected from light; cover IV bottle with foil or dark plastic; follow your institution's policy regarding covering IV tubing; incompatible with bacteriostatic water and saline solution. Administer with an infusion pump.
Norepinephrine Bitartrate	Action:	Constricts blood vessels and increases blood pressure, heart rate, and the force of cardiac contractions.
	Indications:	Acute and severe hypotension not caused by hypovolemia.
	Dosage:	0.5 to 1.0 mcg/min IV (**only route**), titrate infusion to patient's BP; may increase dose to a maximum of 30 mcg/min. Use only with D_5W or D_5NS.
	Precautions:	May cause an increased need for oxygen in myocardium; monitor patient's rhythm continuously for development of dysrhythmias. Since BP can drop very rapidly, monitor vital signs frequently, at least every 2 to 3 minutes. Use with caution in pregnancy and in the elderly. Contraindicated in patients with V Fib, dysrhythmias with rapid heart rates, hypertension, or hypersensitivity to norepinephrine bitartrate. Assess IV site frequently because infiltration may cause death of tissues around the IV site. Incompatible with aminophylline, lidocaine, sodium bicarbonate, and NS solution.
Sodium Bicarbonate	Actions:	Reduces acidosis.
	Indications:	Metabolic acidosis; prolonged cardiac arrest; cardiotoxicity with some drug overdoses; hyperkalemia.
	Dosage:	1 mEq/kg IV; flush with 20 ml NS solution before and after administering medication to reduce possibility of drug interactions. Repeat dose based on arterial blood gas results to reduce possibility of drug interactions.
	Precautions:	Monitor electrolytes, arterial blood gases, and kidney function. Use with caution in pregnancy, in CHF, and in the elderly. Contraindicated in patients with respiratory acidosis or hypersensitivity to sodium bicarbonate. Do **not** mix with any other medication.

Research Medication

This medication is not currently approved by the FDA for **IV administration** in the United States of America, except in research. However, it may be in use in other countries.

Sotalol	Action:	Prolongs absolute refractory period without affecting conduction; suppresses ventricular ectopy when amiodarone, lidocaine, and procainamide have not been effective.
	Indications:	To control supraventricular and ventricular dysrhythmias.
	Dosage:	1 to 1.5 mg/kg IV slowly at 10 mg/min.
	Precautions:	*Must be given slowly*. May cause bradycardia, hypotension, and torsades de pointes. Use with caution in pregnancy, in the elderly, and with medications that prolong QT intervals. Contraindicated in hypersensitivity to sotalol, chronic lung diseases, bradycardia, and second- or third-degree heart blocks.

ADULT TREATMENT GUIDELINES

The treatments for the dysrhythmias and conditions outlined in this section are only general guidelines. They should be used in conjunction with, **not** instead of, your institution's policies and procedures. All treatments should be performed under the guidance of a physician.

As with any dysrhythmia, ongoing assessment of the patient's condition is essential. The patient's tolerance of the dysrhythmia and any subsequent symptoms will help determine appropriate treatment. Patient assessment involves observing the patient's overall condition and monitoring vital signs (blood pressure, pulse, and respiration) frequently. Comparing the patient's actual pulse rate with the heart rate on the monitor allows you to assess the heart's ability to contract in response to the conduction of an electric impulse through the cardiac muscle, and to circulate blood throughout the body to all the body's cells.

In addition to interpreting the dysrhythmia on the monitor screen, it is important to evaluate the ST segments, T waves, and QT intervals. Changes in these components may provide you with clues to potential cardiac problems.

The treatment of an acute coronary syndromes (ACS), such as a myocardial infarction, may vary slightly, depending on changes to the ST segment on a 12-Lead ECG. These changes help classify the increased risks of an MI and are identified as:

1. *STEMI*   ST Elevation Myocardial Infarction
2. *UA/NSTEMI*   Unstable Angina with Non-ST Elevation Myocardial Infarction
3. *NSTEMI*   Non-ST Elevation Myocardial Infarction

Patients who are unable to tolerate a dysrhythmia will be symptomatic or medically unstable, and will show signs and symptoms of poor cardiac output. These signs and symptoms may include cool, clammy skin; hypotension or hypertension; pallor; cyanosis; dyspnea; chest pain not relieved by rest; diaphoresis; dizziness; nausea and/or vomiting; decrease in urinary output, and/or decrease in the level of consciousness.

Any one of these symptoms by itself may not indicate poor cardiac output. However, if these symptoms occur with either bradycardia or tachycardia, it strongly suggests the patient is not tolerating the dysrhythmia, and treatment should be started immediately.

For the purpose of treatment, it is understood that all patients are adult. Anyone wishing to learn pediatric treatment protocols is encouraged to attend a pediatric advanced life support course (PALS).

It is also understood that:

1. All patients are being monitored.
2. No contraindications exist to any treatment protocols.
3. All patients have either intravenous or intraosseous access.
4. Intravenous/intraosseous medications are administered at the port closest to the IV/IO site, followed by a 20 ml flush of IV/IO fluids; then if possible, elevation of that extremity for 10 to 20 seconds. These three actions will promote faster circulation of the medications.
5. All patients are assessed both before and after any treatment or the administration of any medication.
6. All appropriate laboratory tests have been ordered, when available.

Artifact

1. Artifact is not treated.
2. Correct the cause of the artifact to simplify identification of the rhythm.
3. Initiate treatment, if necessary.

Acute Coronary Syndromes/Myocardial Infarction

A. <u>STEMI</u> (ST Elevation Myocardial Infarction): Elevated ST segments with symptoms of injury or death to cardiac muscle.
   1. Assess the patient; be prepared to initiate morphine, oxygen, nitroglycerin, and aspirin (MONA protocol).
   2. Provide oxygen; apply pulse oximetry.
   3. Begin IV fluids.
   4. Give nitroglycerin sublingual or spray for pain; may be given a total of three times, if needed.
   5. Obtain a 12-Lead ECG. Reassess the patient.
   6. If no relief from repeated nitroglycerin, administer morphine IV, titrated to pain relief; consider IV nitroglycerin.
   7. Continue to assess and monitor the patient. Treat any dysrhythmias that occur.
   8. Begin beta-blockers, clopidogrel, heparin (UFH or LMWH).
   9. Once diagnosis of MI has been confirmed, begin fibrinolytic protocol within 12 hours of onset of symptoms (when PCI is not available within a reasonable period of time). Consider oral aspirin and IV heparin, if included in fibrinolytic protocol.
   10. Continued assessment and monitoring of the patient is essential. Transfer patient to the care of a cardiologist in the coronary care unit.

B. <u>UA/NSTEMI</u> (Unstable Angina with Non-ST Elevation Myocardial Infarction): ST depression or inverted T wave with unstable angina indicating cardiac ischemia.
   1. Assess the patient; be prepared to initiate morphine, oxygen, nitroglycerin, and aspirin (MONA protocol).
   2. Provide oxygen; apply pulse oximetry.
   3. Begin IV fluids.
   4. Give nitroglycerin sublingual or spray for pain; may be given a total of three times, if needed.
   5. Obtain a 12-Lead ECG. Reassess the patient.
   6. If no relief from repeated sublingual nitroglycerin, administer morphine IV, titrated to pain relief; consider IV nitroglycerin.
   7. Continue to assess and monitor the patient. Treat any dysrhythmias that occur.
   8. Begin IV nitroglycerin; beta blockers; clopidogeral; heparin (UFH or LMWH), glycoprotein IIb/IIIa inhibitor.
   9. Continued assessment and monitoring of the patient is essential. Transfer patient to the care of a cardiologist in the coronary care unit.

C. <u>NSTEMI</u> (Non-ST Elevation Myocardial Infarction): Normal ST segments or T waves with suspicion of angina
   1. Assess the patient; be prepared to initiate morphine, oxygen, nitroglycerin, and aspirin (MONA protocol).
   2. Provide oxygen; apply pulse oximetry.
   3. Begin IV fluids.
   4. Give nitroglycerin sublingual or spray for pain; may be given a total of three times, if needed.
   5. Obtain a 12-Lead electrocardiograph. Reassess the patient.
   6. If no relief from repeated sublingual nitroglycerin, administer morphine IV, titrated to pain relief; consider IV nitroglycerin.

7. Continue to assess and monitor the patient. Treat any dysrhythmias that occur.
8. Consider admitting to a cardiac monitored bed for observation, while waiting for results of laboratory tests and/or electrocardiographic confirmation of ST changes or MI.

> **NOTE:** If patient symptoms worsen, or if ST segment or electrocardiograph changes indicate cardiac ischemia, treat the patient's condition as an MI and begin reperfusion therapy, if within protocols. Other therapies that may be used include ACE inhibitors, stress tests, or a cardiac catheterization.

Normal Sinus Rhythm and Atrial Dysrhythmias

Normal Sinus Rhythm

1. Normal sinus rhythm does not require treatment.
2. **Remember**, the monitor is **not** the patient. The patient must be assessed, and, if symptomatic, treatment must be initiated.
3. Continue to assess and monitor the patient.

Sinus Bradycardia

1. Assess the patient. If the patient is medically **stable**, continue to observe the patient. If the patient is medically **unstable**, begin treatment.
2. Provide oxygen; apply pulse oximetry.
3. Begin IV fluids.
4. Obtain a 12-Lead ECG. Reassess the patient.
5. An artificial pacemaker (temporary or permanent) may be necessary. Use a transcutaneous or transvenous pacemaker, if available, until a permanent pacemaker is placed.
6. May consider administering atropine while waiting for pacemaker. Reassess the patient; repeat atropine, if necessary.
7. Epinephrine may be administered to patients who do not respond to atropine.
8. Dopamine may be administered for a systolic BP less than 80 mm Hg.
9. Continue to assess and monitor the patient.
10. Reassess the patient. If the dysrhythmia has converted to another rhythm and/or rate, reassess the patient; if necessary, treat the new dysrhythmia.

Sinus Tachycardia

1. Assess the patient. If the patient is medically **stable**, continue to observe the patient. If the patient is medically **unstable**, begin treatment.
2. Determine the cause of the tachycardia:
   a. Fever
      (1) Administer antipyretics, such as aspirin, ibuprofen, or acetaminophen, to lower fever.
      (2) Provide cool to tepid bath.
   b. Anxiety
      (1) Acknowledge the patient's anxiety.
      (2) Offer reassurance in a calm manner.
   c. Pain
      (1) Administer pain medication as ordered.
      (2) Use relaxation techniques.
   d. Hypovolemia
      (1) Replace fluids or blood.
3. Provide oxygen; apply pulse oximetry.
4. Begin IV fluids.

5. Obtain a 12-Lead electrocardiograph. Reassess the patient.
6. Consider using beta-blockers, diltiazem, or digoxin if the patient's HR is greater than 100 but less than 151 beats/min. If HR is greater than 150 beats/min, treat as SVT.
7. Reassess the patient. If the dysrhythmia has converted to another rhythm and/or rate, reassess the patient; if necessary, treat the new dysrhythmia.

Sinus Arrhythmia

1. Assess the patient. If the patient is medically **stable**, continue to observe the patient. If signs of **poor cardiac output** are present, begin treatment.
2. Provide oxygen; apply pulse oximetry.
3. Begin IV fluids.
4. Obtain a 12-Lead electrocardiograph. Reassess the patient.
5. If overall HR is bradycardic, an artificial pacemaker (temporary or permanent) may be necessary. Use a transcutaneous or transvenous pacemaker, if available, until a permanent pacemaker is placed.
6. May consider administering atropine while waiting for pacemaker. Reassess the patient; repeat atropine, if necessary.
7. Epinephrine may be administered to patients who do not respond to atropine.
8. Dopamine may be administered for a systolic BP less than 80 mm Hg.
9. Reassess the patient. If the dysrhythmia has converted to another rhythm and/or rate, reassess the patient; if necessary, treat the new dysrhythmia.

Sinus Exit Block; Sinus Arrest

1. If the sinus exit block or sinus arrest is a new dysrhythmia, observe the patient closely for a change in the cardiac rhythm and/or rate. If the patient is medically **stable**, continue to observe the patient. If signs of **poor cardiac output** are present, begin treatment.
2. Provide oxygen; apply pulse oximetry.
3. Begin IV fluids.
4. Obtain a 12-Lead electrocardiograph. Reassess the patient.
5. Sinus exit block and sinus arrest are both indications of damage or injury to the SA node. If the pauses are frequent or long, the patient may become medically **unstable** and require an artificial pacemaker.
6. May consider administering atropine while waiting for pacemaker. Reassess the patient; repeat atropine, if necessary.
7. Epinephrine may be administered to patients who do not respond to atropine.
8. Dopamine may be administered for a systolic BP less than 80 mm Hg.
9. Reassess the patient. If the dysrhythmia has converted to another rhythm and/or rate, reassess the patient; if necessary, treat the new dysrhythmia.

Premature Atrial Complex

1. Assess the patient. A PAC by itself does not require treatment. If the patient is medically **unstable** or shows signs of poor cardiac output, treat the underlying rhythm and/or rate.
2. If the cause of the PAC is caffeine or nicotine, decrease or eliminate the stimulant in the patient's daily intake.
3. If the PAC is a new occurrence, observe the patient closely for a change in the cardiac rhythm and/or rate.
4. Continue to reassess and monitor the patient.

Paroxysmal Atrial Tachycardia/Paroxysmal Supraventricular Tachycardia; Supraventricular Tachycardia

1. Assess the patient. Even if the patient is medically **stable**, begin treatment. Treatment is usually started, since most patients cannot tolerate this rapid rhythm for prolonged periods of time.
2. Provide oxygen; apply pulse oximetry.
3. Begin IV fluids.
4. May perform vagal stimulation, such as the Valsalva maneuver (have the patient bear down) or carotid massage. Reassess the patient.
5. Obtain a 12-Lead electrocardiograph. Reassess the patient.
6. Administer adenosine.
7. If PAT/PSVT; SVT continues, repeat adenosine at higher dose; may repeat this dose once after 1 to 2 minutes.
8. If PAT/PSVT; SVT continues, monitor vital signs and reassess the patient.
9. If the PAT/PSVT; SVT continues, consider using diltiazem or beta-blockers, to convert the PAT/PSVT; SVT to a normal or more stable rhythm.
10. Reassess the patient.
11. If the patient is medically **unstable**, consider synchronized cardioversion.
12. Reassess the patient. If the dysrhythmia has converted to another rhythm and/or rate, reassess the patient; if necessary, treat the new dysrhythmia.

Atrial Flutter; Atrial Fibrillation

1. Assess the patient. If patient is medically **stable** with heart rate below 150, continue to observe the patient.
2. Provide oxygen; apply pulse oximetry.
3. Begin IV fluids.
4. Obtain a 12-Lead electrocardiograph. Reassess the patient.
5. If overall HR is bradycardic and patient is medically stable, continue to observe the patient. If patient becomes medically **unstable**, an artificial pacemaker (temporary or permanent) may be necessary. Use a transcutaneous or transvenous pacemaker, if available, until a permanent pacemaker is placed.
6. May consider administering atropine while waiting for pacemaker. Reassess the patient; repeat atropine, if necessary.
7. Epinephrine may be administered to patients who do not respond to atropine.
8. Dopamine may be administered for a systolic BP less than 80 mm Hg.
9. Consider diltiazem or beta-blockers, if the patient's HR is greater than 150 beats/min. and patient is medically stable.
10. Consider anticoagulant administration with slow, rapid and uncontrolled ventricular response.
11. Reassess the patient. If the dysrhythmia has converted to another rhythm and/or rate, reassess the patient; if necessary, treat the new dysrhythmia.

Wolff-Parkinson-White Syndrome

1. Assess the patient.
2. Provide oxygen; apply pulse oximetry.
3. Begin IV fluids.
4. Obtain a 12-Lead electrocardiograph. Reassess the patient.
5. If overall HR is bradycardic and patient has no symptoms, continue to observe. If patient becomes **unstable**, an artificial pacemaker (temporary or permanent) may be necessary. Use a transcutaneous or transvenous pacemaker, if available, until a permanent pacemaker is placed.
6. Consider administering atropine while waiting for pacemaker. Reassess the patient; repeat atropine, if necessary.
7. Epinephrine may be administered to patients who do not respond to atropine.
8. Dopamine may be administered for a systolic BP less than 80 mm Hg.
9. If heart rate is greater than 150 beats per min. and patient is stable, consider amiodarone. Do **not** use adenosine, digoxin, diltiazem, or verapamil.

10. Synchronized cardioversion may be indicated if the patient becomes **unstable.**
11. Reassess the patient. If the dysrhythmia has converted to another rhythm and/or rate, reassess the patient; if necessary, treat the new dysrhythmia.

> **NOTE:** In Wolff-Parkinson-White syndrome, if standard drug treatment is not successful, expert consultation is advised, for possible radio frequency catheter ablation therapy.

Junctional Dysrhythmias

Junctional Dysrhythmia

1. Assess the patient. If the patient is medically **stable,** continue observing him or her.
2. If the patient is medically **unstable,** begin treatment, following appropriate junctional guidelines.

Junctional Bradycardia Dysrhythmia

1. Assess the patient. If the patient is medically **stable,** continue to observe the patient. If the patient is medically unstable, begin treatment.
2. Provide oxygen; apply pulse oximetry.
3. Begin IV infusion.
4. Obtain a 12-Lead electrocardiograph. Reassess the patient.
5. An artificial pacemaker (temporary or permanent) may be necessary. Use a transcutaneous or transvenous pacemaker, if available, until a permanent pacemaker is placed.
6. Consider administering atropine while waiting for pacemaker. Reassess the patient; repeat atropine, if necessary.
7. Epinephrine may be administered to patients who do not respond to atropine.
8. Dopamine may be administered for a systolic BP less than 80 mm Hg.
9. Reassess the patient. If the dysrhythmia has converted to another rhythm and/or rate, reassess the patient; if necessary, treat the new dysrhythmia.

Accelerated Junctional Dysrhythmia; Junctional Tachycardia Dysrhythmia

1. Assess the patient. If the patient is medically **stable,** continue to observe the patient. If the patient is medically **unstable,** begin treatment.
2. Determine the cause of the tachycardia:
   a. Fever
      (1) Administer antipyretics, such as aspirin, ibuprofen or acetaminophen, to lower fever.
      (2) Provide cool to tepid bath.
   b. Anxiety
      (1) Acknowledge the patient's anxiety.
      (2) Offer reassurance in a calm manner.
   c. Pain
      (1) Administer pain medication as ordered.
      (2) Use relaxation techniques.
   d. Hypovolemia
      (1) Replace fluids or blood.
   e. Consider digoxin toxicity
3. Provide oxygen; apply pulse oximetry.
4. Begin IV fluids.
5. Obtain a 12-Lead electrocardiograph. Reassess the patient.
6. If the HR is greater than 150 beats/min, treat as PAT/PSVT; SVT.
7. Synchronized cardioversion may be indicated if the patient becomes **unstable.**
8. Reassess the patient. If the dysrhythmia has converted to another rhythm and/or rate, reassess the patient; if necessary, treat the new dysrhythmia.

Premature Junctional Complex

1. Assess the patient. PJCs are not treated unless the patient becomes medically unstable.
2. If the cause of the PJC is caffeine or nicotine, decrease or eliminate the stimulant in the patient's daily intake.
3. If the PJCs are a new occurrence, observe the patient closely for a change in the cardiac rhythm and/or rate.
4. If necessary, treat the underlying rhythm and/or HR according to the patient's symptoms.
5. Reassess the patient. If the dysrhythmia has converted to another rhythm and/or rate, reassess the patient; if necessary, treat the new dysrhythmia.

Wandering Junctional Pacemaker Dysrhythmia; Wandering Atrial Pacemaker Dysrhythmia

1. Assess the patient.
2. Provide oxygen; apply pulse oximetry.
3. Begin IV fluids.
4. Obtain a 12-Lead electrocardiograph. Reassess the patient.
5. If overall HR is bradycardic, and patient is medically **stable**, continue to observe. If patient becomes medically **unstable**, an artificial pacemaker (temporary or permanent) may be necessary. Use a transcutaneous or transvenous pacemaker, if available, until a permanent pacemaker is placed.
6. Consider administering atropine while waiting for pacemaker. Reassess the patient; repeat atropine, if necessary.
7. Epinephrine may be administered to patients who do not respond to atropine.
8. Dopamine may be administered for a systolic BP less than 80 mm Hg.
9. Consider using vagal stimulation; if patient's heart rate is greater than 150 beats/min, treat as SVT.
10. Synchronized cardioversion may be indicated if patient becomes unstable.
11. Reassess the patient. If the dysrhythmia has converted to another rhythm and/or rate, reassess the patient; if necessary, treat the new dysrhythmia.

Heart Blocks

First-Degree Heart Block

1. Assess the patient. A first-degree block by itself does not require treatment.
2. If the first-degree block is a new occurrence, observe the patient closely for a change in the cardiac rhythm and/or rate.
3. If the patient is medically **unstable** or is showing signs of poor cardiac output, treat the underlying rhythm and/or rate.
4. Continue to reassess and monitor the patient.
5. Reassess the patient. If the dysrhythmia has converted to another rhythm and/or rate, reassess the patient; if necessary, treat the new dysrhythmia.

Second-Degree Heart Block, Type I (Mobitz I, Wenckebach)

1. Assess the patient. A second-degree heart block, type I, by itself does not usually require treatment.
2. If the second-degree heart block, type I is a new occurrence, observe the patient closely for a change in the cardiac rhythm and/or rate. This dysrhythmia could be the result of an acute myocardial infarction (MI).
3. Provide oxygen; apply pulse oximetry.
4. Begin IV fluids.
5. Obtain a 12-Lead electrocardiograph. Reassess the patient.
6. If overall HR is bradycardic, and patient is **stable**, continue to observe. If patient becomes medically **unstable**, an artificial pacemaker (temporary or permanent) may be necessary. Use a transcutaneous or transvenous pacemaker, if available, until a permanent pacemaker is placed.

7. Consider administering atropine while waiting for pacemaker. Reassess the patient; repeat atropine, if necessary.
8. Epinephrine may be administered to patients who do not respond to atropine.
9. Dopamine may be administered for a systolic BP less than 80 mm Hg.
10. Reassess the patient. If the dysrhythmia has converted to another rhythm and/ or rate, reassess the patient; if necessary, treat the new dysrhythmia.

Second-Degree Heart Block, Type II (Mobitz II); Third-Degree Heart Block (Complete Heart Block, Complete AV Dissociation)

1. Assess the patient. Remember, this may become a lethal dysrhythmia. If the patient is medically **stable**, continue to observe the patient. If the patient is medically **unstable** or is showing signs of poor cardiac output, treatment should be started immediately.
2. Provide oxygen; apply pulse oximetry.
3. Begin IV fluids. Reassess the patient.
4. Obtain a 12-Lead electrocardiograph. Reassess the patient.
5. If overall HR is bradycardic, a transcutaneous pacemaker should be applied immediately. Reassess the patient. Consider atropine while waiting for pacemaker.
6. Consider dopamine or epinephrine infusion while waiting for pacemaker.
7. Reassess the patient. If the dysrhythmia has converted to another rhythm and/ or rate, reassess the patient; if necessary, treat the new dysrhythmia.

Bundle Branch Block

1. Assess the patient. A bundle branch block by itself does not require treatment.
2. If the bundle branch block is a new occurrence, this could indicate an acute myocardial infarction (MI). Observe the patient closely for a change in the cardiac rhythm and/or rate.
3. If the patient is medically **unstable** and is showing signs of poor cardiac output, treat the underlying rhythm and/or rate.
4. Continue to monitor and reassess the patient.

Ventricular Dysrhythmias

Premature Ventricular Complex

1. Assess the patient. If patient is medically **stable** continue to observe. Begin treatment if the patient is showing signs of poor cardiac output or if any of the following **"danger signals"** are present:
   a. More than six PVCs in 1 minute
   b. Bigeminy
   c. Multifocal PVCs
   d. R on T phenomenon
   e. Run of V Tach
2. Provide oxygen; apply pulse oximetry.
3. Begin IV fluids.
4. Obtain a 12-Lead electrocardiograph. Reassess the patient.
5. If the rate is bradycardic, and patient is medically **stable**, continue to observe. If patient becomes medically **unstable**, administer atropine. Reassess the patient; repeat atropine, if necessary.
6. If heart rate is greater than 150 beats per minute, and patient is stable, administer lidocaine.
7. Reassess the patient.
8. If the patient becomes medically **unstable**, consider synchronized cardioversion.
9. If lidocaine has controlled the PVCs and the patient has a pulse, start a continuous lidocaine infusion.
10. Reassess the patient. If the dysrhythmia has converted to another rhythm and/ or rate, reassess the patient; if necessary, treat the new dysrhythmia.

Ventricular Tachycardia

1. Assess the patient. Remember, this may be a lethal dysrhythmia. If the patient has a pulse and is in **stable** condition, begin treatment.
2. Provide oxygen; apply pulse oximetry.
3. Start IV fluids. Reassess the patient.
4. Administer amiodarone.
5. Obtain a 12-Lead electrocardiograph. Reassess the patient.
6. Start an amiodarone infusion, if the amiodarone has controlled the VT and the patient has a pulse.
7. Reassess the patient. If amiodarone did not control the VT, or if the patient becomes unstable, consider synchronized cardioversion.
8. If the patient does not have a pulse **or** loses the pulse at any time during treatment, begin CPR and follow the treatment guidelines for V Fib, which is also the treatment for *pulseless ventricular tachycardia.*
9. Reassess the patient. If the dysrhythmia has converted to another rhythm and/ or rate, reassess the patient; if necessary, treat the new dysrhythmia.

Torsades de Pointes

Torsades de pointes may result from a prolonged QT interval. Amiodarone, lidocaine, procainamide, and quinidine may **all** prolong QT intervals.

1. Assess the patient
2. Provide oxygen; apply pulse oximetry.
3. Begin IV fluids. Reassess the patient.
4. Obtain electrolyte panel and treat abnormal levels.
5. Obtain a 12-Lead electrocardiograph. Reassess the patient.
6. If the patient is medically **stable**, magnesium sulfate may be used. Reassess the patient.
7. If patient becomes medically **unstable**, consider synchronized cardioversion.
8. If the patient does not have a pulse **or** loses the pulse at any time during treatment, begin CPR and follow the treatment guidelines for V Fib/pulseless VT, which is also the treatment for pulseless torsades de pointes.
9. Reassess the patient. If the dysrhythmia has converted to another rhythm and/ or rate, reassess the patient; if necessary, treat the new dysrhythmia.

Ventricular Fibrillation; Pulseless Ventricular Tachycardia; Pulseless Torsades de Pointes

1. Assess the patient. Remember to check lead placement as some types of artifact can mimic these types of dysrhythmias. If the dysrhythmia is V Fib, pulseless V Tach, or pulseless torsades de pointes, remember that these are **lethal** dysrhythmias. Treatment must be started immediately.
2. Begin CPR using 100% oxygen by bag-mask device. (Continue CPR **except** during defibrillation.)
3. Defibrillate immediately; deliver one shock and immediately resume CPR for two minutes, at five cycles of 30 compressions to 2 breaths.
4. Intubate the patient and begin IV fluids as soon as possible.
5. Reassess the patient and check the rhythm.
6. If no change, defibrillate immediately; deliver one shock and immediately resume CPR for two minutes, at five cycles of 30 compressions to 2 breaths.
7. During CPR deliver epinephrine or give vasopressin **one time only,** to replace the <u>first</u> <u>or</u> <u>second</u> dose of epinephrine.
8. Reassess the patient and check the rhythm.
9. If no change, defibrillate immediately; deliver one shock and immediately resume CPR for two minutes, at five cycles of 30 compressions to 2 breaths.

10. During CPR consider amiodarone or lidocaine; if rhythm is known to be torsades de pointes, give magnesium sulfate (one time only).
11. Continue to repeat steps 5 through 10.
12. Once the patient has a pulse, start a continuous infusion of the medication that was successful in ending the pulseless VT, V Fib, or pulseless torsades de pointes.
13. When the rhythm and/or rate changes, reassess the patient; treat the new dysrhythmia, if necessary.

Idioventricular Dysrhythmia; Agonal Dysrhythmia (Dying Heart)

1. Assess the patient. Remember, these are **lethal** dysrhythmias, and treatment must be started immediately.
2. If pulseless, treat as pulseless electrical activity (PEA).
3. If patient has a pulse, treat as **unstable** second-degree heart block, type II.
4. Reassess the patient. If the dysrhythmia has converted to another rhythm and/or rate, reassess the patient; if necessary, treat the new dysrhythmia.

Asystole; Pulseless Electrical Activity; Ventricular Standstill

1. Assess the patient. Remember, these are **lethal** dysrhythmias, and treatment **must** be started immediately.
2. Check lead placement. Confirm asystole in two different monitor leads (for example, Lead II and MCL_1).
3. Begin CPR, using 100% oxygen via bag-mask.
4. Intubate and begin IV fluids as soon as possible.
5. While continuing CPR, administer epinephrine every three to five minutes, per protocol. Vasopressin **one time only** can be given to replace either the first or second dose of epinephrine. Reassess the patient after each medication. Consider up to 3 doses of atropine, alternating with epinephrine, if monitor shows a heart rate less than 60.
6. If unable to distinguish between fine V Fib and asystole, treat as V Fib.
7. If the cardiac dysrhythmia and/or rate changes, treat the new dysrhythmia, if necessary.
8. Consider possible causes:
   a. Hypovolemia—give fluid replacement; reassess the patient.
   b. Hypoxia—increase ventilations and oxygen; reassess the patient.
   c. Cardiac tamponade—physician performs pericardiocentesis; reassess the patient.
   d. Tension pneumothorax—perform needle decompression; reassess the patient.
   e. Acidosis—give oxygen, obtain arterial blood gas values (ABGs); evaluate and treat appropriately.
   f. Hypokalemia or hyperkalemia—obtain electrolyte panel and treat accordingly.
   g. Hypothermia—assess patient for low body temperature and treat accordingly.
   h. Hypoglycemia—perform finger stick and treat appropriately.
   i. Cardiac muscle is too damaged to contract, no treatment available.
   j. Assess patient for any of the following additional causes:
      (1) Drug overdose
      (2) Coronary thrombosis (ACS)
      (3) Pulmonary thrombosis (embolism)
      (4) Trauma

Funny Looking Beats

Escape Beats

1. Assess the patient. Escape beats by themselves do not require treatment.
2. If the escape beat is a new occurrence, observe the patient closely for a change in the cardiac rhythm and/or rate.
3. If the patient is medically **unstable** or is showing signs of poor cardiac output, treat the underlying rhythm and/or rate.
4. Continue to reassess and monitor the patient.

Aberrantly Conducted Beats

1. Assess the patient. Aberrantly conducted beats (complexes) by themselves do not require treatment.
2. If the aberrantly conducted complex is a new occurrence, observe the patient closely for a change in the cardiac rhythm and/or rate.
3. If the patient is medically **unstable** or is showing signs of poor cardiac output, treat the underlying rhythm and/or rate.
4. Continue to assess and monitor the patient.

Pacemaker Rhythms

1. Assess the patient. If the patient is medically unstable, treat the underlying rhythm and/or rate.
2. If the pacemaker is malfunctioning (not pacing), the pacemaker must be repaired or replaced. A transcutaneous or transvenous pacemaker may be used temporarily until the permanent pacemaker is repaired or replaced.
3. Provide oxygen; apply pulse oximetry.
4. Start IV fluids.
5. Reassure the patient by giving frequent explanations of the procedures being performed and by acting in a calm manner.
6. Continue to reassess and monitor the patient.

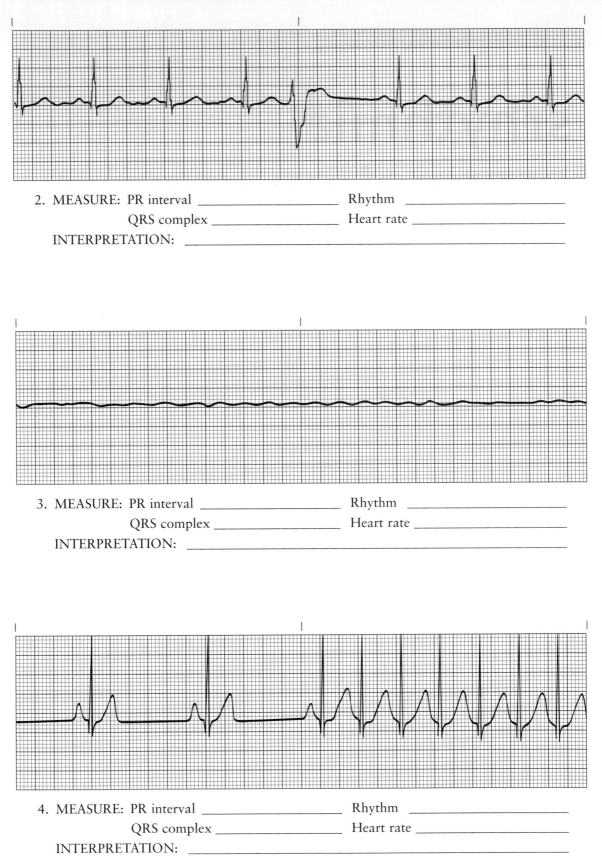

2. MEASURE: PR interval _____ Rhythm _____

                  QRS complex _____ Heart rate _____

       INTERPRETATION: _____

3. MEASURE: PR interval _____ Rhythm _____

                  QRS complex _____ Heart rate _____

       INTERPRETATION: _____

4. MEASURE: PR interval _____ Rhythm _____

                  QRS complex _____ Heart rate _____

       INTERPRETATION: _____

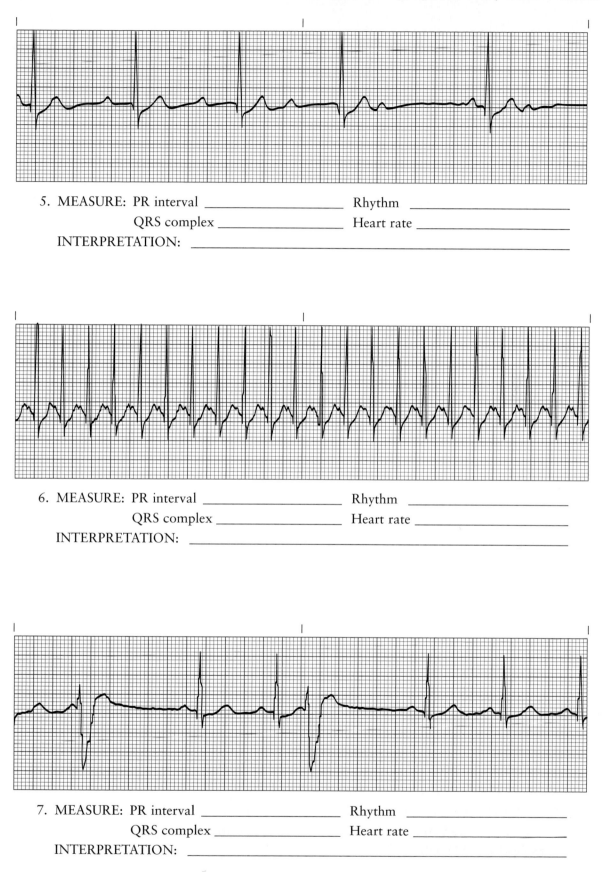

5. MEASURE: PR interval _____ Rhythm _____

            QRS complex _____ Heart rate _____

  INTERPRETATION: _____

6. MEASURE: PR interval _____ Rhythm _____

            QRS complex _____ Heart rate _____

  INTERPRETATION: _____

7. MEASURE: PR interval _____ Rhythm _____

            QRS complex _____ Heart rate _____

  INTERPRETATION: _____

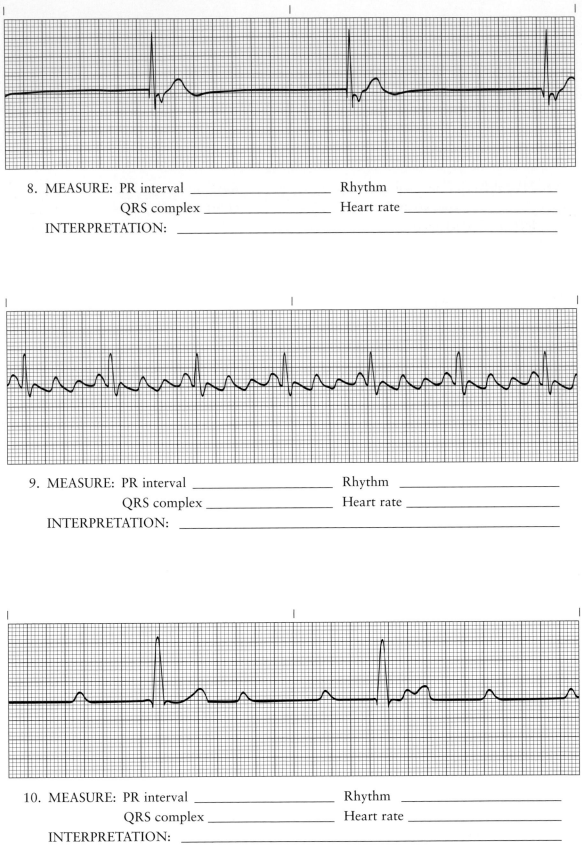

8. MEASURE: PR interval _____ Rhythm _____

   QRS complex _____ Heart rate _____

   INTERPRETATION: _____

9. MEASURE: PR interval _____ Rhythm _____

   QRS complex _____ Heart rate _____

   INTERPRETATION: _____

10. MEASURE: PR interval _____ Rhythm _____

   QRS complex _____ Heart rate _____

   INTERPRETATION: _____

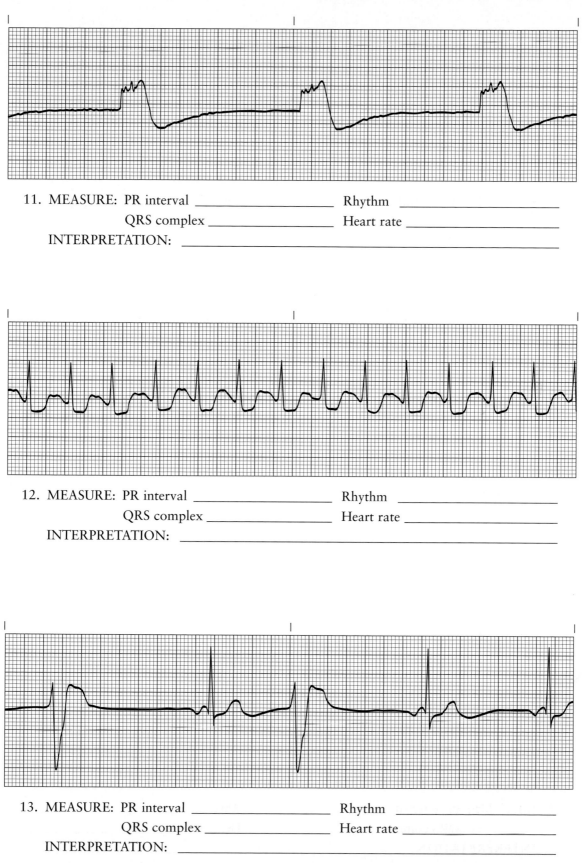

11. MEASURE: PR interval _____   Rhythm _____

    QRS complex _____   Heart rate _____

    INTERPRETATION: _____

12. MEASURE: PR interval _____   Rhythm _____

    QRS complex _____   Heart rate _____

    INTERPRETATION: _____

13. MEASURE: PR interval _____   Rhythm _____

    QRS complex _____   Heart rate _____

    INTERPRETATION: _____

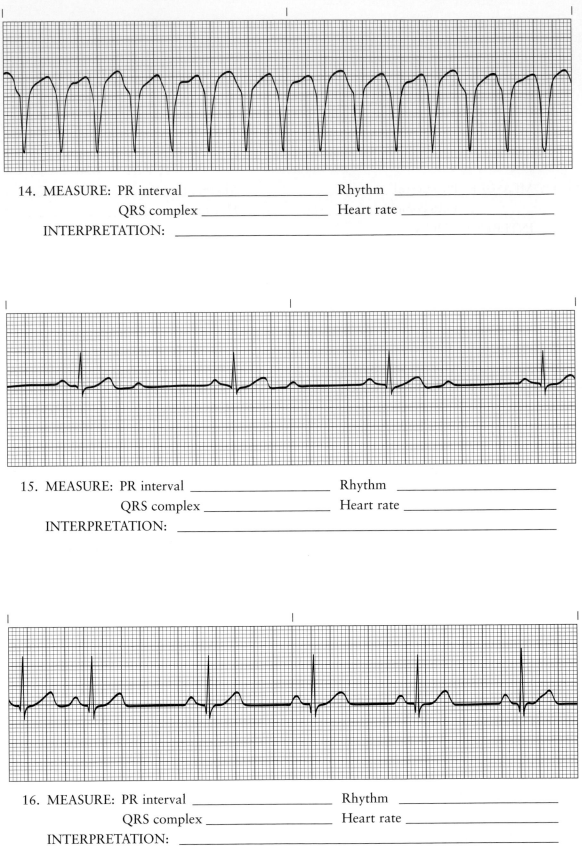

14. MEASURE: PR interval _____ Rhythm _____

                   QRS complex _____ Heart rate _____

        INTERPRETATION: _____

15. MEASURE: PR interval _____ Rhythm _____

                   QRS complex _____ Heart rate _____

        INTERPRETATION: _____

16. MEASURE: PR interval _____ Rhythm _____

                   QRS complex _____ Heart rate _____

        INTERPRETATION: _____

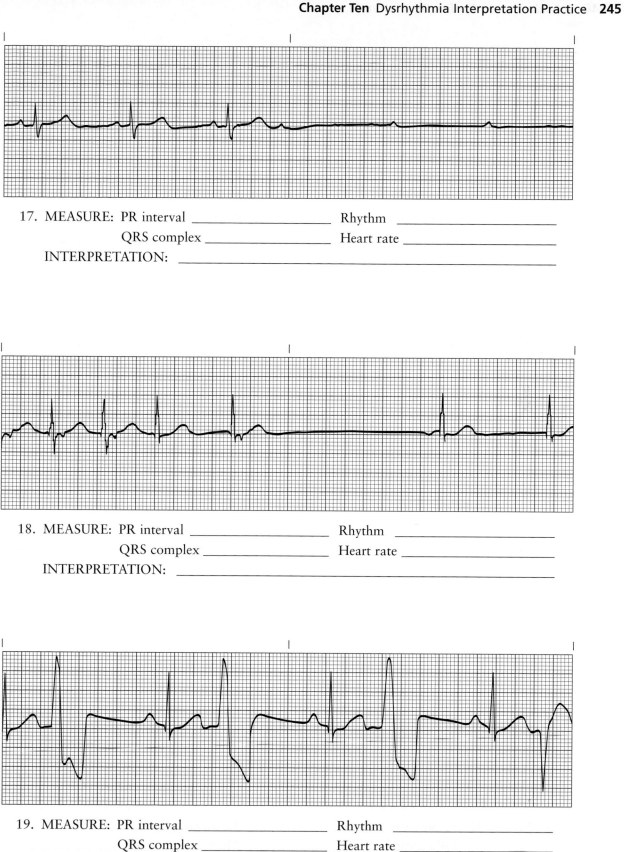

17. MEASURE: PR interval _____ Rhythm _____

    QRS complex _____ Heart rate _____

    INTERPRETATION: _____

18. MEASURE: PR interval _____ Rhythm _____

    QRS complex _____ Heart rate _____

    INTERPRETATION: _____

19. MEASURE: PR interval _____ Rhythm _____

    QRS complex _____ Heart rate _____

    INTERPRETATION: _____

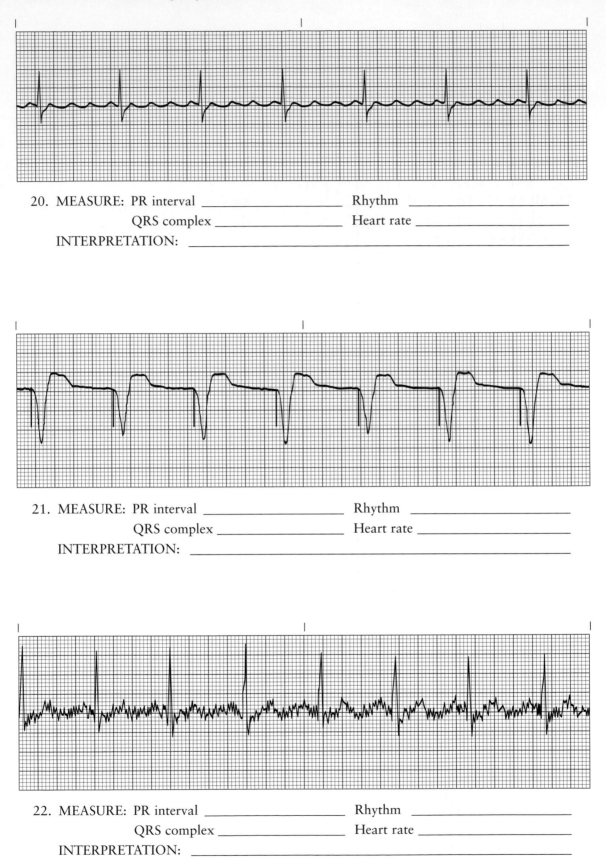

20. MEASURE: PR interval _____   Rhythm _____

                    QRS complex _____   Heart rate _____

        INTERPRETATION: _____

21. MEASURE: PR interval _____   Rhythm _____

                    QRS complex _____   Heart rate _____

        INTERPRETATION: _____

22. MEASURE: PR interval _____   Rhythm _____

                    QRS complex _____   Heart rate _____

        INTERPRETATION: _____

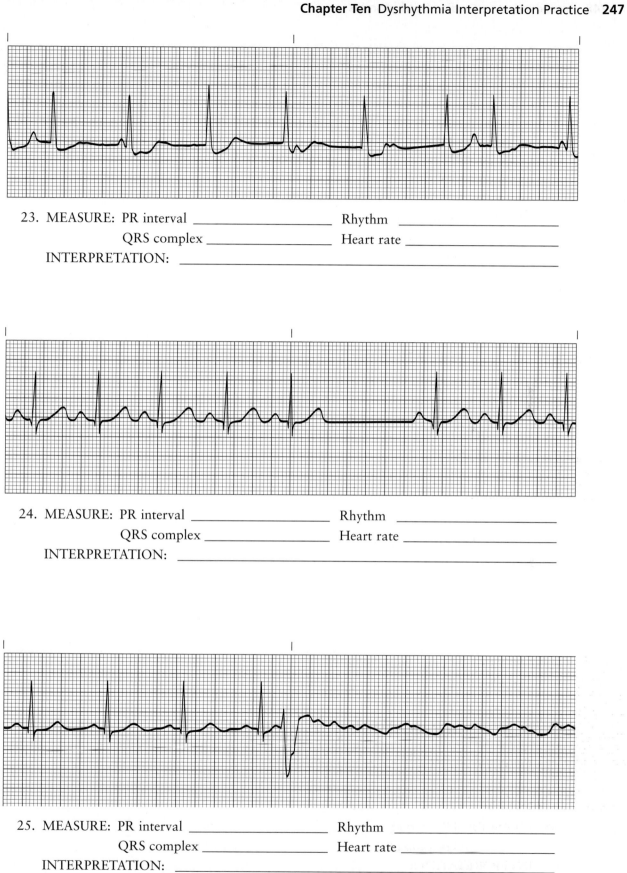

23. MEASURE: PR interval _____   Rhythm _____

       QRS complex _____   Heart rate _____

   INTERPRETATION: _____

24. MEASURE: PR interval _____   Rhythm _____

       QRS complex _____   Heart rate _____

   INTERPRETATION: _____

25. MEASURE: PR interval _____   Rhythm _____

       QRS complex _____   Heart rate _____

   INTERPRETATION: _____

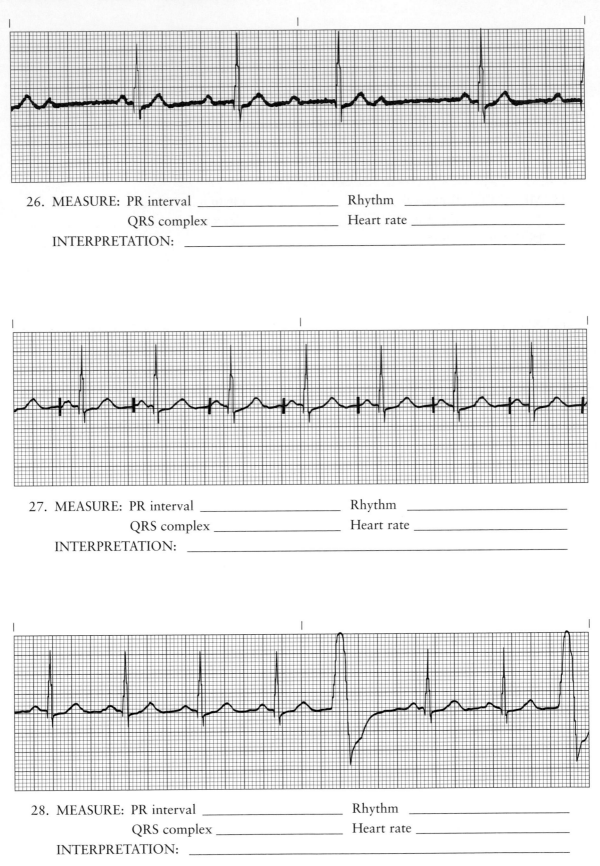

26. MEASURE: PR interval _____ Rhythm _____

    QRS complex _____ Heart rate _____

    INTERPRETATION: _____

27. MEASURE: PR interval _____ Rhythm _____

    QRS complex _____ Heart rate _____

    INTERPRETATION: _____

28. MEASURE: PR interval _____ Rhythm _____

    QRS complex _____ Heart rate _____

    INTERPRETATION: _____

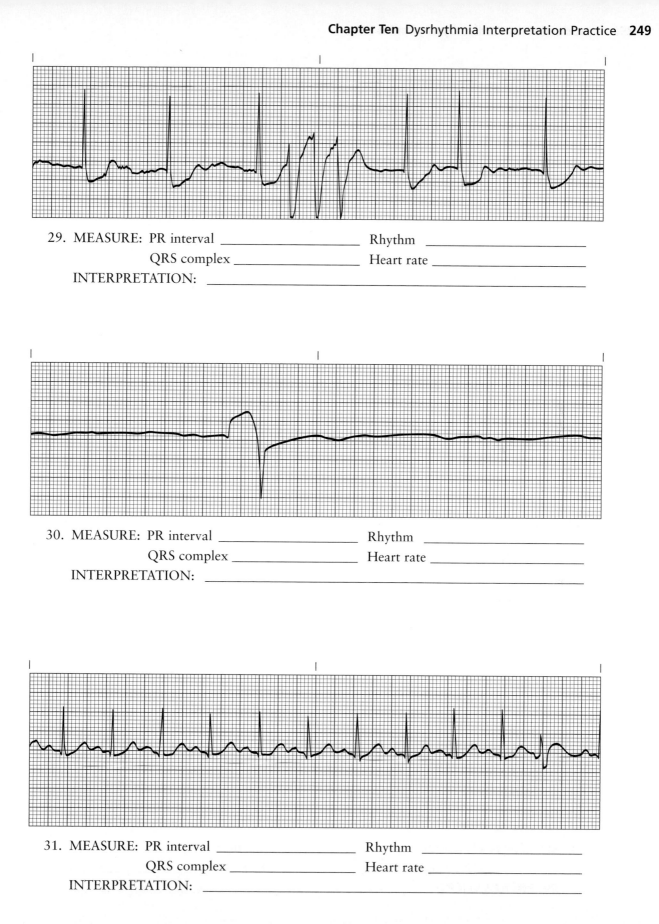

29. MEASURE: PR interval _____ Rhythm _____

QRS complex _____ Heart rate _____

INTERPRETATION: _____

30. MEASURE: PR interval _____ Rhythm _____

QRS complex _____ Heart rate _____

INTERPRETATION: _____

31. MEASURE: PR interval _____ Rhythm _____

QRS complex _____ Heart rate _____

INTERPRETATION: _____

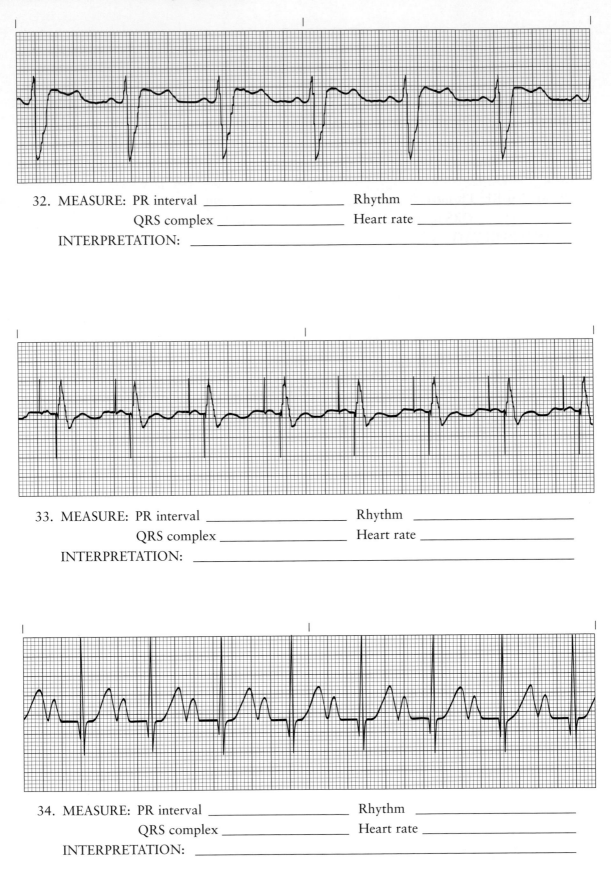

32. MEASURE: PR interval _____   Rhythm _____

                QRS complex _____   Heart rate _____

      INTERPRETATION: _____

33. MEASURE: PR interval _____   Rhythm _____

                QRS complex _____   Heart rate _____

      INTERPRETATION: _____

34. MEASURE: PR interval _____   Rhythm _____

                QRS complex _____   Heart rate _____

      INTERPRETATION: _____

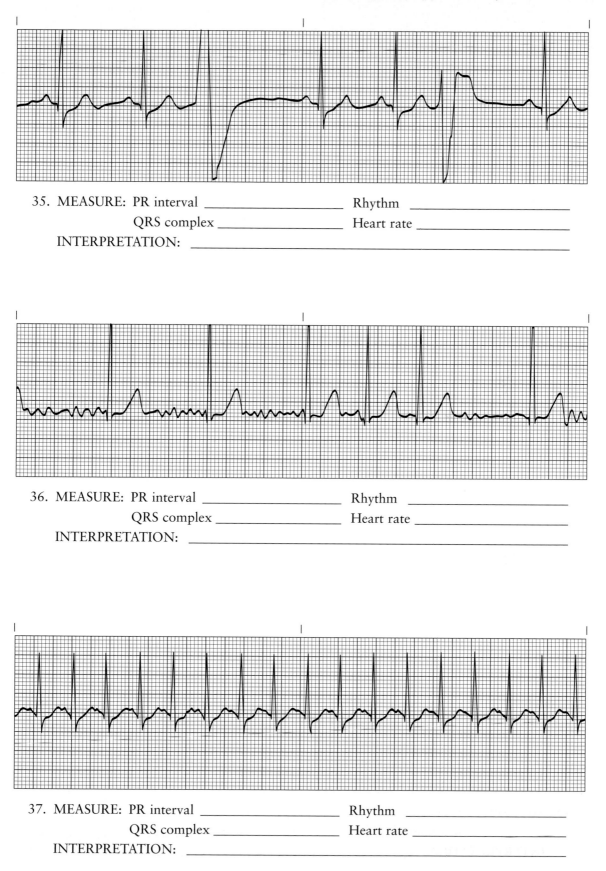

35. MEASURE: PR interval _____ Rhythm _____
    QRS complex _____ Heart rate _____
    INTERPRETATION: _____

36. MEASURE: PR interval _____ Rhythm _____
    QRS complex _____ Heart rate _____
    INTERPRETATION: _____

37. MEASURE: PR interval _____ Rhythm _____
    QRS complex _____ Heart rate _____
    INTERPRETATION: _____

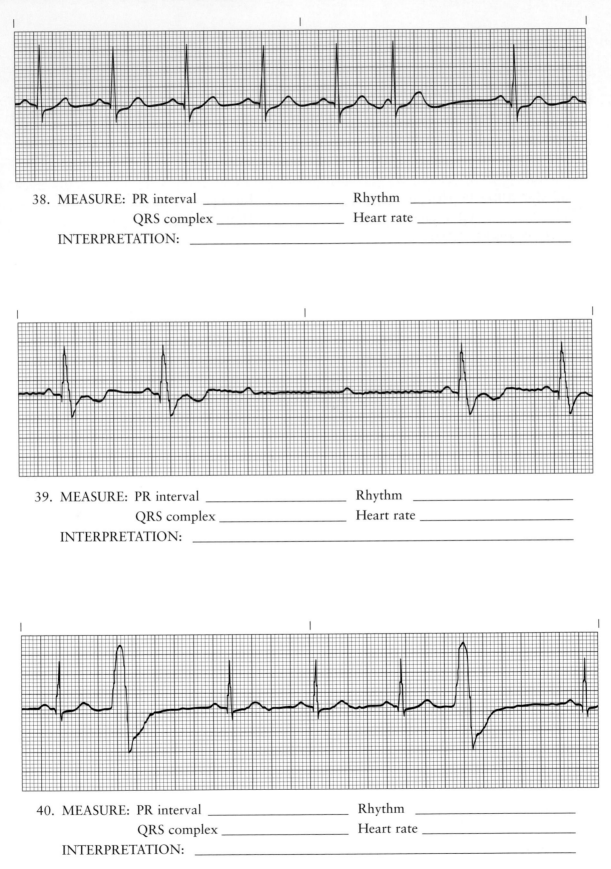

38. MEASURE: PR interval _____ Rhythm _____

               QRS complex _____ Heart rate _____

INTERPRETATION: _____

39. MEASURE: PR interval _____ Rhythm _____

               QRS complex _____ Heart rate _____

INTERPRETATION: _____

40. MEASURE: PR interval _____ Rhythm _____

               QRS complex _____ Heart rate _____

INTERPRETATION: _____

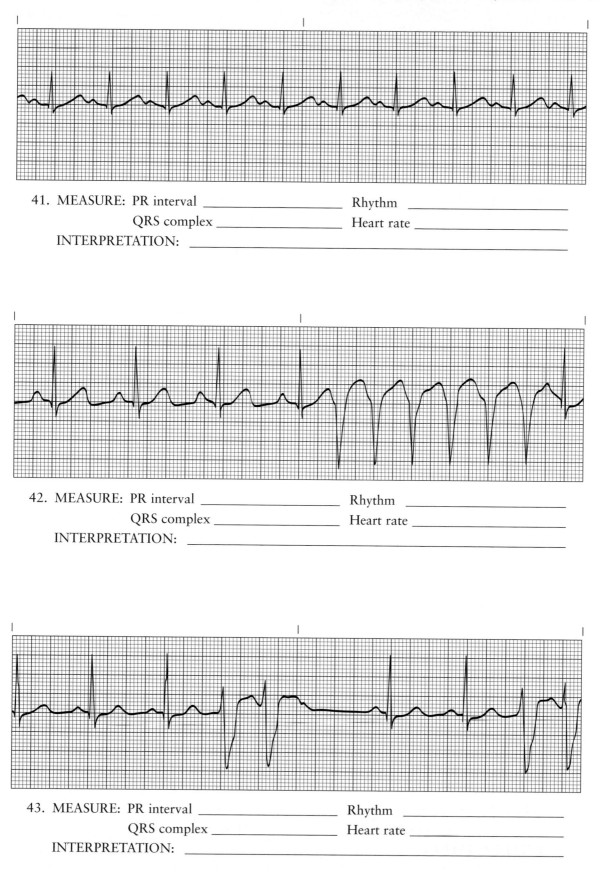

41. MEASURE: PR interval _____ Rhythm _____

                 QRS complex _____ Heart rate _____

    INTERPRETATION: _____

42. MEASURE: PR interval _____ Rhythm _____

                 QRS complex _____ Heart rate _____

    INTERPRETATION: _____

43. MEASURE: PR interval _____ Rhythm _____

                 QRS complex _____ Heart rate _____

    INTERPRETATION: _____

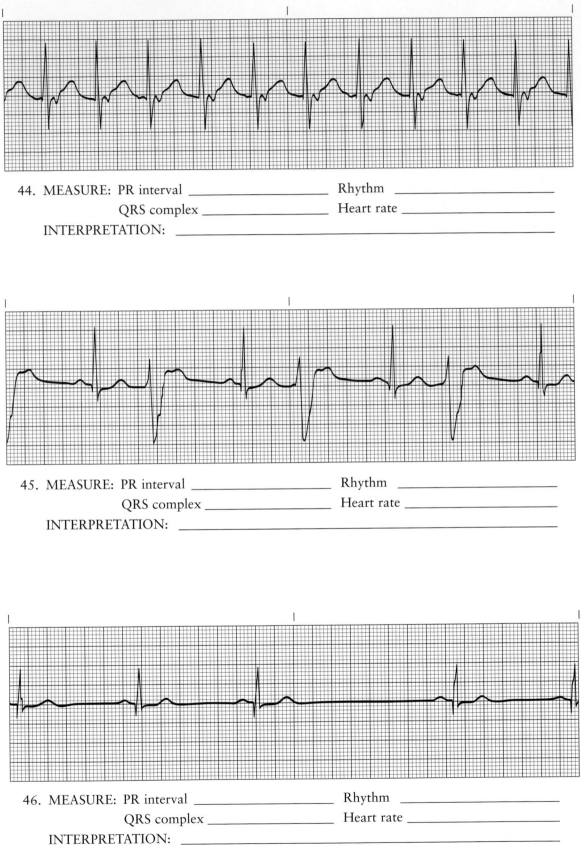

44. MEASURE: PR interval _____ Rhythm _____

                  QRS complex _____ Heart rate _____

    INTERPRETATION: _____

45. MEASURE: PR interval _____ Rhythm _____

                  QRS complex _____ Heart rate _____

    INTERPRETATION: _____

46. MEASURE: PR interval _____ Rhythm _____

                  QRS complex _____ Heart rate _____

    INTERPRETATION: _____

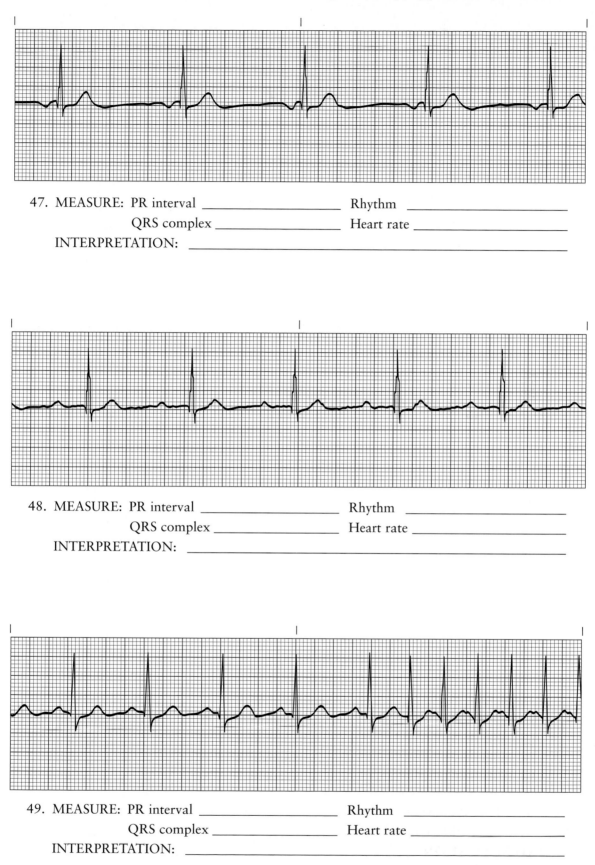

47. MEASURE: PR interval _____   Rhythm _____

           QRS complex _____   Heart rate _____

     INTERPRETATION: _____

48. MEASURE: PR interval _____   Rhythm _____

           QRS complex _____   Heart rate _____

     INTERPRETATION: _____

49. MEASURE: PR interval _____   Rhythm _____

           QRS complex _____   Heart rate _____

     INTERPRETATION: _____

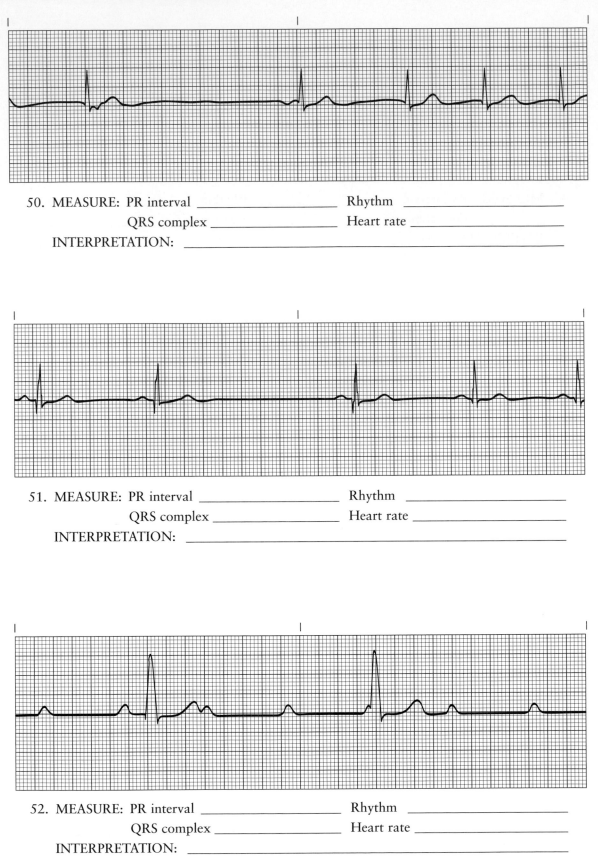

50. MEASURE: PR interval _____ Rhythm _____

                  QRS complex _____ Heart rate _____

     INTERPRETATION: _____

51. MEASURE: PR interval _____ Rhythm _____

                  QRS complex _____ Heart rate _____

     INTERPRETATION: _____

52. MEASURE: PR interval _____ Rhythm _____

                  QRS complex _____ Heart rate _____

     INTERPRETATION: _____

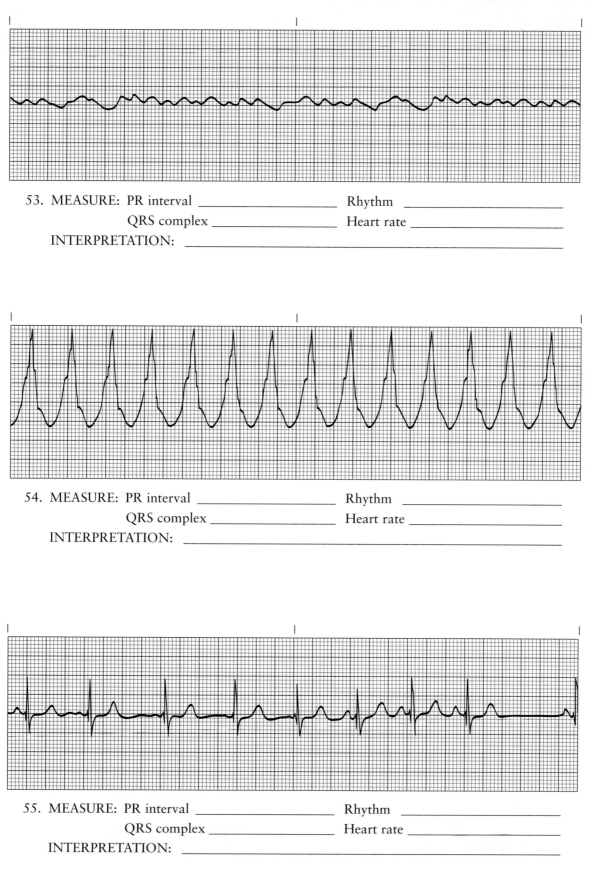

53. MEASURE: PR interval _____ Rhythm _____

QRS complex _____ Heart rate _____

INTERPRETATION: _____

54. MEASURE: PR interval _____ Rhythm _____

QRS complex _____ Heart rate _____

INTERPRETATION: _____

55. MEASURE: PR interval _____ Rhythm _____

QRS complex _____ Heart rate _____

INTERPRETATION: _____

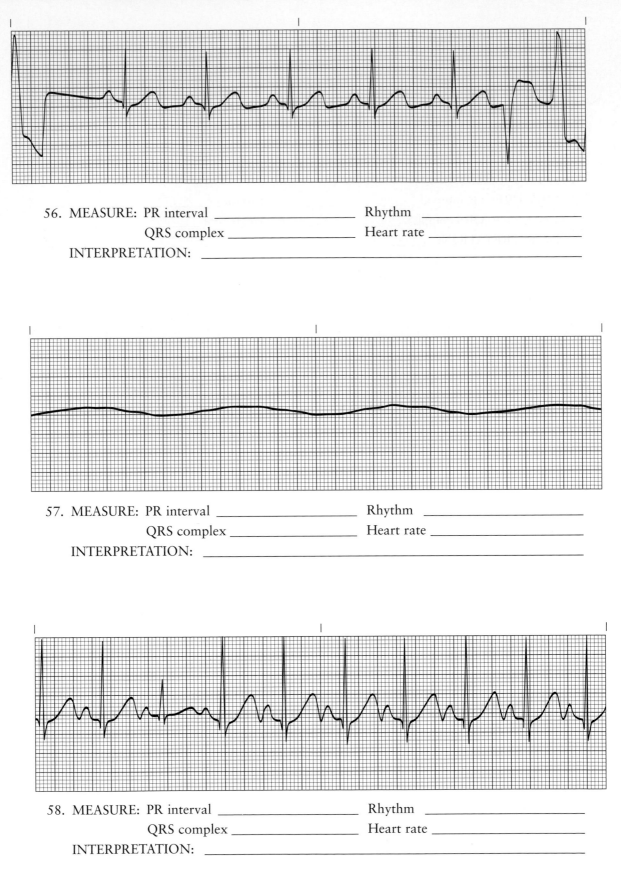

56. MEASURE: PR interval _____ Rhythm _____

                    QRS complex _____ Heart rate _____

          INTERPRETATION: _____

57. MEASURE: PR interval _____ Rhythm _____

                    QRS complex _____ Heart rate _____

          INTERPRETATION: _____

58. MEASURE: PR interval _____ Rhythm _____

                    QRS complex _____ Heart rate _____

          INTERPRETATION: _____

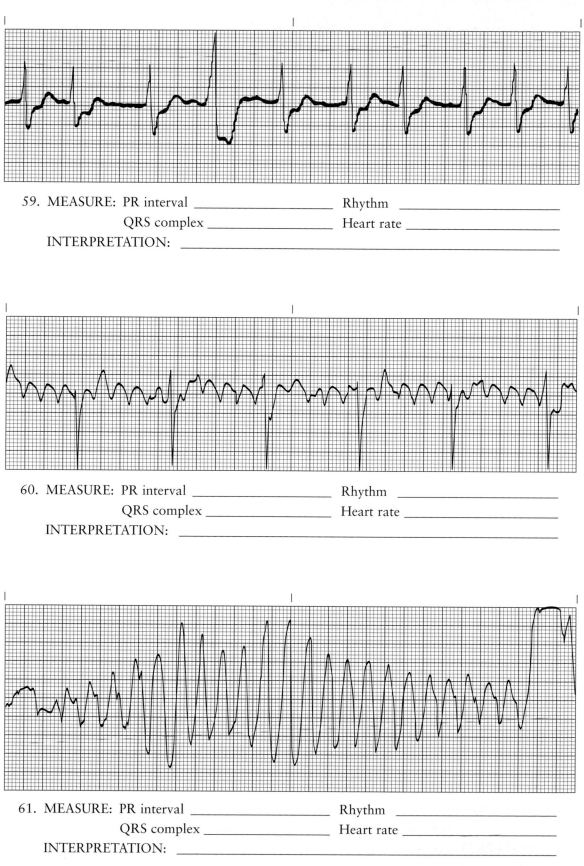

59. MEASURE: PR interval _____ Rhythm _____

             QRS complex _____ Heart rate _____

    INTERPRETATION: _____

60. MEASURE: PR interval _____ Rhythm _____

             QRS complex _____ Heart rate _____

    INTERPRETATION: _____

61. MEASURE: PR interval _____ Rhythm _____

             QRS complex _____ Heart rate _____

    INTERPRETATION: _____

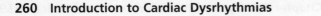

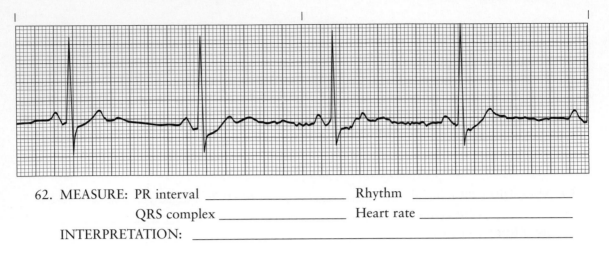

62. MEASURE: PR interval _____ Rhythm _____

                 QRS complex _____ Heart rate _____

           INTERPRETATION: _____

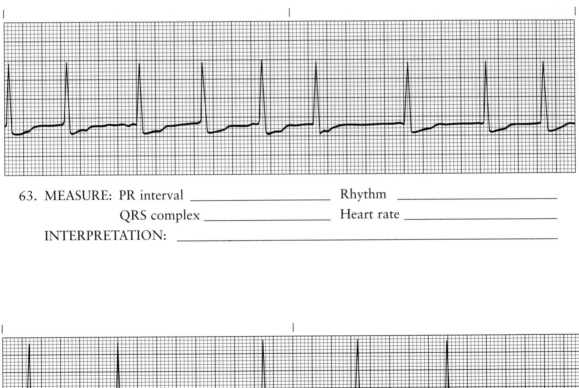

63. MEASURE: PR interval _____ Rhythm _____

                 QRS complex _____ Heart rate _____

           INTERPRETATION: _____

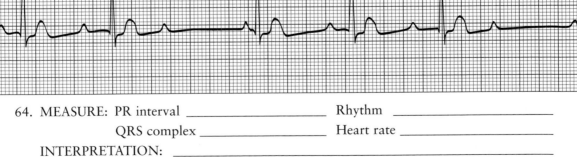

64. MEASURE: PR interval _____ Rhythm _____

                 QRS complex _____ Heart rate _____

           INTERPRETATION: _____

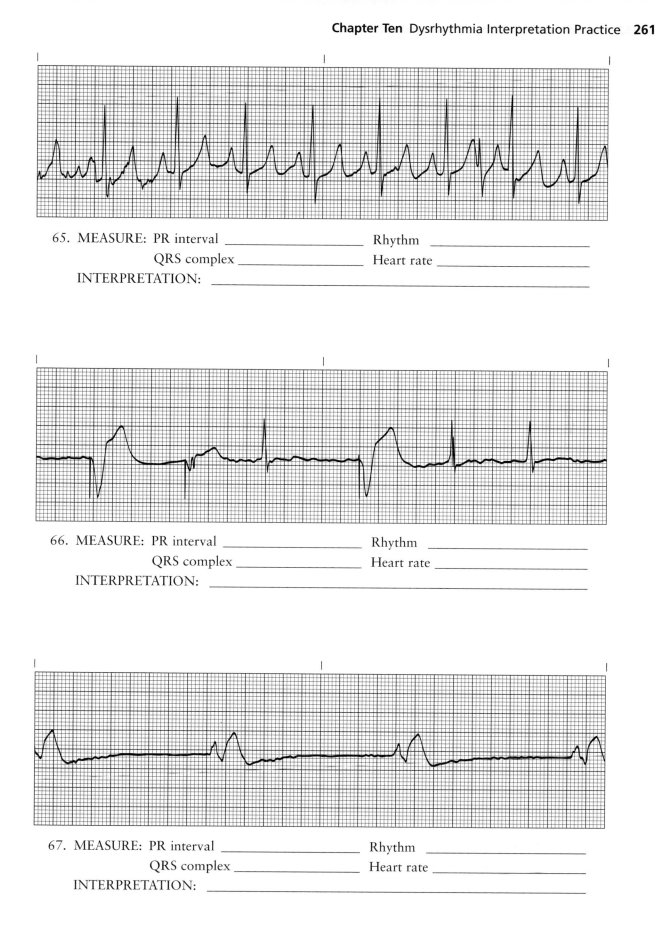

65. MEASURE: PR interval _____ Rhythm _____

                QRS complex _____ Heart rate _____

    INTERPRETATION: _____

66. MEASURE: PR interval _____ Rhythm _____

                QRS complex _____ Heart rate _____

    INTERPRETATION: _____

67. MEASURE: PR interval _____ Rhythm _____

                QRS complex _____ Heart rate _____

    INTERPRETATION: _____

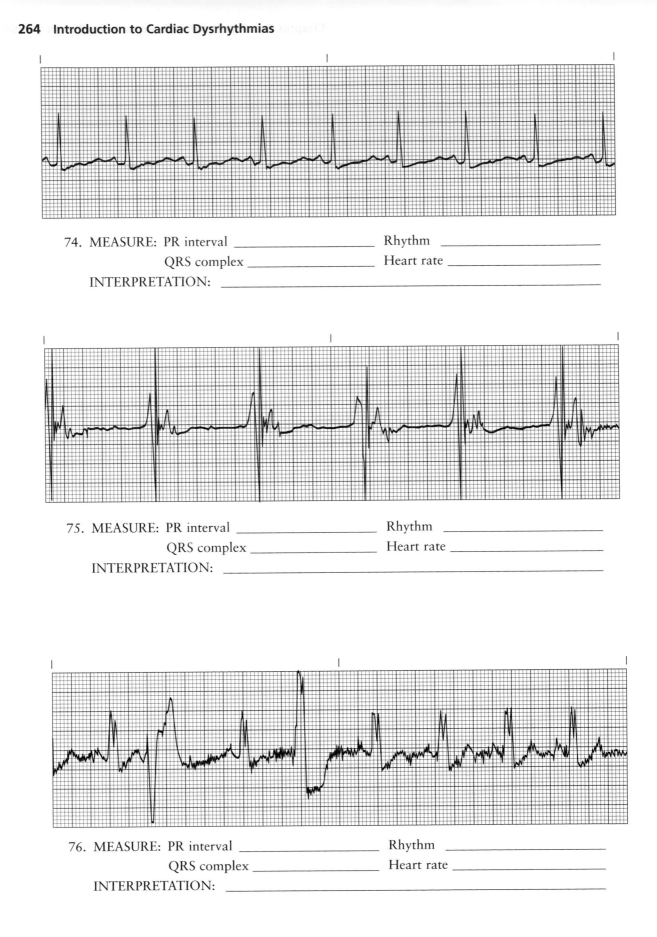

74. MEASURE: PR interval _____ Rhythm _____

QRS complex _____ Heart rate _____

INTERPRETATION: _____

75. MEASURE: PR interval _____ Rhythm _____

QRS complex _____ Heart rate _____

INTERPRETATION: _____

76. MEASURE: PR interval _____ Rhythm _____

QRS complex _____ Heart rate _____

INTERPRETATION: _____

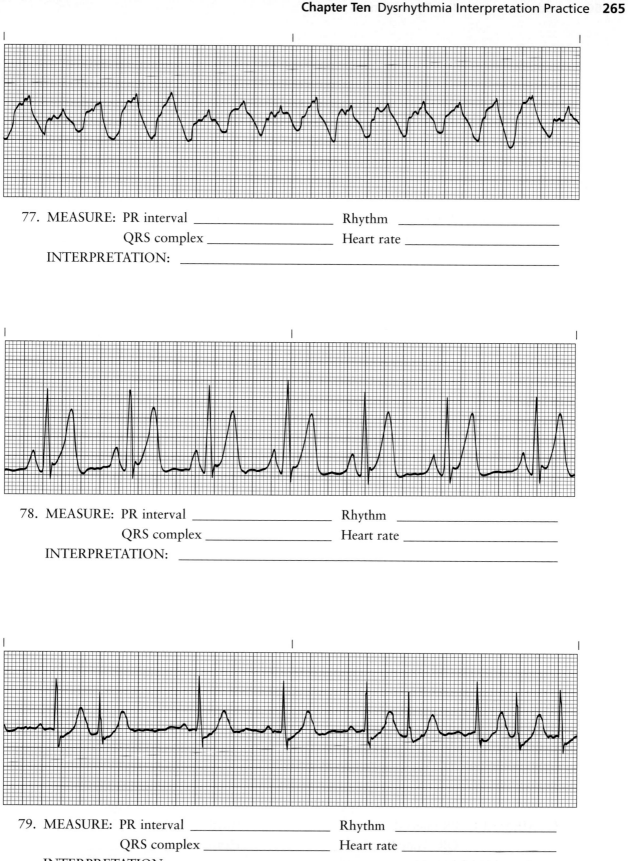

77. MEASURE: PR interval _____   Rhythm _____

QRS complex _____   Heart rate _____

INTERPRETATION: _____

78. MEASURE: PR interval _____   Rhythm _____

QRS complex _____   Heart rate _____

INTERPRETATION: _____

79. MEASURE: PR interval _____   Rhythm _____

QRS complex _____   Heart rate _____

INTERPRETATION: _____

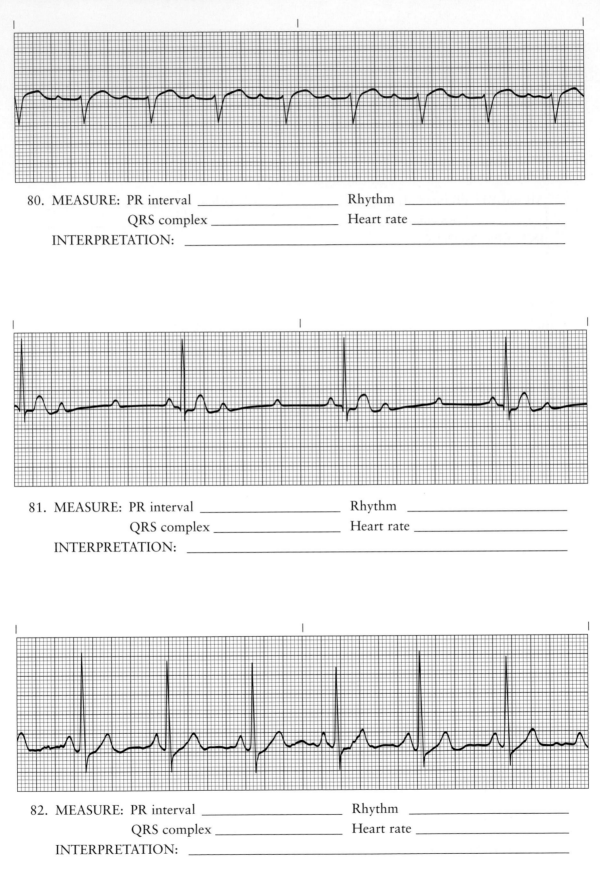

80. MEASURE: PR interval _____ Rhythm _____

QRS complex _____ Heart rate _____

INTERPRETATION: _____

81. MEASURE: PR interval _____ Rhythm _____

QRS complex _____ Heart rate _____

INTERPRETATION: _____

82. MEASURE: PR interval _____ Rhythm _____

QRS complex _____ Heart rate _____

INTERPRETATION: _____

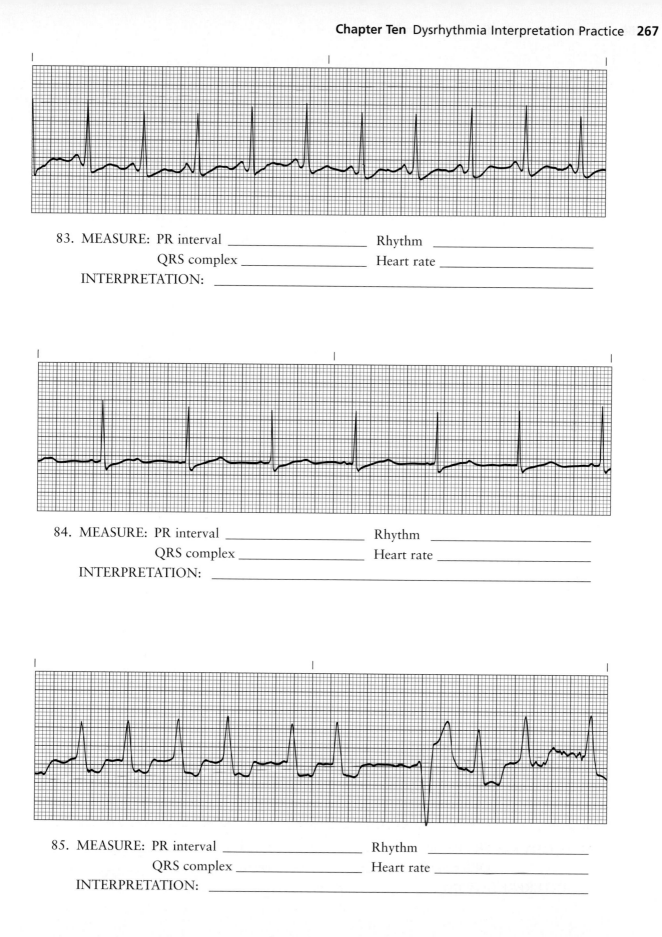

83. MEASURE: PR interval _____   Rhythm _____

             QRS complex _____   Heart rate _____

      INTERPRETATION: _____

84. MEASURE: PR interval _____   Rhythm _____

             QRS complex _____   Heart rate _____

      INTERPRETATION: _____

85. MEASURE: PR interval _____   Rhythm _____

             QRS complex _____   Heart rate _____

      INTERPRETATION: _____

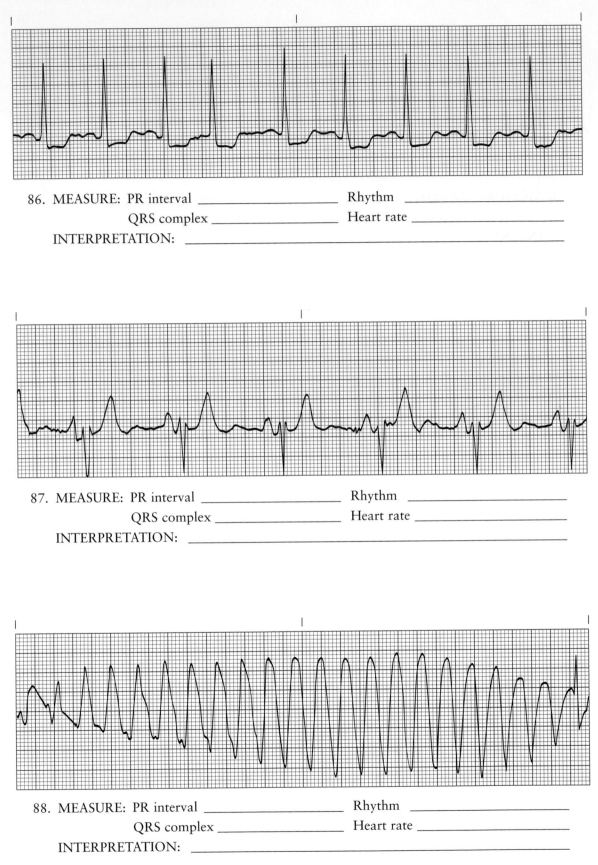

86. MEASURE: PR interval _____   Rhythm _____

QRS complex _____   Heart rate _____

INTERPRETATION: _____

87. MEASURE: PR interval _____   Rhythm _____

QRS complex _____   Heart rate _____

INTERPRETATION: _____

88. MEASURE: PR interval _____   Rhythm _____

QRS complex _____   Heart rate _____

INTERPRETATION: _____

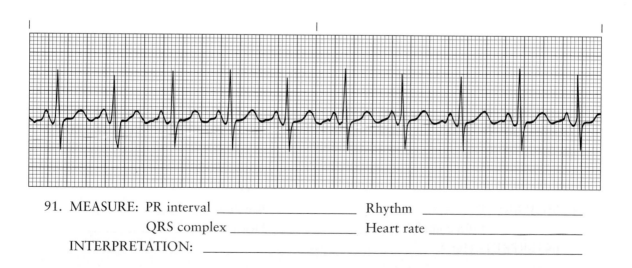

89. MEASURE: PR interval _____   Rhythm _____

                  QRS complex _____   Heart rate _____

    INTERPRETATION: _____

90. MEASURE: PR interval _____   Rhythm _____

                  QRS complex _____   Heart rate _____

    INTERPRETATION: _____

91. MEASURE: PR interval _____   Rhythm _____

                  QRS complex _____   Heart rate _____

    INTERPRETATION: _____

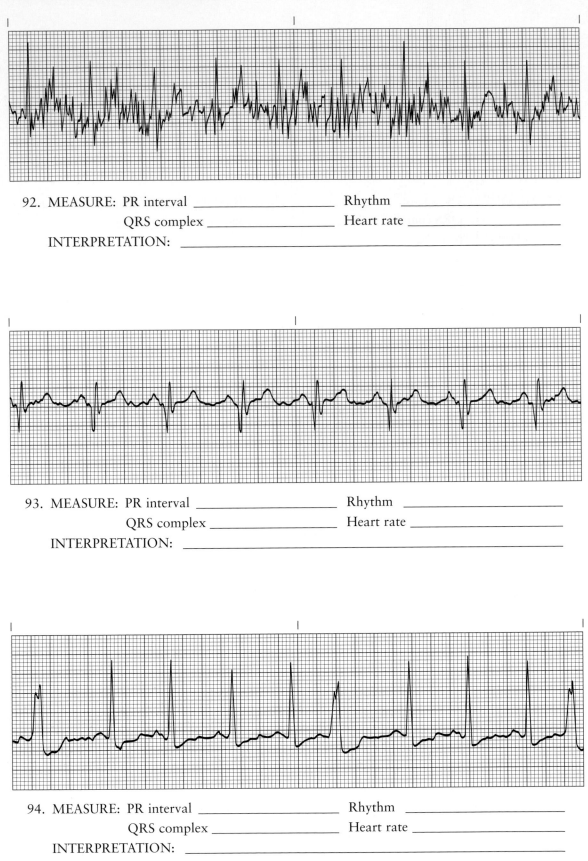

92. MEASURE: PR interval _____ Rhythm _____

                QRS complex _____ Heart rate _____

      INTERPRETATION: _____

93. MEASURE: PR interval _____ Rhythm _____

                QRS complex _____ Heart rate _____

      INTERPRETATION: _____

94. MEASURE: PR interval _____ Rhythm _____

                QRS complex _____ Heart rate _____

      INTERPRETATION: _____

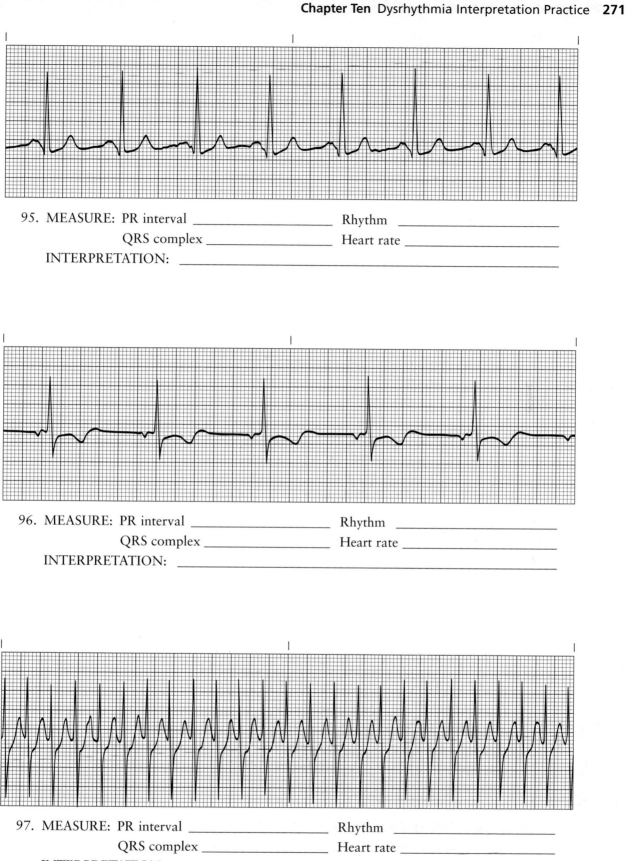

95. MEASURE: PR interval _____   Rhythm _____

              QRS complex _____   Heart rate _____

     INTERPRETATION: _____

96. MEASURE: PR interval _____   Rhythm _____

              QRS complex _____   Heart rate _____

     INTERPRETATION: _____

97. MEASURE: PR interval _____   Rhythm _____

              QRS complex _____   Heart rate _____

     INTERPRETATION: _____

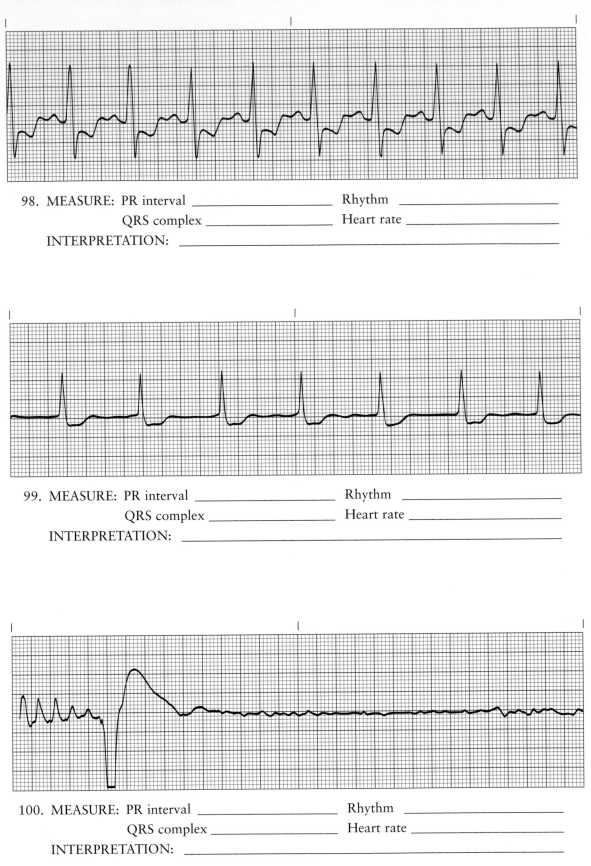

98. MEASURE: PR interval _____ Rhythm _____

            QRS complex _____ Heart rate _____

     INTERPRETATION: _____

99. MEASURE: PR interval _____ Rhythm _____

            QRS complex _____ Heart rate _____

     INTERPRETATION: _____

100. MEASURE: PR interval _____ Rhythm _____

             QRS complex _____ Heart rate _____

      INTERPRETATION: _____

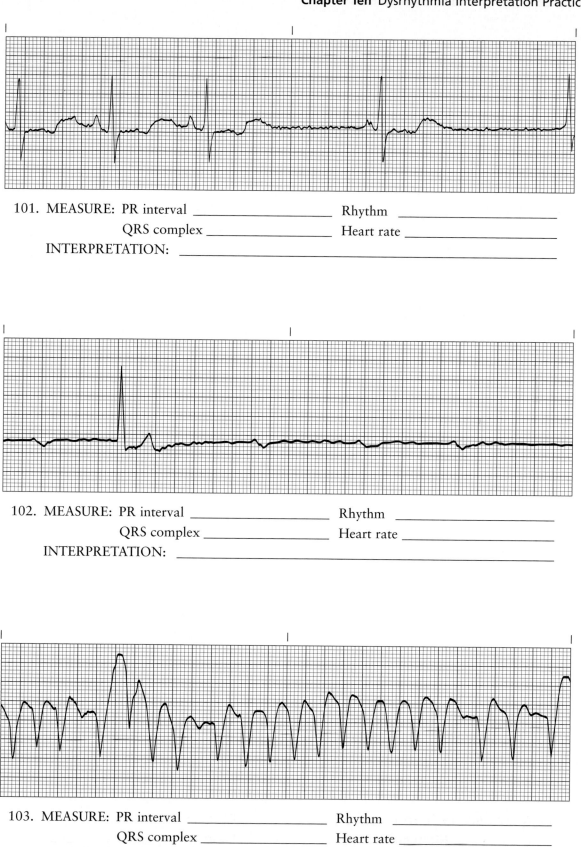

101. MEASURE: PR interval _____ Rhythm _____

            QRS complex _____ Heart rate _____

    INTERPRETATION: _____

102. MEASURE: PR interval _____ Rhythm _____

            QRS complex _____ Heart rate _____

    INTERPRETATION: _____

103. MEASURE: PR interval _____ Rhythm _____

            QRS complex _____ Heart rate _____

    INTERPRETATION: _____

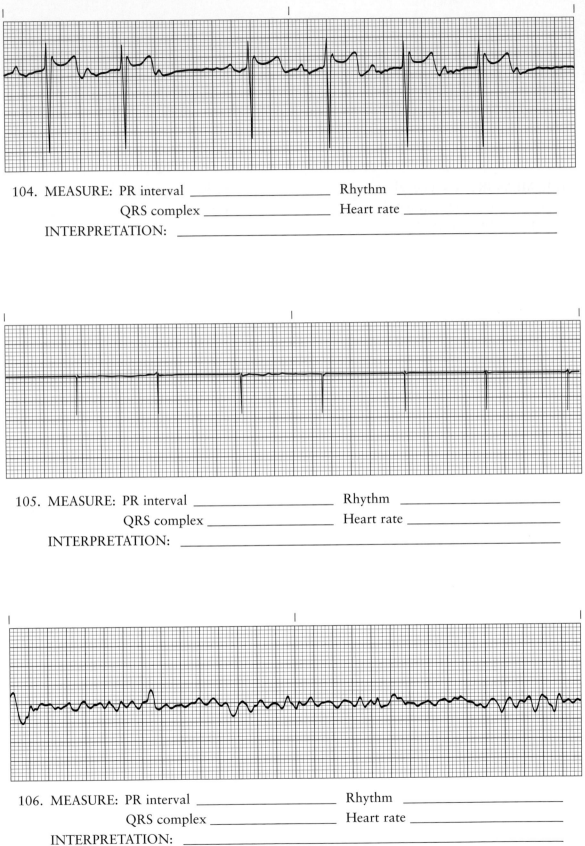

104. MEASURE: PR interval _____   Rhythm _____

       QRS complex _____   Heart rate _____

       INTERPRETATION: _____

105. MEASURE: PR interval _____   Rhythm _____

       QRS complex _____   Heart rate _____

       INTERPRETATION: _____

106. MEASURE: PR interval _____   Rhythm _____

       QRS complex _____   Heart rate _____

       INTERPRETATION: _____

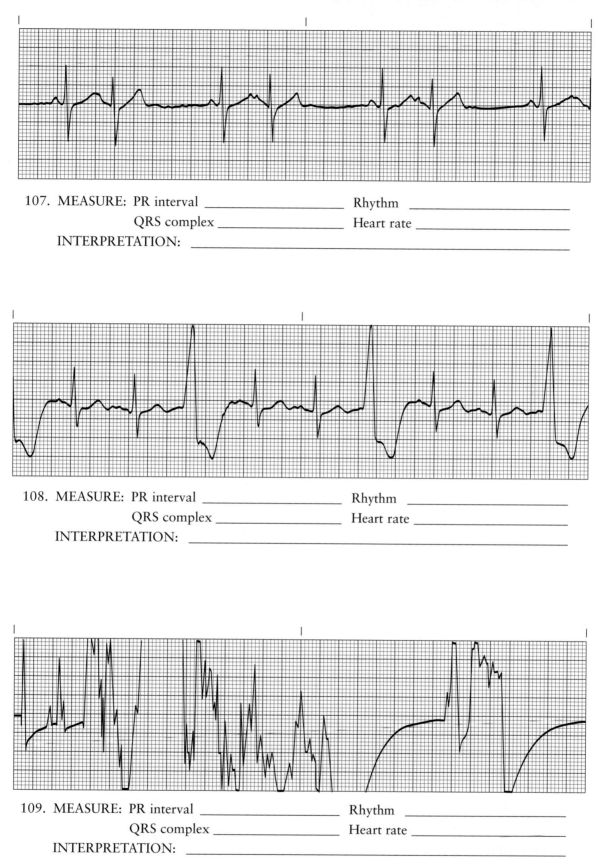

107. MEASURE: PR interval _____ Rhythm _____

             QRS complex _____ Heart rate _____

      INTERPRETATION: _____

108. MEASURE: PR interval _____ Rhythm _____

             QRS complex _____ Heart rate _____

      INTERPRETATION: _____

109. MEASURE: PR interval _____ Rhythm _____

             QRS complex _____ Heart rate _____

      INTERPRETATION: _____

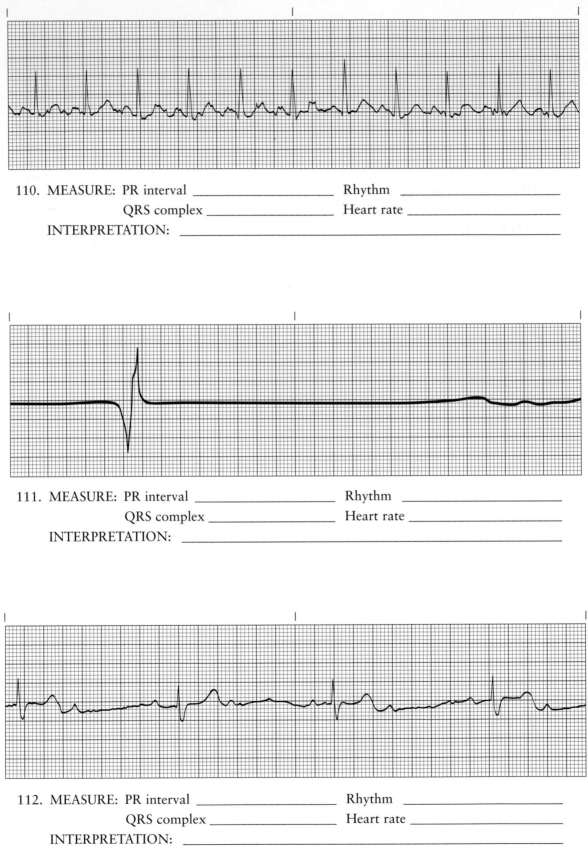

110. MEASURE: PR interval _____ Rhythm _____

QRS complex _____ Heart rate _____

INTERPRETATION: _____

111. MEASURE: PR interval _____ Rhythm _____

QRS complex _____ Heart rate _____

INTERPRETATION: _____

112. MEASURE: PR interval _____ Rhythm _____

QRS complex _____ Heart rate _____

INTERPRETATION: _____

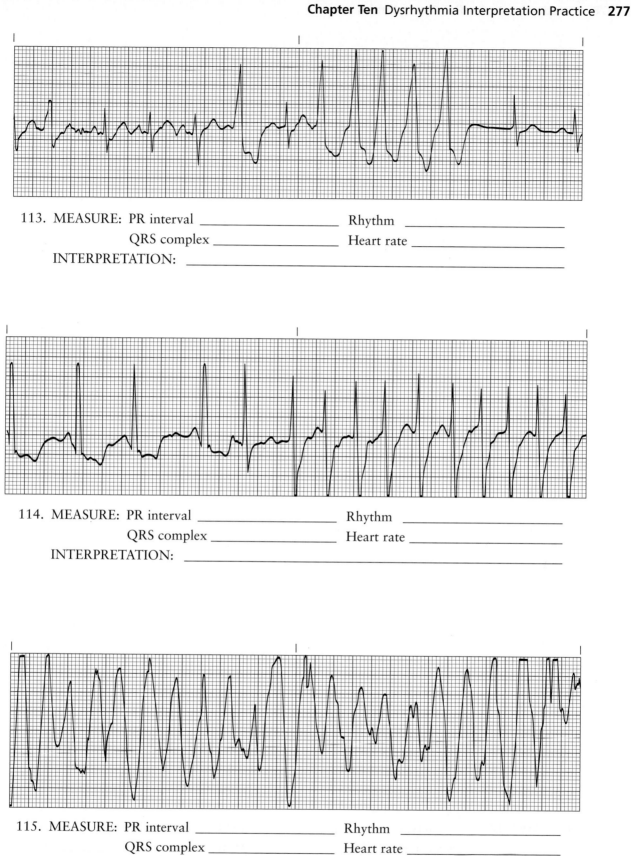

113. MEASURE: PR interval _____ Rhythm _____

QRS complex _____ Heart rate _____

INTERPRETATION: _____

114. MEASURE: PR interval _____ Rhythm _____

QRS complex _____ Heart rate _____

INTERPRETATION: _____

115. MEASURE: PR interval _____ Rhythm _____

QRS complex _____ Heart rate _____

INTERPRETATION: _____

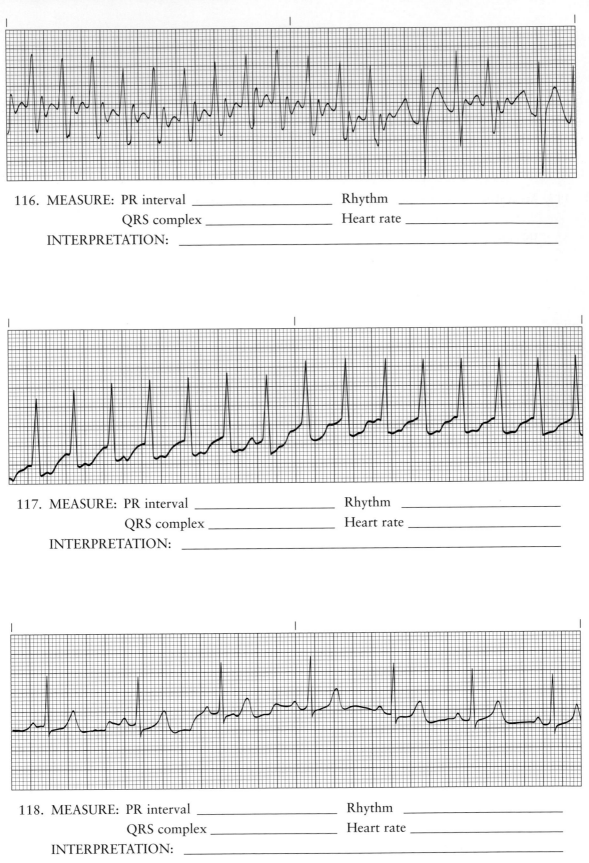

116. MEASURE: PR interval _____ Rhythm _____

  QRS complex _____ Heart rate _____

  INTERPRETATION: _____

117. MEASURE: PR interval _____ Rhythm _____

  QRS complex _____ Heart rate _____

  INTERPRETATION: _____

118. MEASURE: PR interval _____ Rhythm _____

  QRS complex _____ Heart rate _____

  INTERPRETATION: _____

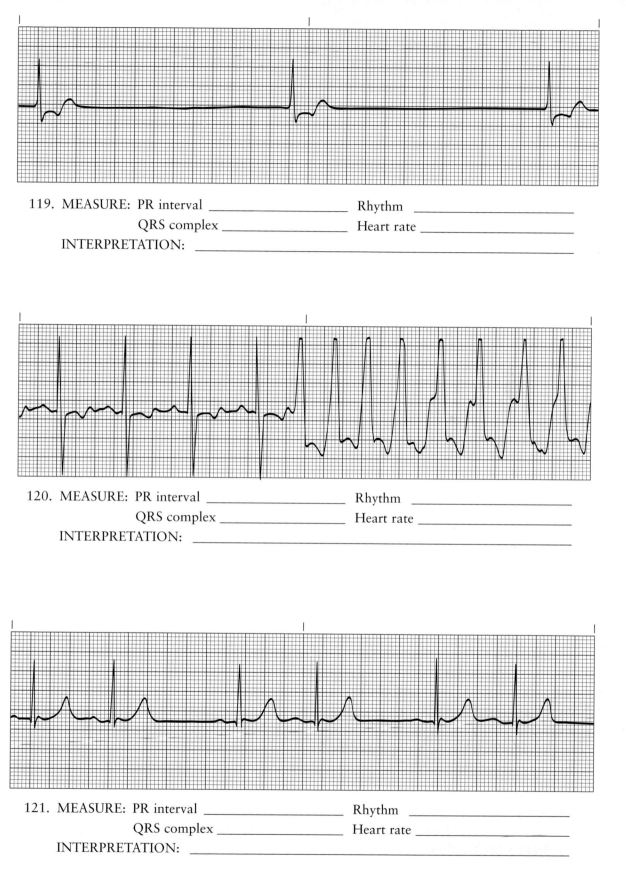

119. MEASURE: PR interval _____ Rhythm _____

QRS complex _____ Heart rate _____

INTERPRETATION: _____

120. MEASURE: PR interval _____ Rhythm _____

QRS complex _____ Heart rate _____

INTERPRETATION: _____

121. MEASURE: PR interval _____ Rhythm _____

QRS complex _____ Heart rate _____

INTERPRETATION: _____

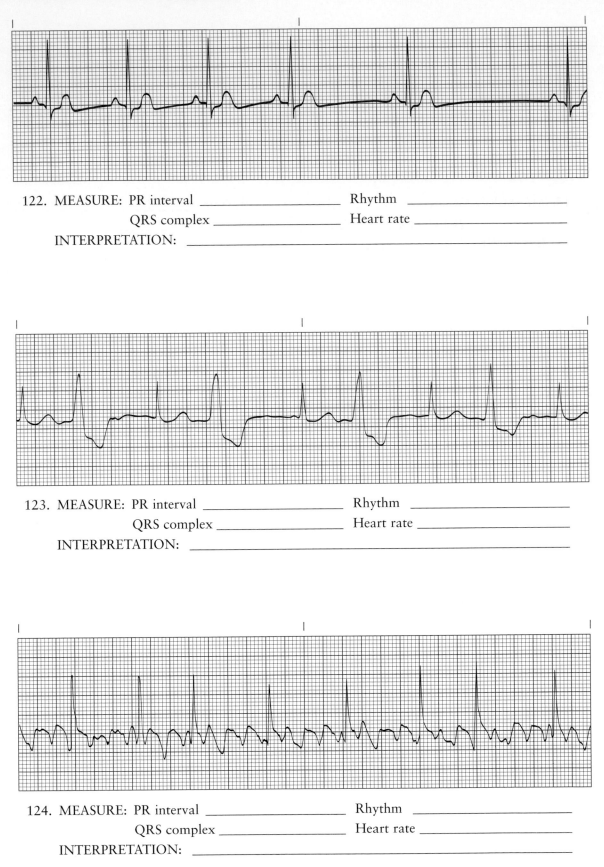

122. MEASURE: PR interval _____ Rhythm _____

     QRS complex _____ Heart rate _____

     INTERPRETATION: _____

123. MEASURE: PR interval _____ Rhythm _____

     QRS complex _____ Heart rate _____

     INTERPRETATION: _____

124. MEASURE: PR interval _____ Rhythm _____

     QRS complex _____ Heart rate _____

     INTERPRETATION: _____

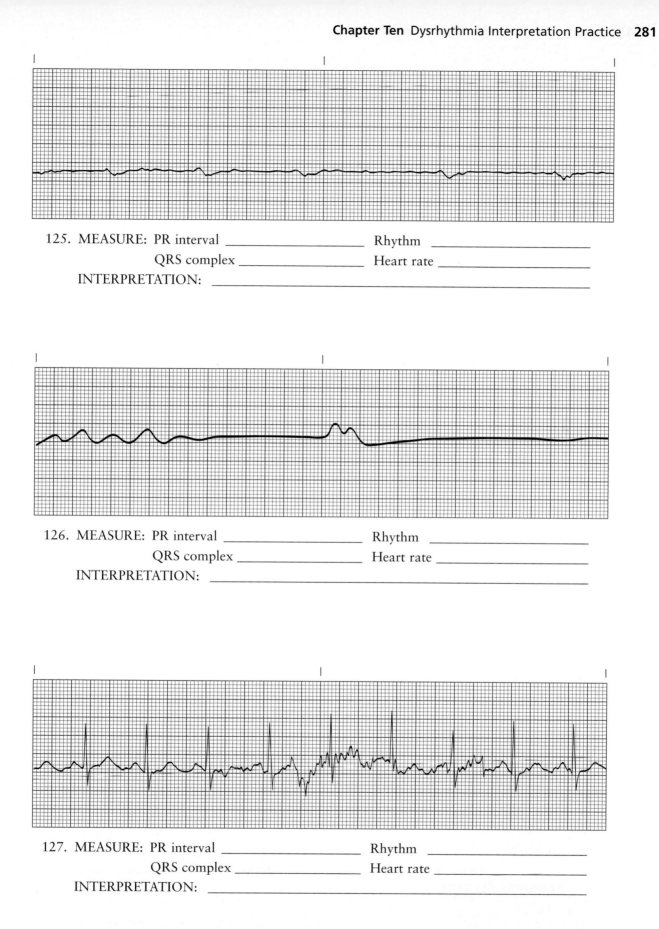

125. MEASURE: PR interval _____   Rhythm _____

              QRS complex _____   Heart rate _____

     INTERPRETATION: _____

126. MEASURE: PR interval _____   Rhythm _____

              QRS complex _____   Heart rate _____

     INTERPRETATION: _____

127. MEASURE: PR interval _____   Rhythm _____

              QRS complex _____   Heart rate _____

     INTERPRETATION: _____

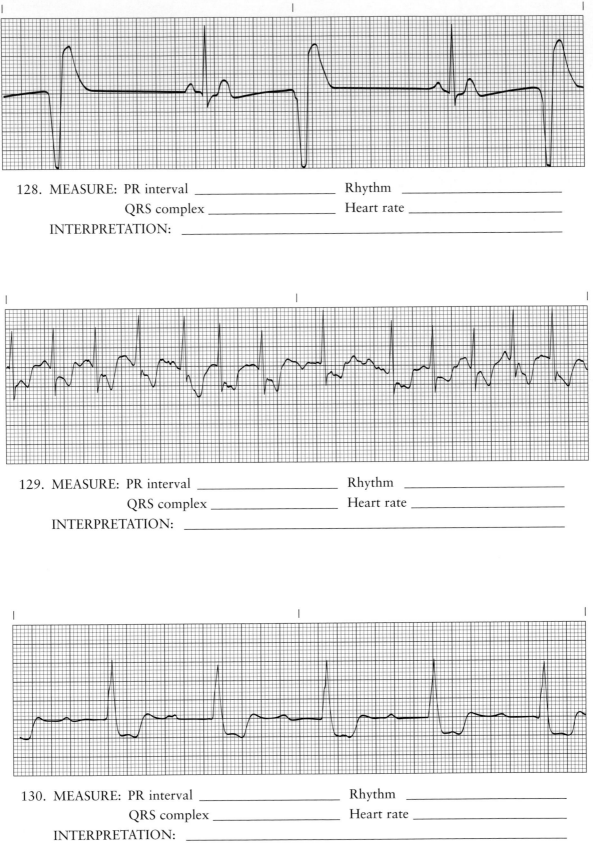

128. MEASURE: PR interval _____ Rhythm _____

QRS complex _____ Heart rate _____

INTERPRETATION: _____

129. MEASURE: PR interval _____ Rhythm _____

QRS complex _____ Heart rate _____

INTERPRETATION: _____

130. MEASURE: PR interval _____ Rhythm _____

QRS complex _____ Heart rate _____

INTERPRETATION: _____

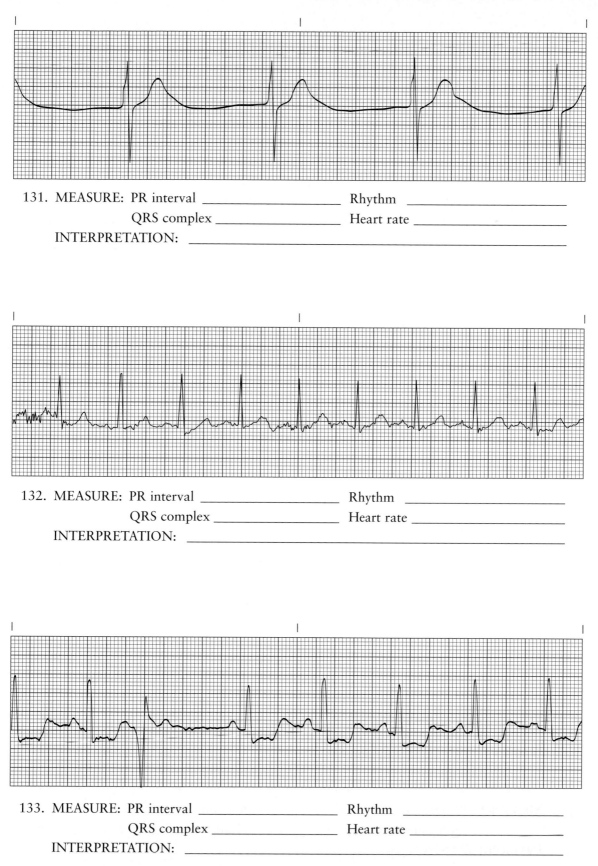

131. MEASURE: PR interval _____ Rhythm _____

                  QRS complex _____ Heart rate _____

    INTERPRETATION: _____

132. MEASURE: PR interval _____ Rhythm _____

                  QRS complex _____ Heart rate _____

    INTERPRETATION: _____

133. MEASURE: PR interval _____ Rhythm _____

                  QRS complex _____ Heart rate _____

    INTERPRETATION: _____

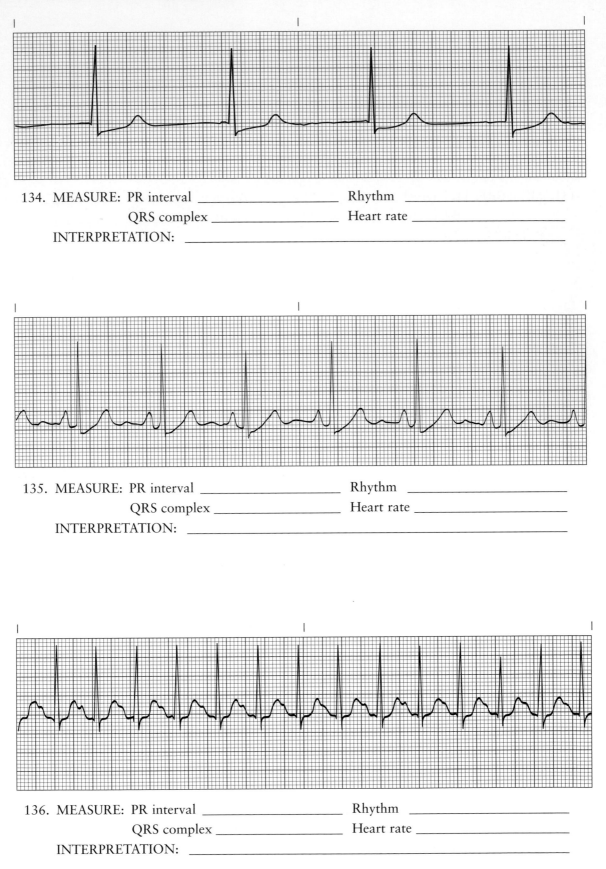

134. MEASURE: PR interval _____   Rhythm _____

                 QRS complex _____   Heart rate _____

INTERPRETATION: _____

135. MEASURE: PR interval _____   Rhythm _____

                 QRS complex _____   Heart rate _____

INTERPRETATION: _____

136. MEASURE: PR interval _____   Rhythm _____

                 QRS complex _____   Heart rate _____

INTERPRETATION: _____

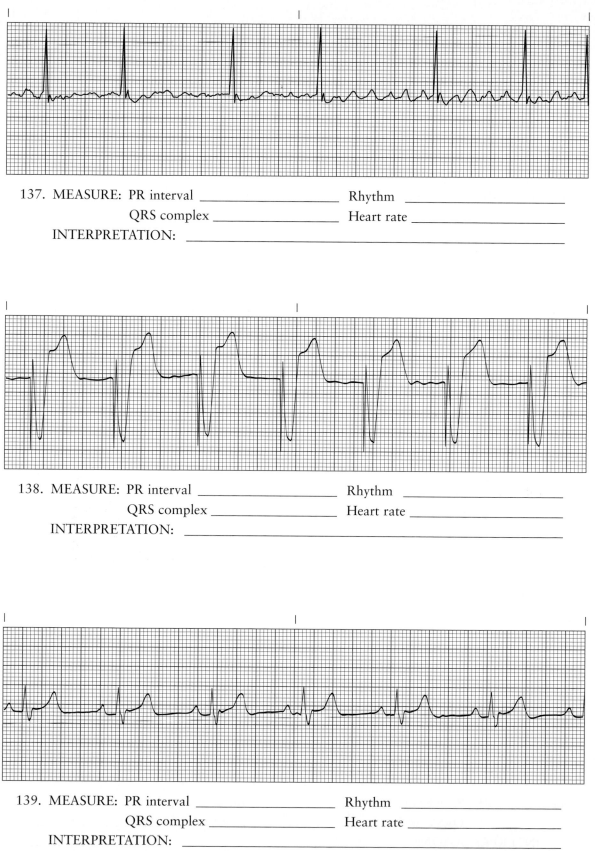

137. MEASURE: PR interval _____ Rhythm _____

QRS complex _____ Heart rate _____

INTERPRETATION: _____

138. MEASURE: PR interval _____ Rhythm _____

QRS complex _____ Heart rate _____

INTERPRETATION: _____

139. MEASURE: PR interval _____ Rhythm _____

QRS complex _____ Heart rate _____

INTERPRETATION: _____

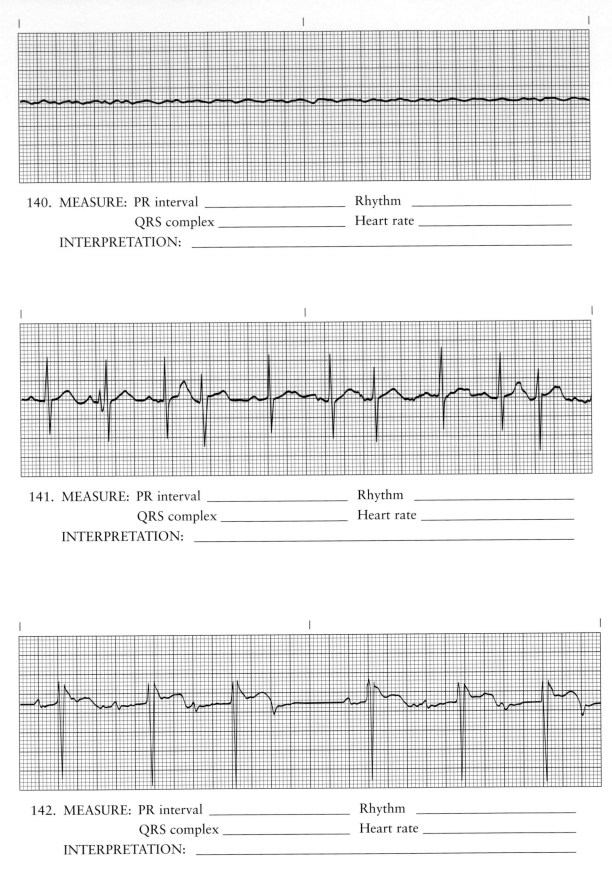

140. MEASURE: PR interval _____ Rhythm _____

                     QRS complex _____ Heart rate _____

                     INTERPRETATION: _____

141. MEASURE: PR interval _____ Rhythm _____

                     QRS complex _____ Heart rate _____

                     INTERPRETATION: _____

142. MEASURE: PR interval _____ Rhythm _____

                     QRS complex _____ Heart rate _____

                     INTERPRETATION: _____

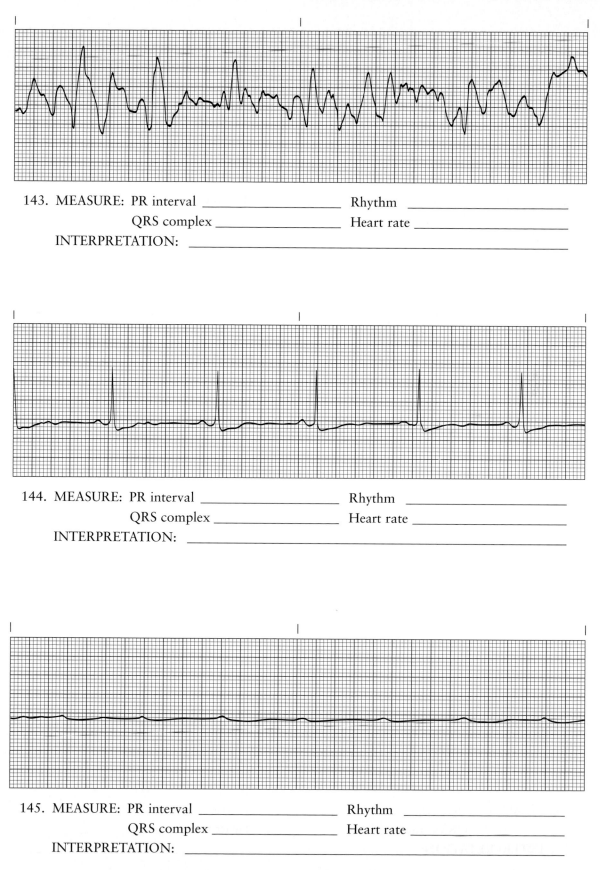

143. MEASURE: PR interval _____   Rhythm _____

             QRS complex _____   Heart rate _____

    INTERPRETATION: _____

144. MEASURE: PR interval _____   Rhythm _____

             QRS complex _____   Heart rate _____

    INTERPRETATION: _____

145. MEASURE: PR interval _____   Rhythm _____

             QRS complex _____   Heart rate _____

    INTERPRETATION: _____

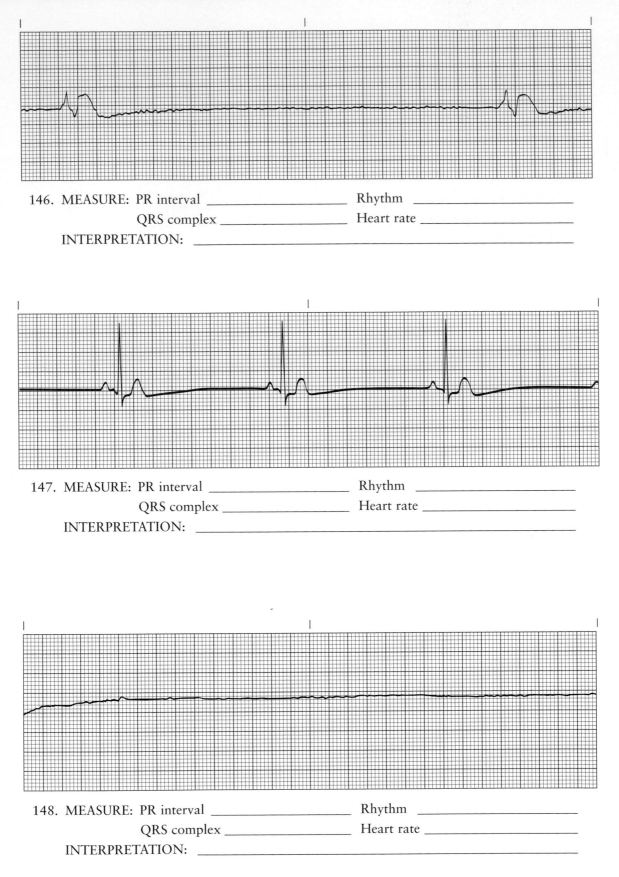

146. MEASURE: PR interval _____ Rhythm _____

     QRS complex _____ Heart rate _____

  INTERPRETATION: _____

147. MEASURE: PR interval _____ Rhythm _____

     QRS complex _____ Heart rate _____

  INTERPRETATION: _____

148. MEASURE: PR interval _____ Rhythm _____

     QRS complex _____ Heart rate _____

  INTERPRETATION: _____

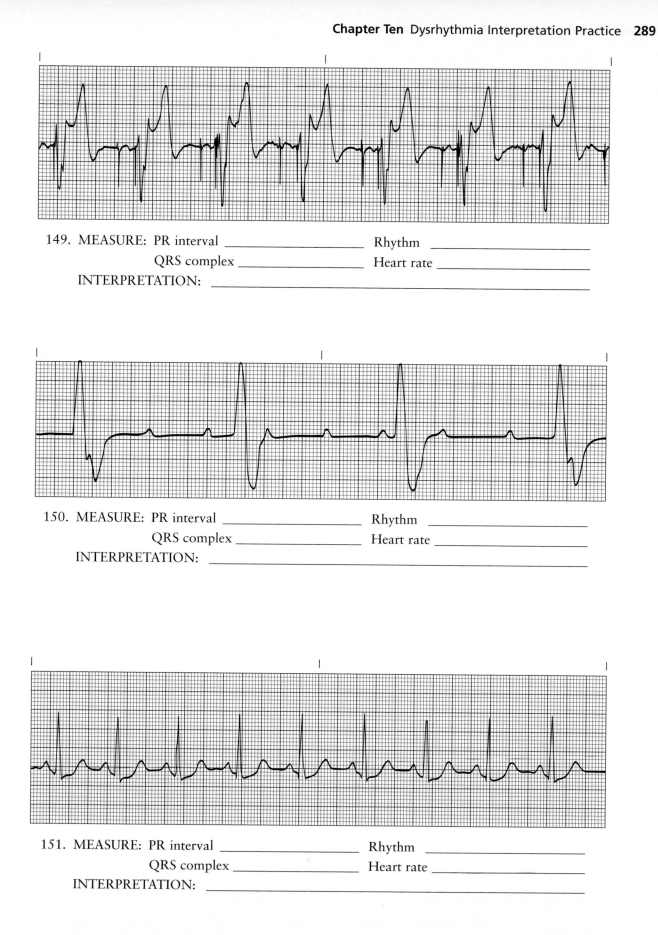

149. MEASURE: PR interval _____ Rhythm _____

QRS complex _____ Heart rate _____

INTERPRETATION: _____

150. MEASURE: PR interval _____ Rhythm _____

QRS complex _____ Heart rate _____

INTERPRETATION: _____

151. MEASURE: PR interval _____ Rhythm _____

QRS complex _____ Heart rate _____

INTERPRETATION: _____

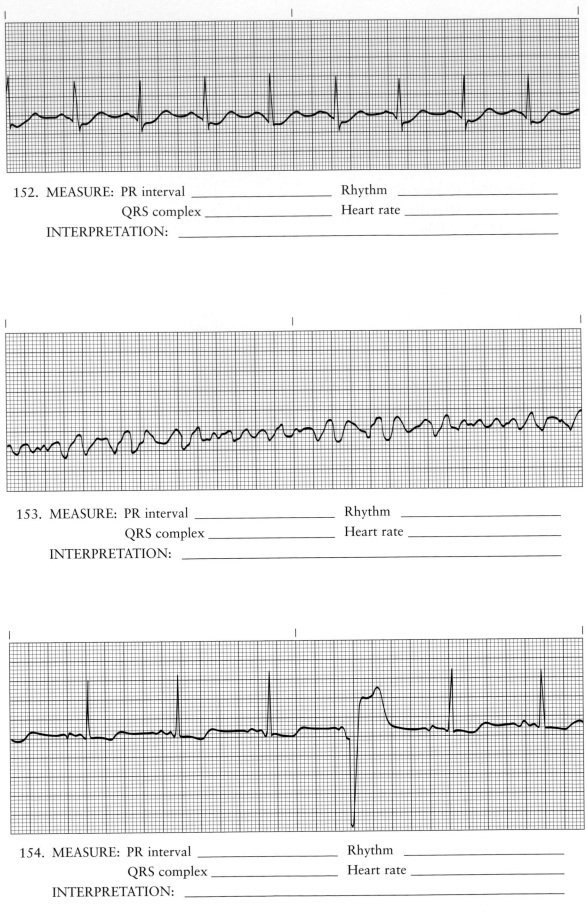

152. MEASURE: PR interval _____   Rhythm _____

QRS complex _____   Heart rate _____

INTERPRETATION: _____

153. MEASURE: PR interval _____   Rhythm _____

QRS complex _____   Heart rate _____

INTERPRETATION: _____

154. MEASURE: PR interval _____   Rhythm _____

QRS complex _____   Heart rate _____

INTERPRETATION: _____

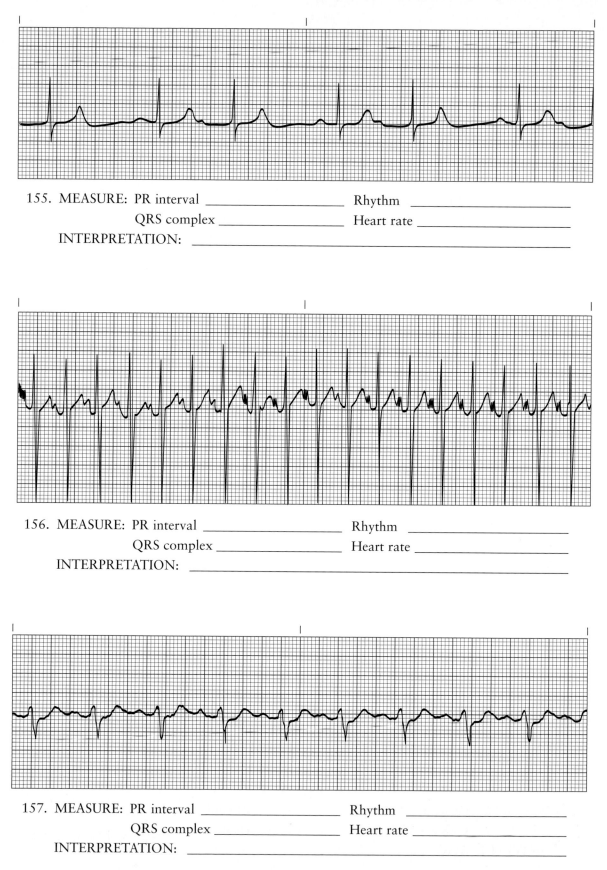

155. MEASURE: PR interval _____ Rhythm _____

QRS complex _____ Heart rate _____

INTERPRETATION: _____

156. MEASURE: PR interval _____ Rhythm _____

QRS complex _____ Heart rate _____

INTERPRETATION: _____

157. MEASURE: PR interval _____ Rhythm _____

QRS complex _____ Heart rate _____

INTERPRETATION: _____

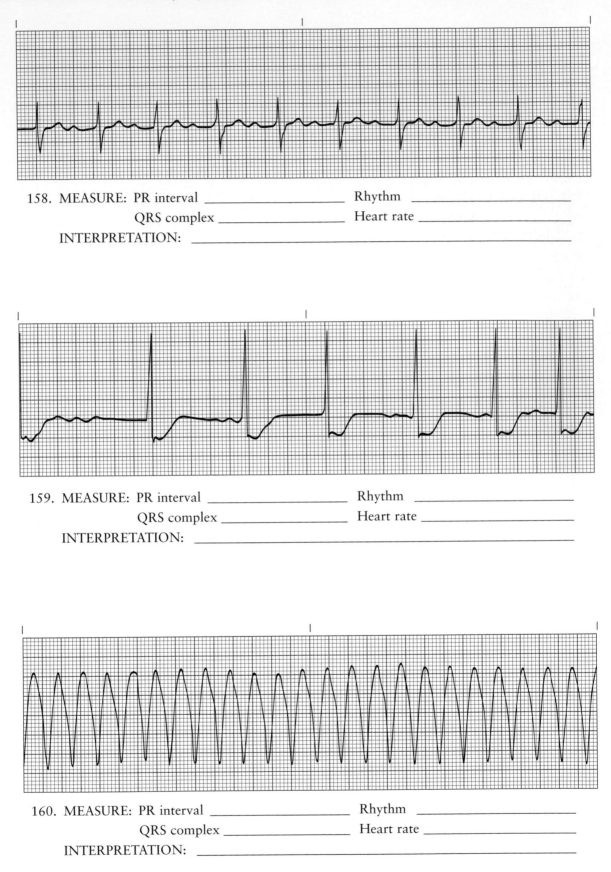

158. MEASURE: PR interval _____   Rhythm _____

QRS complex _____   Heart rate _____

INTERPRETATION: _____

159. MEASURE: PR interval _____   Rhythm _____

QRS complex _____   Heart rate _____

INTERPRETATION: _____

160. MEASURE: PR interval _____   Rhythm _____

QRS complex _____   Heart rate _____

INTERPRETATION: _____

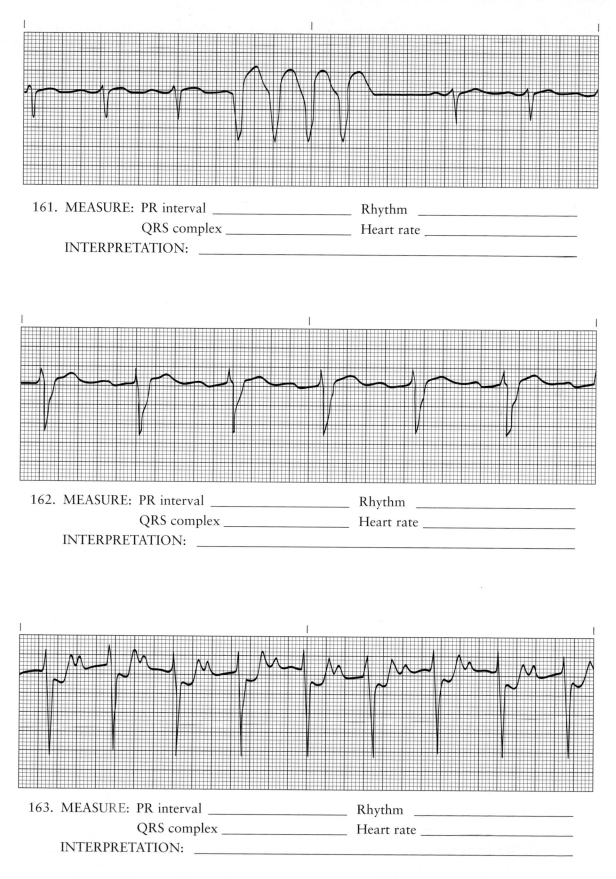

161. MEASURE: PR interval _____ Rhythm _____

QRS complex _____ Heart rate _____

INTERPRETATION: _____

162. MEASURE: PR interval _____ Rhythm _____

QRS complex _____ Heart rate _____

INTERPRETATION: _____

163. MEASURE: PR interval _____ Rhythm _____

QRS complex _____ Heart rate _____

INTERPRETATION: _____

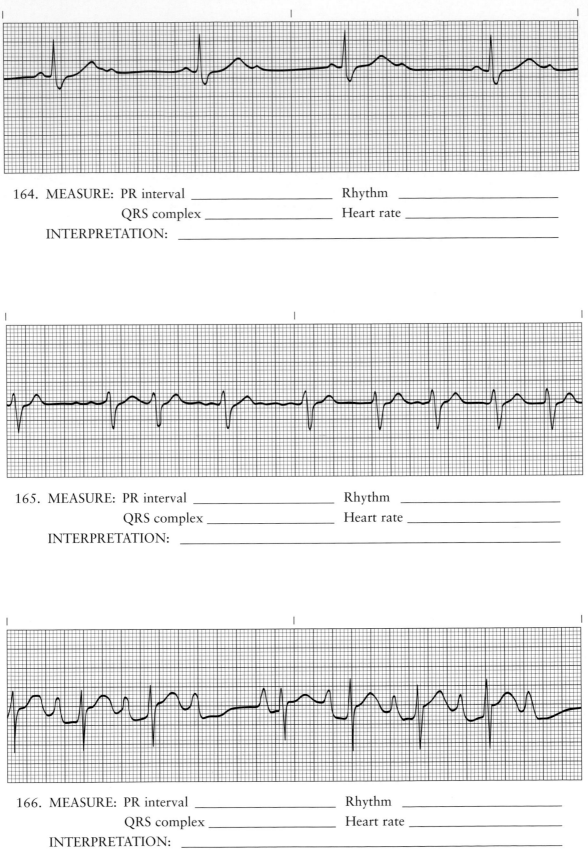

164. MEASURE: PR interval _____ Rhythm _____

QRS complex _____ Heart rate _____

INTERPRETATION: _____

165. MEASURE: PR interval _____ Rhythm _____

QRS complex _____ Heart rate _____

INTERPRETATION: _____

166. MEASURE: PR interval _____ Rhythm _____

QRS complex _____ Heart rate _____

INTERPRETATION: _____

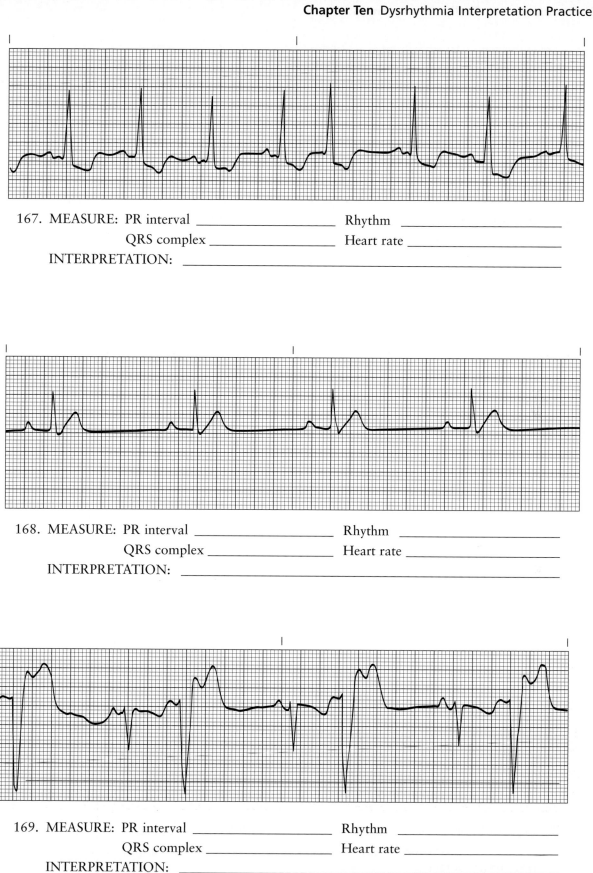

167. MEASURE: PR interval _____ Rhythm _____

                    QRS complex _____ Heart rate _____

     INTERPRETATION: _____

168. MEASURE: PR interval _____ Rhythm _____

                    QRS complex _____ Heart rate _____

     INTERPRETATION: _____

169. MEASURE: PR interval _____ Rhythm _____

                    QRS complex _____ Heart rate _____

     INTERPRETATION: _____

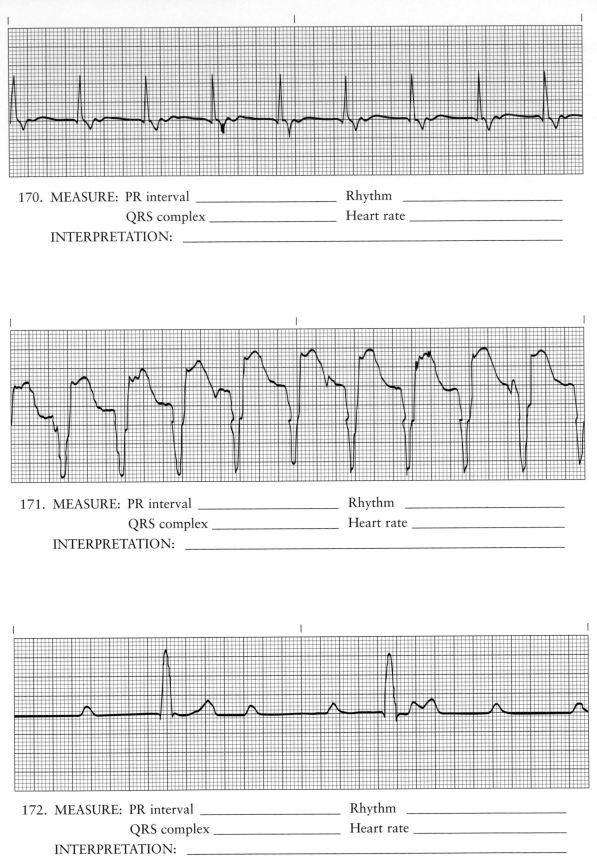

170. MEASURE: PR interval _____ Rhythm _____

                QRS complex _____ Heart rate _____

      INTERPRETATION: _____

171. MEASURE: PR interval _____ Rhythm _____

                QRS complex _____ Heart rate _____

      INTERPRETATION: _____

172. MEASURE: PR interval _____ Rhythm _____

                QRS complex _____ Heart rate _____

      INTERPRETATION: _____

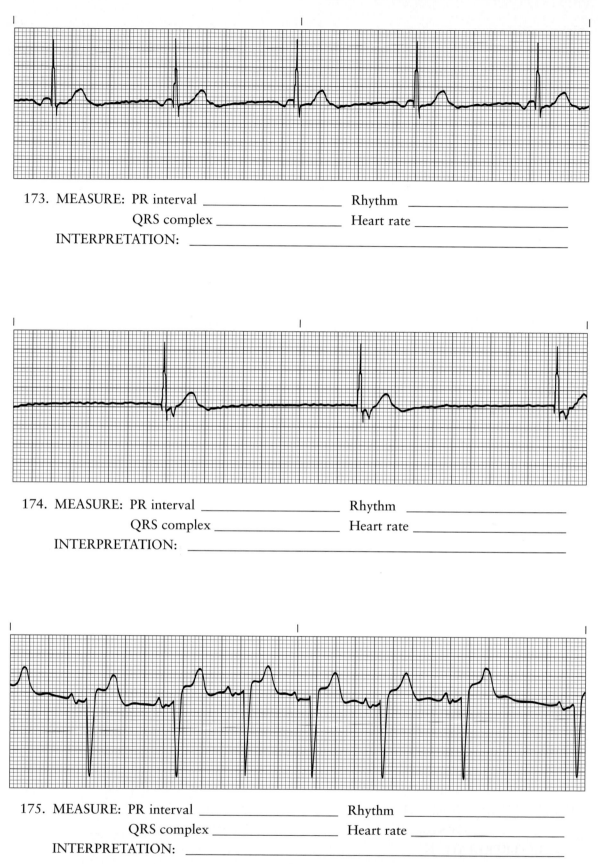

173. MEASURE: PR interval _____ Rhythm _____

QRS complex _____ Heart rate _____

INTERPRETATION: _____

174. MEASURE: PR interval _____ Rhythm _____

QRS complex _____ Heart rate _____

INTERPRETATION: _____

175. MEASURE: PR interval _____ Rhythm _____

QRS complex _____ Heart rate _____

INTERPRETATION: _____

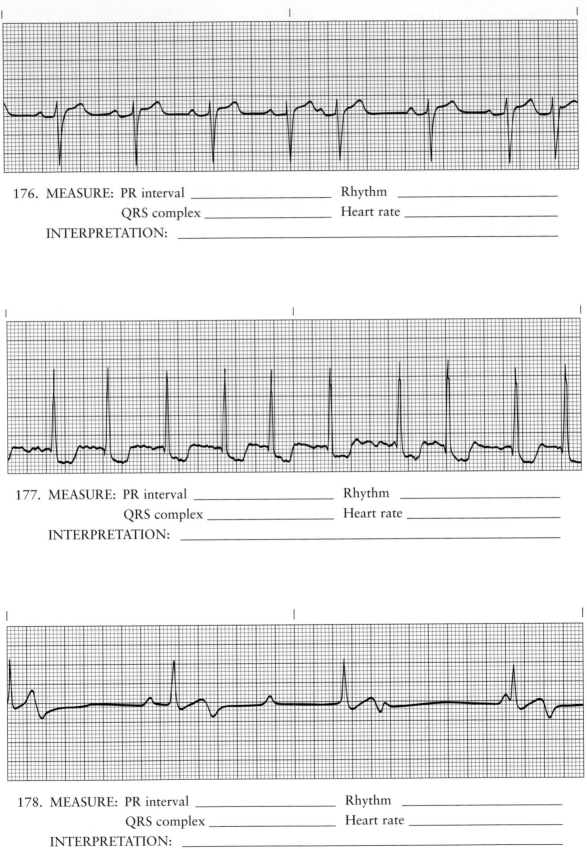

176. MEASURE: PR interval _____ Rhythm _____

QRS complex _____ Heart rate _____

INTERPRETATION: _____

177. MEASURE: PR interval _____ Rhythm _____

QRS complex _____ Heart rate _____

INTERPRETATION: _____

178. MEASURE: PR interval _____ Rhythm _____

QRS complex _____ Heart rate _____

INTERPRETATION: _____

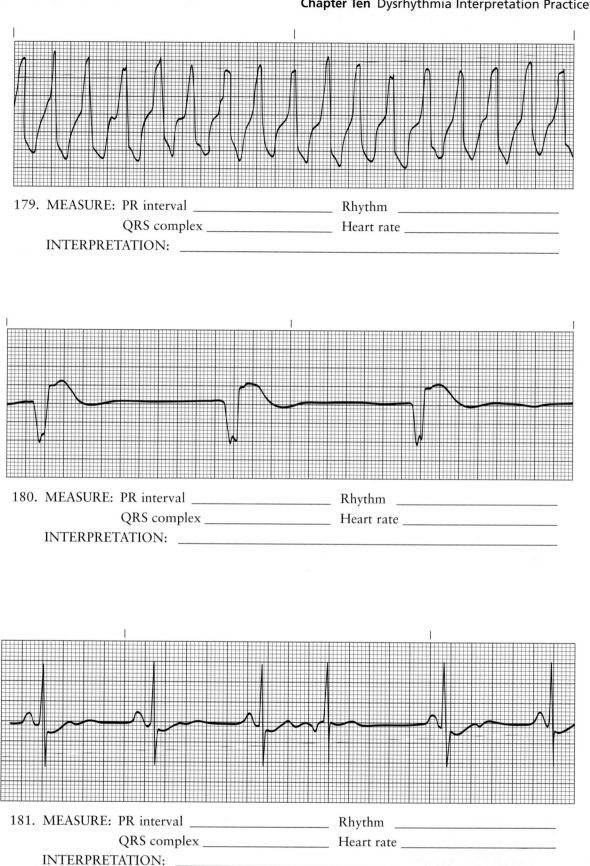

179. MEASURE: PR interval _____   Rhythm _____

QRS complex _____   Heart rate _____

INTERPRETATION: _____

180. MEASURE: PR interval _____   Rhythm _____

QRS complex _____   Heart rate _____

INTERPRETATION: _____

181. MEASURE: PR interval _____   Rhythm _____

QRS complex _____   Heart rate _____

INTERPRETATION: _____

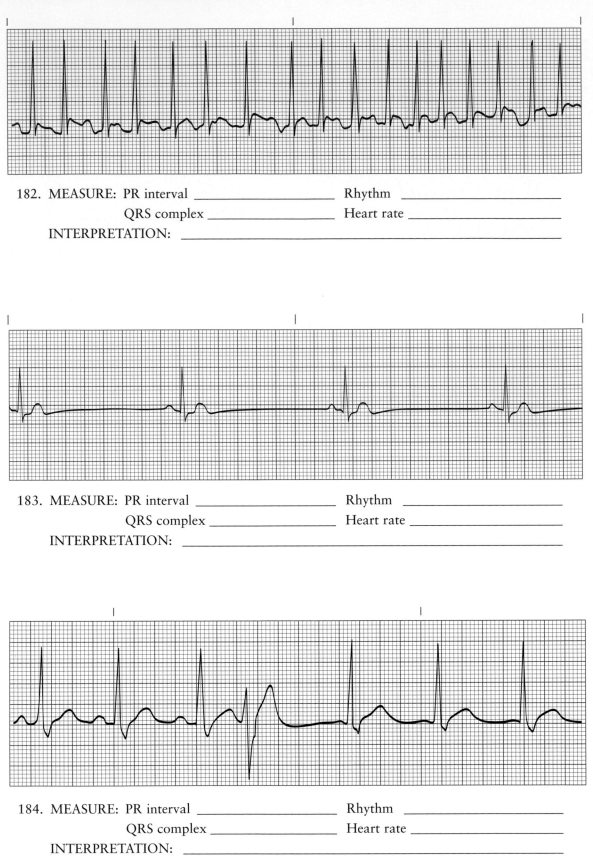

182. MEASURE: PR interval _____   Rhythm _____

     QRS complex _____   Heart rate _____

     INTERPRETATION: _____

183. MEASURE: PR interval _____   Rhythm _____

     QRS complex _____   Heart rate _____

     INTERPRETATION: _____

184. MEASURE: PR interval _____   Rhythm _____

     QRS complex _____   Heart rate _____

     INTERPRETATION: _____

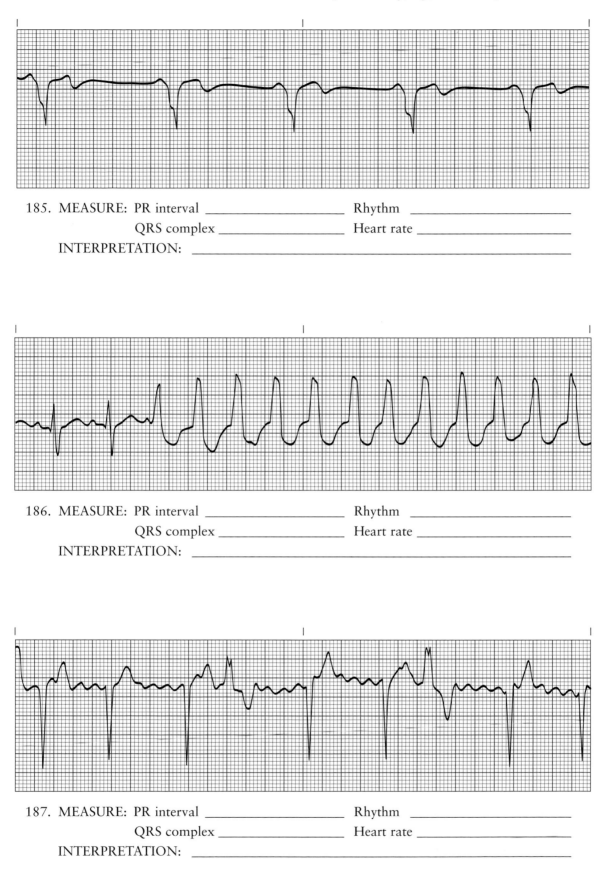

185. MEASURE: PR interval _____ Rhythm _____

QRS complex _____ Heart rate _____

INTERPRETATION: _____

186. MEASURE: PR interval _____ Rhythm _____

QRS complex _____ Heart rate _____

INTERPRETATION: _____

187. MEASURE: PR interval _____ Rhythm _____

QRS complex _____ Heart rate _____

INTERPRETATION: _____

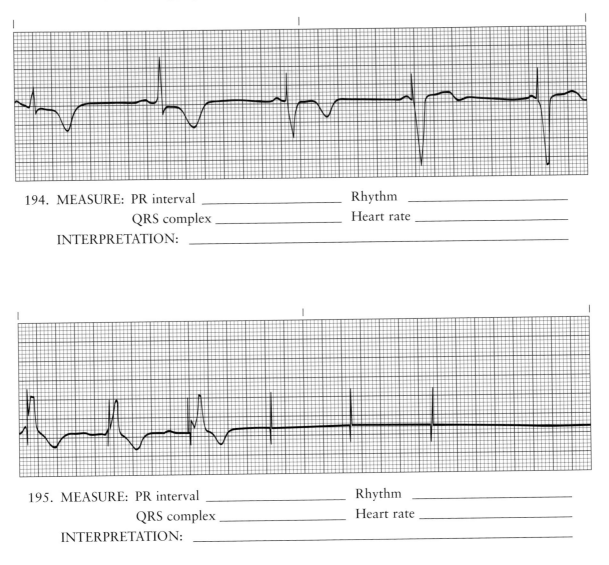

194. MEASURE: PR interval _____ Rhythm _____

               QRS complex _____ Heart rate _____

    INTERPRETATION: _____

195. MEASURE: PR interval _____ Rhythm _____

               QRS complex _____ Heart rate _____

    INTERPRETATION: _____

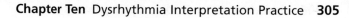

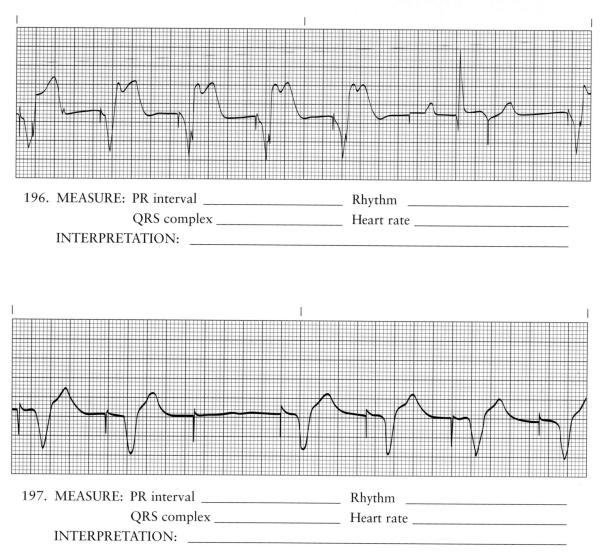

196. MEASURE: PR interval _____ Rhythm _____

               QRS complex _____ Heart rate _____

     INTERPRETATION: _____

197. MEASURE: PR interval _____ Rhythm _____

               QRS complex _____ Heart rate _____

     INTERPRETATION: _____

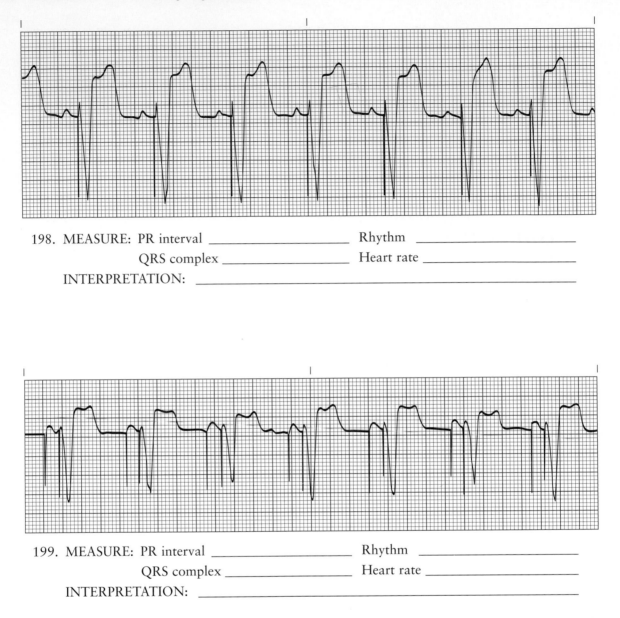

198. MEASURE: PR interval _____ Rhythm _____

                QRS complex _____ Heart rate _____

      INTERPRETATION: _____

199. MEASURE: PR interval _____ Rhythm _____

                QRS complex _____ Heart rate _____

      INTERPRETATION: _____

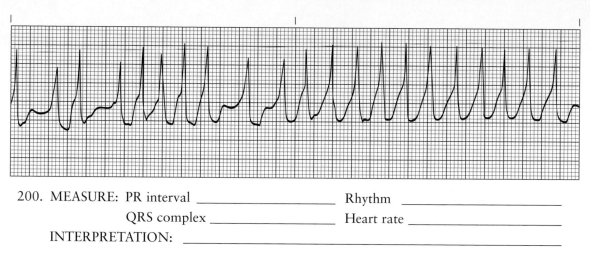

200. MEASURE: PR interval _____ Rhythm _____

                QRS complex _____ Heart rate _____

    INTERPRETATION: _____

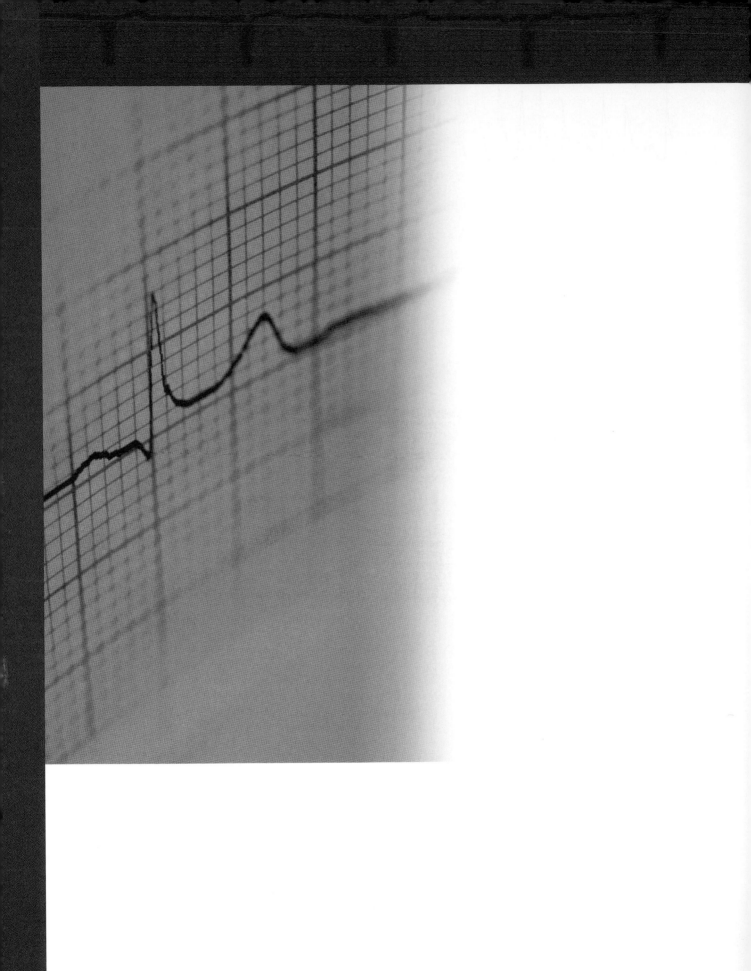

CHAPTER 11

Case Studies

This chapter uses case studies/clinical scenarios to help you "put it all together." They are an excellent way to learn and remember new material. They also increase your ability to relate signs and symptoms to patient care, and to recognize potential patient problems.

The case studies involve you in medical situations, giving examples of how patient assessment, dysrhythmia identification, medications, and procedures all contribute to the treatment of the patient.

The treatments used in these case studies are based on the guidelines of the American Heart Association, as listed in Chapter 9. Remember that these are only general guidelines and should be used in conjunction with, **not** instead of, the policies and procedures of your institution. All treatment **must** be performed under the guidance of a physician. Only properly trained individuals should administer medications or treatments.

To use these case studies, first assess the patient, next identify the dysrhythmia, and then determine the appropriate treatment, based on your findings. Keep in mind that all patients must be assessed initially, as well as before and after each medication or treatment. This will help you evaluate the patient's tolerance of the dysrhythmia and their response to the medications or treatments.

Assessing the patient for poor cardiac output involves more than taking the blood pressure, heart rate, and looking at the monitor screen. It also includes evaluating the patient's respirations, skin temperature, and level of consciousness. This can be done by talking to, looking at, listening to, and touching the patient. To learn the proper way to evaluate patients, consider attending a physical assessment course.

For the purpose of this chapter, it is understood that:

- All patients are adult.
- All patients are either on a cardiac monitor or will soon be placed on a cardiac monitor.
- No contraindications exist to any of the treatment protocols.
- All patients are being assessed both before and after each medication or treatment.
- After the administration of any medication, all intravenous or intraosseous lines are flushed with 20 ml of IV/IO solution; then, if possible, the extremity is elevated for 10 to 20 seconds.
- All appropriate laboratory tests have been ordered, when available.

We encourage you to use these case studies and to also make up additional situations. Just as interpreting rhythm strips becomes easier with practice, so will patient assessments and treatments.

Case Study 1

You are caring for a 26-year-old patient on the telemetry unit who complains that her heart is "racing" and "pounding" in her chest. The cardiac monitor shows the rhythm seen in Figure 11-1.

Fig. 11-1

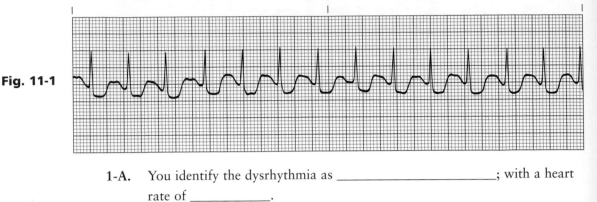

1-A. You identify the dysrhythmia as _____; with a heart rate of _____.

As you enter her room to assess the patient, you notice several empty coffee cups and soda cans scattered around the room. The patient is pacing back and forth, and is unable to sit still for long. The patient's vital signs are BP 136/84, pulse 140, and respiratory rate (RR) of 26.

As you talk with the patient, she admits to being very anxious about waiting for the results of tests that had been completed that morning.

1-B. Your next actions include:

1. _____
2. _____
3. _____
4. _____

You see that the patient appears less anxious and is now able to relax in bed. The cardiac monitor now displays the rhythm shown in Figure 11-2.

Fig. 11-2

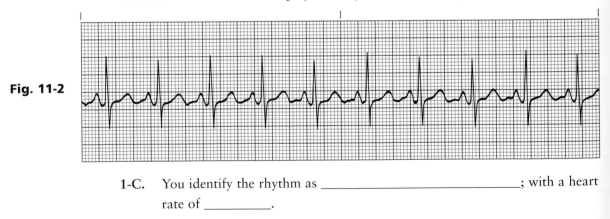

1-C. You identify the rhythm as _____; with a heart rate of _____.

You reassess the patient and find BP 128/72, pulse 100, and RR 20. You continue to monitor the patient for any further changes.

Case Study 2

A 70-kg patient is brought to the emergency department by his co-worker. The patient states that he has been having occasional dizzy spells for a few days and today he fainted. The cardiac monitor shows the dysrhythmia seen in Figure 11-3. You assess the patient and find signs of poor cardiac output, including pale, cool, clammy skin; mild chest pain; light-headedness; mild nausea; slight shortness of breath. Vital signs are BP 92/46, pulse 40, and RR 22.

Fig. 11-3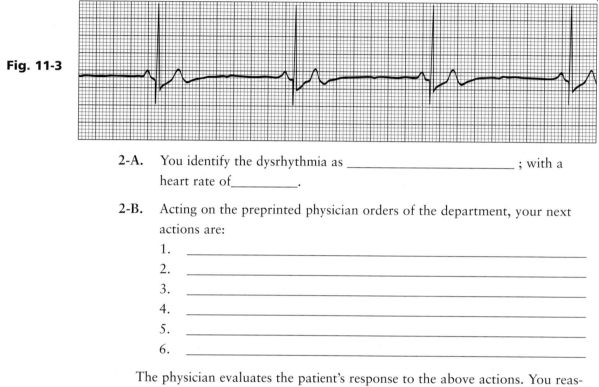

2-A.   You identify the dysrhythmia as _____ ; with a heart rate of_____.

2-B.   Acting on the preprinted physician orders of the department, your next actions are:

1. _____
2. _____
3. _____
4. _____
5. _____
6. _____

The physician evaluates the patient's response to the above actions. You reassess the patient and find a slight improvement. The chest pain, shortness of breath, and nausea are decreased. Vital signs are BP 96/52, pulse 46, and RR 20. There is no change in the dysrhythmia.

2-C.   The physician orders you to repeat _____.

2-D.   Because there is no change in the dysrhythmia or the patient's condition, the physician initiates the use of a(n) _____.

2-E.   While awaiting the equipment, consider _____.

The patient shows immediate signs of improvement. His skin is now pink, warm, and dry. He denies any nausea, chest pain, or shortness of breath. Vital signs are BP 106/68, pulse 70, and RR 18.

The cardiac monitor shows the rhythm seen in Figure 11-4.

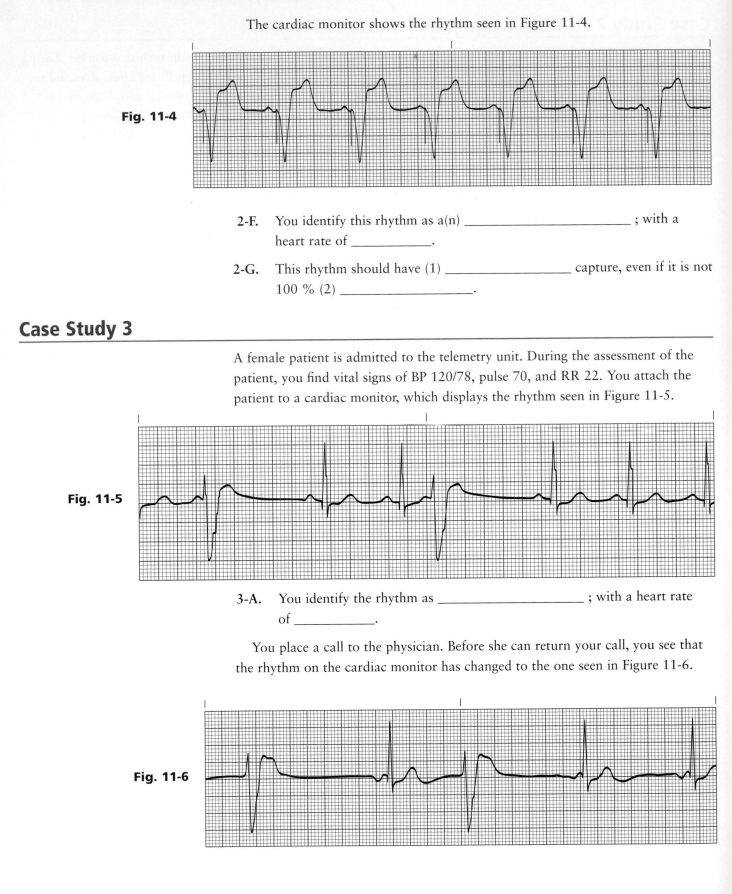

Fig. 11-4

2-F.   You identify this rhythm as a(n) _____ ; with a heart rate of _____.

2-G.   This rhythm should have (1) _____ capture, even if it is not 100 % (2) _____.

Case Study 3

A female patient is admitted to the telemetry unit. During the assessment of the patient, you find vital signs of BP 120/78, pulse 70, and RR 22. You attach the patient to a cardiac monitor, which displays the rhythm seen in Figure 11-5.

Fig. 11-5

3-A.   You identify the rhythm as _____ ; with a heart rate of _____.

You place a call to the physician. Before she can return your call, you see that the rhythm on the cardiac monitor has changed to the one seen in Figure 11-6.

Fig. 11-6

3-B. You identify the dysrhythmia as _____ ; with a heart rate of _____.

3-C. Following the unit's preprinted physician orders, you initiate the following:

1. _____
2. _____
3. _____
4. _____

You reassess the patient and find her vital signs to be BP 104/60, pulse 50, and RR 26. The patient is pale, cool, clammy, and anxious.

3-D. You immediately_____.

> **NOTE:** Remember, after administering **any** IV/IO medication, flush the line with 20 ml of IV/IO fluids and elevate the extremity.

The patient's skin is now warm and dry and she appears less anxious. The BP is now 110/70, pulse 80, and RR 22. The cardiac monitor displays the rhythm seen in Figure 11-7.

Fig. 11-7

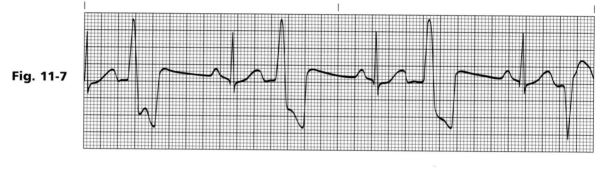

3-E. You interpret the dysrhythmia as _____; with a heart rate of_____.

3-F. The physician arrives and orders _____.

Since this medication controls the PVC's, a continuous IV infusion of the same medication is started.

You continue to monitor the patient for any signs of poor cardiac output or change in the rhythm, especially for any of the "danger signs" for PVCs.

3-G. These danger signs (besides poor cardiac output) include:

1. _____
2. _____
3. _____
4. _____
5. _____

Case Study 4

A patient is admitted to the emergency department. You assess the patient and find he is pale, cool, sweaty, and complaining of chest pain. His vital signs include BP 100/50, pulse 170, and RR 26. The cardiac monitor shows the rhythm as seen in Figure 11-8.

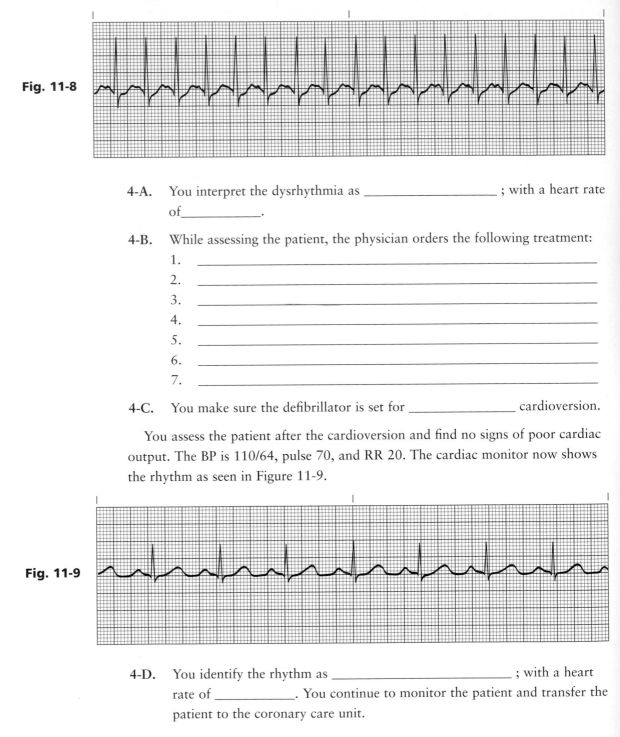

Fig. 11-8

4-A.   You interpret the dysrhythmia as _____ ; with a heart rate of_____.

4-B.   While assessing the patient, the physician orders the following treatment:

1.   _____
2.   _____
3.   _____
4.   _____
5.   _____
6.   _____
7.   _____

4-C.   You make sure the defibrillator is set for _____ cardioversion.

You assess the patient after the cardioversion and find no signs of poor cardiac output. The BP is 110/64, pulse 70, and RR 20. The cardiac monitor now shows the rhythm as seen in Figure 11-9.

Fig. 11-9

4-D.   You identify the rhythm as _____ ; with a heart rate of _____. You continue to monitor the patient and transfer the patient to the coronary care unit.

Case Study 5

During a 5K run, a 27-year-old man is brought to the first-aid station, complaining of weakness and dizziness. You find he is warm, pale, and sweaty with BP 138/82, pulse 100 to 110, and RR 26 on the initial assessment. He denies any pain. You attach him to a cardiac monitor, which displays the rhythm seen in Figure 11-10.

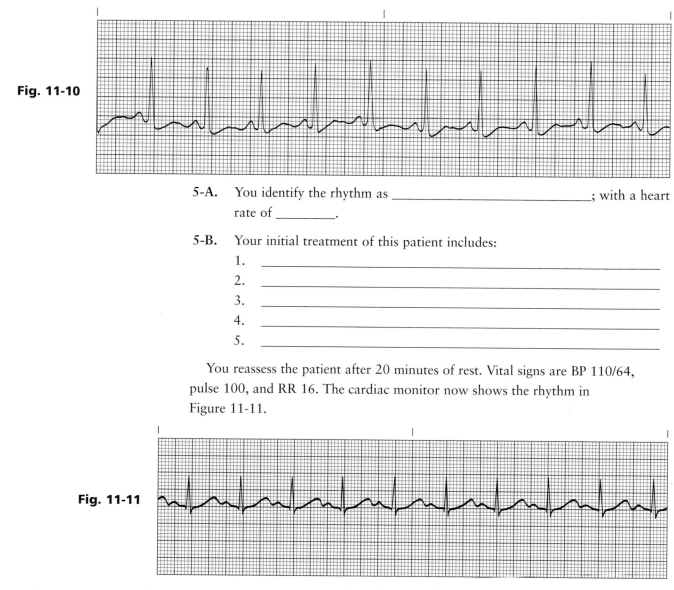

Fig. 11-10

Fig. 11-11

5-A.   You identify the rhythm as _____; with a heart rate of _____.

5-B.   Your initial treatment of this patient includes:

   1. _____

   2. _____

   3. _____

   4. _____

   5. _____

You reassess the patient after 20 minutes of rest. Vital signs are BP 110/64, pulse 100, and RR 16. The cardiac monitor now shows the rhythm in Figure 11-11.

5-C.   You identify the rhythm as _____; with a heart rate of _____.

Because of the prolonged QT intervals, you notify the patient's physician, who recommends transportation to the emergency department for evaluation.

Case Study 6

A patient is waiting for admission to the hospital after being treated in the emergency department for a drug overdose. He has an IV infusion and is receiving oxygen. The cardiac monitor shows a new rhythm as seen in Figure 11-12.

Fig. 11-12

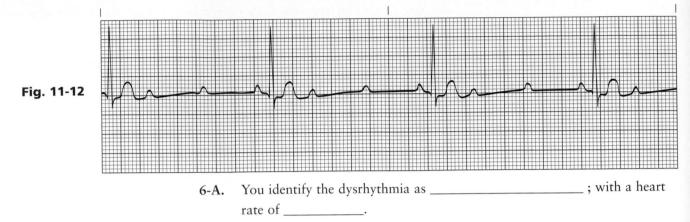

6-A.   You identify the dysrhythmia as _____ ; with a heart rate of _____.

The patient has a BP 100/48, pulse 40, and RR 22 and is pale, clammy, and lethargic. You notify the physician and begin the following preprinted physician orders as the physician re-evaluates the patient:

6-B.   1.   _____

2.   _____

3.   _____

4.   _____

The cardiac monitor suddenly shows the dysrhythmia seen in Figure 11-13.

Fig. 11-13

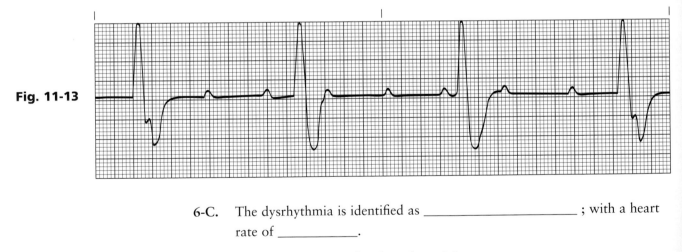

6-C.   The dysrhythmia is identified as _____ ; with a heart rate of _____.

6-D.   The physician immediately orders a(n) _____.

The patient's cardiac output improves as his heart rate increases as a result of this treatment. The patient is admitted to the cardiac care unit.

Case Study 7

You are watching the cardiac monitors in the unit and notice that one patient has an episode of R on T phenomenon. The cardiac monitor now shows the rhythm seen in Figure 11-14.

Fig. 11-14

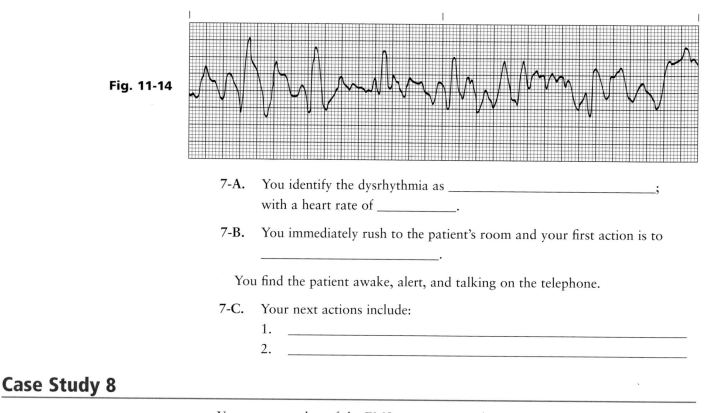

7-A. You identify the dysrhythmia as _____;
     with a heart rate of _____.

7-B. You immediately rush to the patient's room and your first action is to

     _____.

You find the patient awake, alert, and talking on the telephone.

7-C. Your next actions include:
     1. _____
     2. _____

Case Study 8

You are a member of the EMS agency responding to a 9-1-1 call for an unresponsive male. When you arrive at the scene, you assess the patient, as another crewmember attaches the patient to a cardiac monitor. You see the rhythm shown in Figure 11-15.

Fig. 11-15

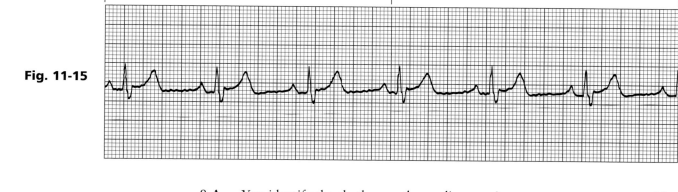

8-A. You identify the rhythm on the cardiac monitor as _____; with a heart rate of _____. However, you find no vital signs during your assessment.

8-B.   You correctly identify the dysrhythmia as _____.

8-C.   You and your crew immediately begin the following treatments:

1.   _____

2.   _____

3.   _____

4.   _____

5.   _____

6.   _____

7.   _____

8.   _____

After transporting the patient to the nearest hospital, the emergency physician assesses the patient.

8-D.   The physician decides to perform pericardiocentesis to relieve a(n)

_____.

8-E.   List three causes of PEA, and include the treatment:

1.   _____ ;   _____

2.   _____ ;   _____

3.   _____ ;   _____

After the procedure, the patient's dysrhythmia converts to that seen in Figure 11-16.

Fig. 11-16
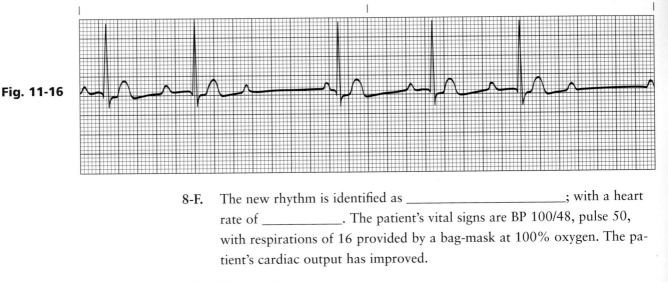

8-F.   The new rhythm is identified as _____; with a heart rate of _____. The patient's vital signs are BP 100/48, pulse 50, with respirations of 16 provided by a bag-mask at 100% oxygen. The patient's cardiac output has improved.

8-G.   You continue to _____.

The patient is transferred to the cardiac care unit for further treatment.

Case Study 9

A patient's cardiac monitor on your unit suddenly shows the dysrhythmia seen in Figure 11-17. He has an IV infusion and is receiving oxygen.

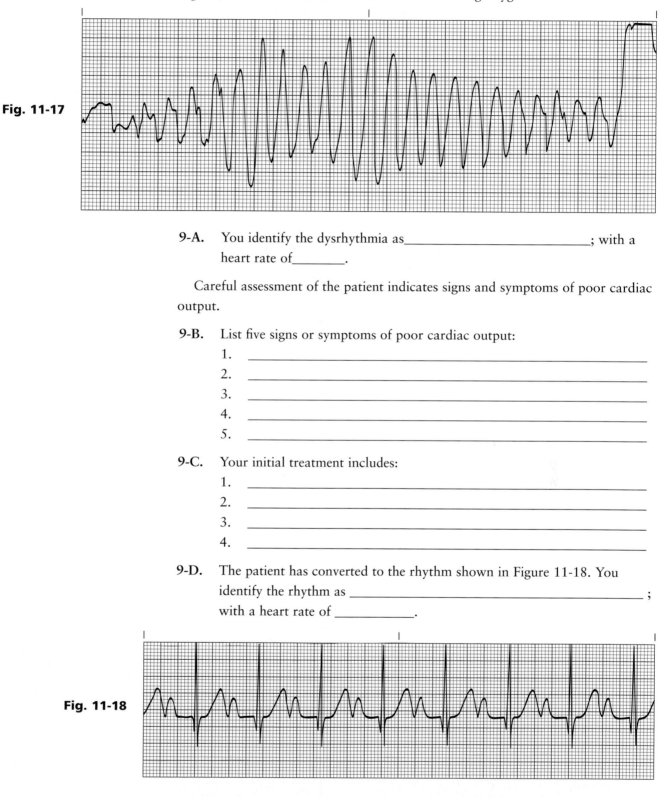

Fig. 11-17

9-A. You identify the dysrhythmia as_____; with a heart rate of_____.

Careful assessment of the patient indicates signs and symptoms of poor cardiac output.

9-B. List five signs or symptoms of poor cardiac output:

1. _____
2. _____
3. _____
4. _____
5. _____

9-C. Your initial treatment includes:

1. _____
2. _____
3. _____
4. _____

9-D. The patient has converted to the rhythm shown in Figure 11-18. You identify the rhythm as _____ ; with a heart rate of _____.

Fig. 11-18

The patient's condition has improved and he no longer has signs of poor cardiac output. You continue to monitor the patient and his cardiac rhythm.

Case Study 10

A patient returns to the cardiac care unit after a minor procedure. He has an IV infusing and is receiving oxygen at 2 L/min by nasal cannula. On assessment, the patient is awake, oriented, and talking about how well he feels. Vital signs are BP 118/88, pulse 50, and RR 20. There is a new dysrhythmia on the cardiac monitor screen; see Figure11-19.

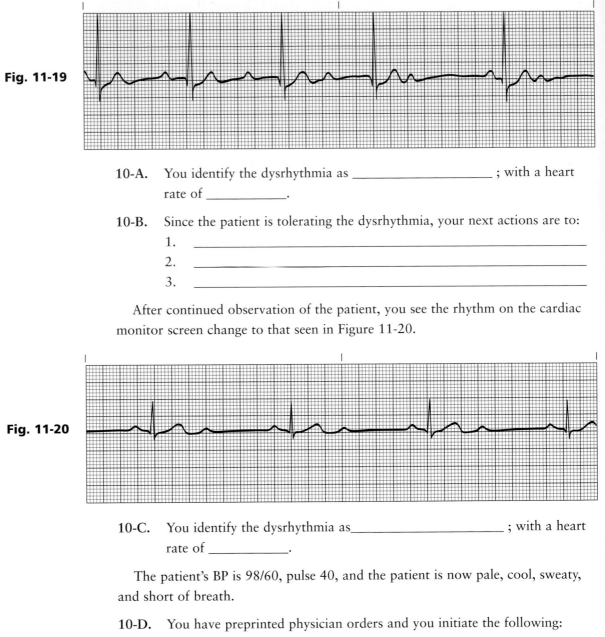

Fig. 11-19

10-A. You identify the dysrhythmia as _____ ; with a heart rate of _____.

10-B. Since the patient is tolerating the dysrhythmia, your next actions are to:

1. _____
2. _____
3. _____

After continued observation of the patient, you see the rhythm on the cardiac monitor screen change to that seen in Figure 11-20.

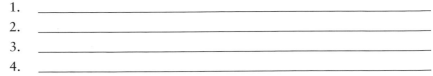

Fig. 11-20

10-C. You identify the dysrhythmia as_____ ; with a heart rate of _____.

The patient's BP is 98/60, pulse 40, and the patient is now pale, cool, sweaty, and short of breath.

10-D. You have preprinted physician orders and you initiate the following:

1. _____
2. _____
3. _____
4. _____

10-E. **After this treatment,** the cardiac dysrhythmia has converted to a(n) _____; with a heart rate of _____; see Figure 11-21.

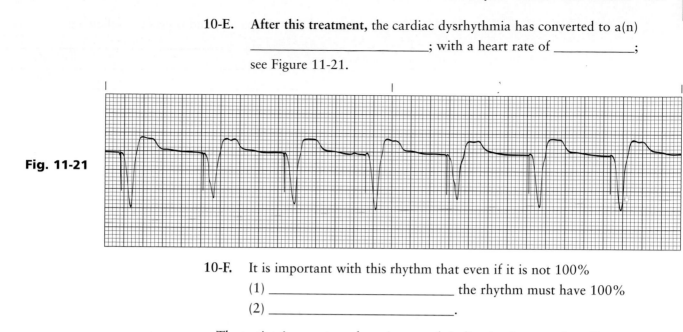

Fig. 11-21

10-F. It is important with this rhythm that even if it is not 100%
(1) _____ the rhythm must have 100%
(2) _____.

The patient's symptoms have improved, indicating improved cardiac output with BP 108/72, pulse 100, and RR 22. You continue to monitor and observe the patient.

Case Study 11

A 52-year-old man, weighing 100 kg, is brought to the emergency department, complaining of pressure in the middle of his chest, difficulty breathing, and nausea. You find his vital signs are BP 110/60, pulse 80, and RR 22. The patient is pale, cool, and diaphoretic.

11-A. These are indications of poor _____.

11-B. The patient is connected to a cardiac monitor. You identify the dysrhythmia in Figure 11-22 as _____; with a heart rate of _____.

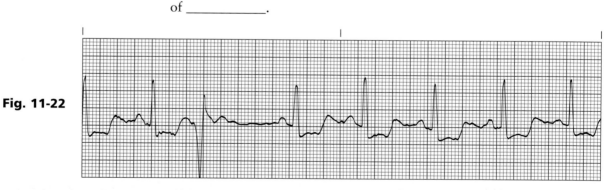

Fig. 11-22

11-C. The physician evaluates the patient and orders the following:

1. _____

2. _____

3. _____

4. _____

As you are completing these orders, the patient suddenly slumps over. You quickly assess the patient and find no vital signs. The cardiac monitor now shows the rhythm seen in Figure 11-23.

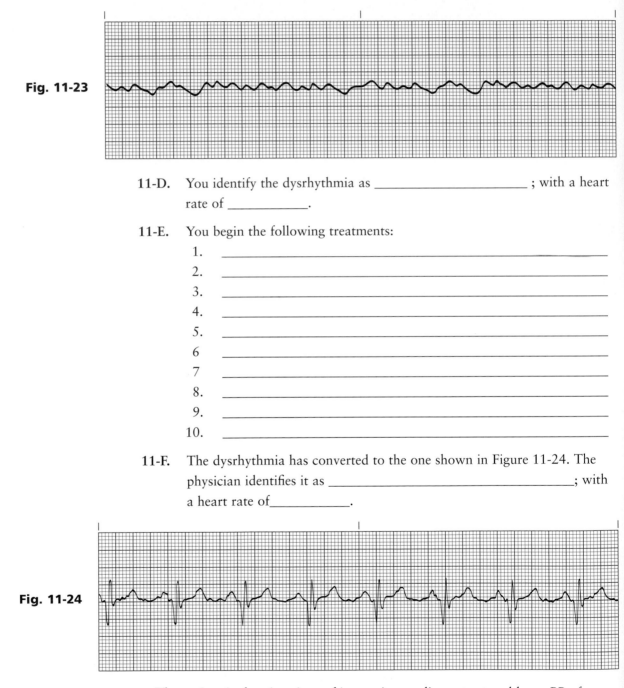

Fig. 11-23

11-D. You identify the dysrhythmia as _____ ; with a heart rate of _____.

11-E. You begin the following treatments:

1. _____

2. _____

3. _____

4. _____

5. _____

6 _____

7 _____

8. _____

9. _____

10. _____

11-F. The dysrhythmia has converted to the one shown in Figure 11-24. The physician identifies it as _____ ; with a heart rate of_____.

Fig. 11-24

The patient is showing signs of improving cardiac output and has a BP of 96/56, pulse of 80, and continues to have respirations of 16, assisted by the use of a bag-mask device. The patient is transferred to the cardiac care unit while you continue to reassess him.

Case Study 12

You come on duty and study the monitors. You observe the dysrhythmia shown in Figure 11-25 on one of the cardiac monitors.

Fig. 11-25

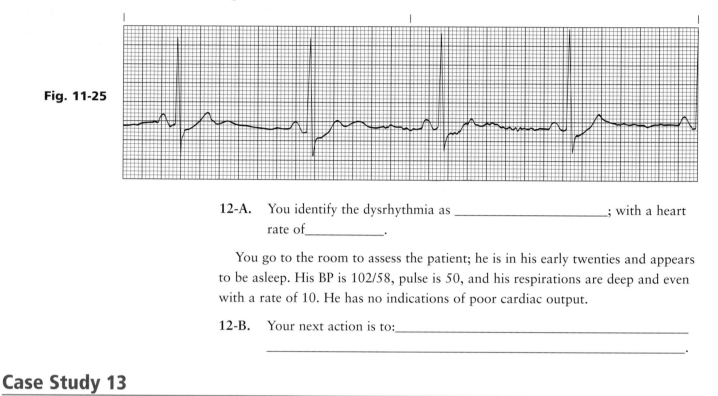

12-A. You identify the dysrhythmia as _____; with a heart rate of_____.

You go to the room to assess the patient; he is in his early twenties and appears to be asleep. His BP is 102/58, pulse is 50, and his respirations are deep and even with a rate of 10. He has no indications of poor cardiac output.

12-B. Your next action is to:_____

_____.

Case Study 13

A 56-year-old woman is brought to the emergency department complaining of episodes of a "racing heart." Her vital signs are stable, and she shows no signs of poor cardiac output. When connected to a cardiac monitor, she has the rhythm shown in Figure 11-26.

Fig. 11-26

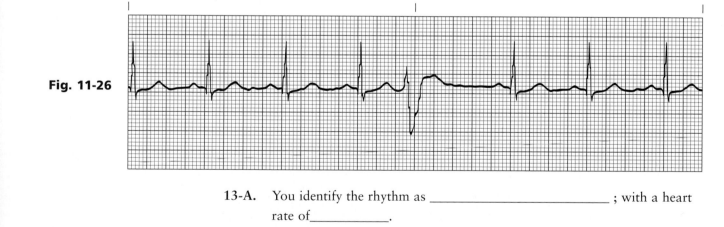

13-A. You identify the rhythm as _____ ; with a heart rate of_____.

As you continue your assessment, the patient suddenly complains of dizziness, shortness of breath, and mild chest pain. She is now pale and clammy, and her vital signs are BP 94/50, pulse 220, and RR 28.

The cardiac monitor shows the change in rhythm seen in Figure 11-27.

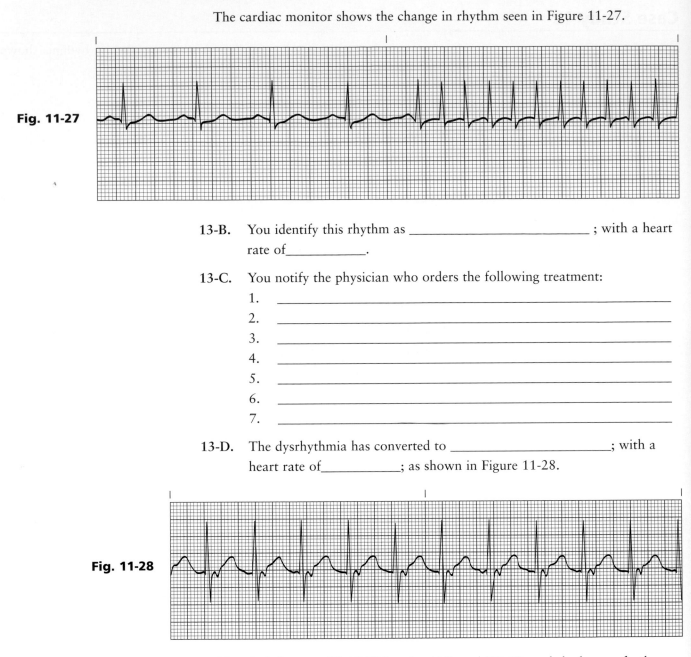

Fig. 11-27

13-B.   You identify this rhythm as _____ ; with a heart rate of_____.

13-C.   You notify the physician who orders the following treatment:

1.   _____

2.   _____

3.   _____

4.   _____

5.   _____

6.   _____

7.   _____

13-D.   The dysrhythmia has converted to _____; with a heart rate of_____; as shown in Figure 11-28.

Fig. 11-28

Her vital signs are BP 106/54, pulse 110, and RR 22, and she has no further signs of poor cardiac output. The patient continues to be monitored while being transferred to the cardiac care unit.

Case Study 14

You respond with the EMS agency to a man complaining of chest pains. When you arrive, you find the patient lying on the bed. He is pale, cool, and clammy, is short of breath, and has mild chest pains with BP 92/48, pulse 50 and irregular, and RR 26.

14-A.   These are signs of _____.

14-B.   You attach the cardiac monitor and identify the rhythm shown in Figure 11-29 as _____; with a heart rate of _____.

Fig. 11-29

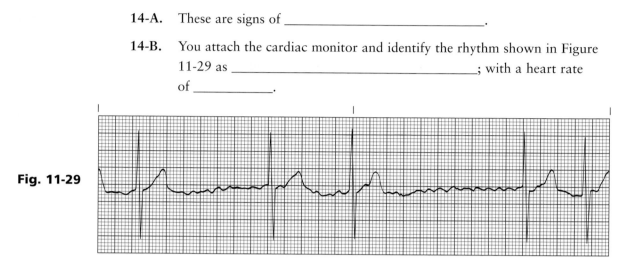

14-C.   You call a report to the hospital and start your preprinted physician orders that include:

1. _____
2. _____
3. _____
4. _____
5. _____
6. _____

You continue to assess the patient while transporting him to the emergency department. His symptoms of poor cardiac output improve, BP 105/60, pulse 76, and RR 20, and his skin is pink, warm, and dry. After arriving at the hospital, the patient is transferred to the emergency department's monitor. The patient complains that "it felt like his heart stopped for just a second then started up again." The cardiac monitor is now showing the rhythm seen in Figure 11-30.

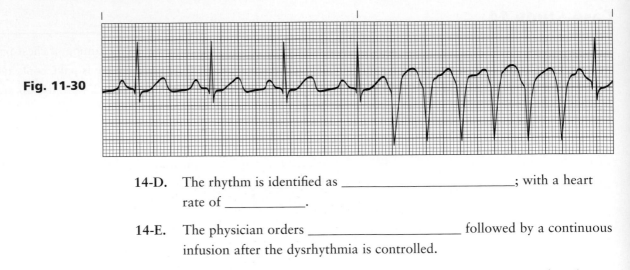

Fig. 11-30

14-D. The rhythm is identified as _____; with a heart rate of _____.

14-E. The physician orders _____ followed by a continuous infusion after the dysrhythmia is controlled.

Vital signs are BP 110/70, pulse 76, and RR 22. The patient is transferred to the cardiac care unit.

Case Study 15

A 45-year-old man is brought to the emergency department by his wife. The patient complains of indigestion, lasting 2 to 3 hours, which was not relieved by antacids. He also complains that his shoulders feel heavy and his jaw is beginning to ache. His wife states that earlier, he had been sweating a lot and vomited twice.

On your assessment, the patient is clammy, pale, nauseated, slightly short of breath, and is now complaining of chest pain. Vital signs are BP 122/75, pulse 70, and RR 24.

15-A. You identify the rhythm on the cardiac monitor (Figure 11-31) as _____; with a heart rate of_____.

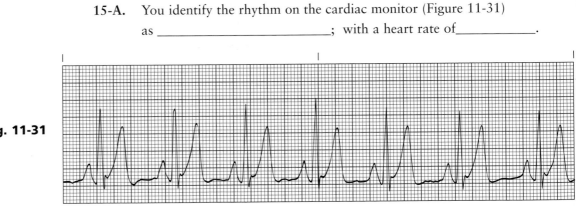

Fig. 11-31

15-B. Because your department has preprinted physician orders for the STEMI protocol, you begin the following treatments:

1. _____
2. _____
3. _____
4. _____

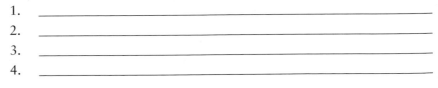
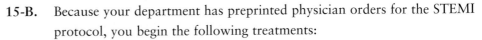

The physician enters the treatment room and examines the patient. You reassess the patient and find no change in the patient's condition, vital signs, or in his cardiac rhythm. The physician orders you to continue following the preprinted physician orders.

15-C. You have repeated the (1) _____ tablets two times without success. You administer a titrated dose of (2)_____ to control the pain.

You reassess the patient. He continues to complain of pain and shortness of breath. Vital signs are now BP 152/94, pulse 92, and RR of 26. You increase the oxygen to 4 L/min.

15-D. While the ECG is being completed, you prepare to administer an infusion of nitroglycerin using an _____, as ordered by the physician.

You reassess the patient after the infusion is started and find that the pain has decreased and the vital signs are now BP 110/78, pulse 82, and RR 20.

15-E. The physician has determined that the patient is having an acute myocardial infarction. After determining that there are no contraindications, the physician decides to begin _____.

Following hospital policy, you begin treatment by starting a continuous heparin infusion, administering a bolus of heparin and giving aspirin, unless already administered, while another nurse prepares the ordered medication.

15-F. You continue to _____ and _____ the patient and his cardiac rhythm.

The patient is transferred to the care of a cardiologist and is moved to the cardiac care unit.

Case Study 16

Your ambulance is called to the scene of a 70-kg man who complains of dizziness and difficulty breathing. On assessment, his vital signs are BP 92/46, pulse 40, and RR 26.

16-A. The cardiac monitor shows _____ ; with a heart rate of_____; see Figure 11-32.

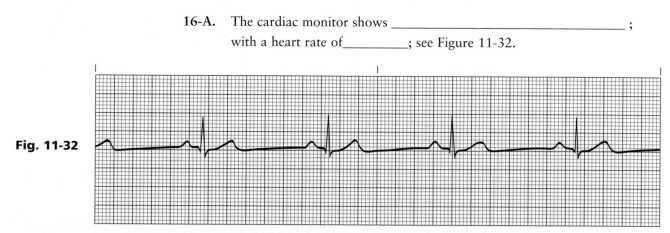

Fig. 11-32

16-B. You follow the preprinted physician orders of your institution, and begin the following treatments:

1. _____

2. _____

3. _____

4. _____

After 5 minutes, you reassess the patient and find BP 102/60, pulse 50, and RR 20. The patient states it is easier to breathe now and that he is less dizzy.

16-C. You identify the dysrhythmia now seen on the monitor as _____; with a heart rate of _____; see Figure 11-33.

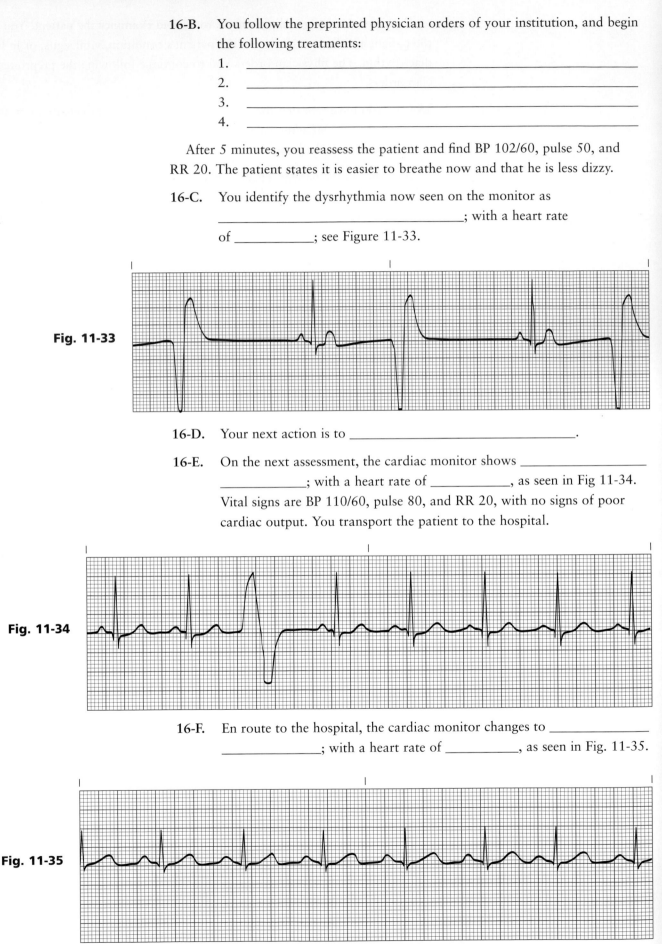

Fig. 11-33

16-D. Your next action is to _____.

16-E. On the next assessment, the cardiac monitor shows _____ _____; with a heart rate of _____, as seen in Fig 11-34. Vital signs are BP 110/60, pulse 80, and RR 20, with no signs of poor cardiac output. You transport the patient to the hospital.

Fig. 11-34

16-F. En route to the hospital, the cardiac monitor changes to _____ _____; with a heart rate of _____, as seen in Fig. 11-35.

Fig. 11-35

16-G. The patient's condition is stable. The cardiac monitor now shows

_____; with a heart rate of _____, as seen

in Figure 11-36.

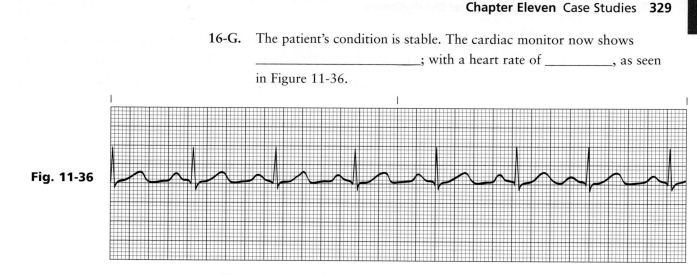

Fig. 11-36

The patient's vital signs are BP 112/70, pulse 70-80, and RR 20. You continue

transporting to the emergency department.

Case Study 17

While on duty in the emergency department triage, a woman enters and asks for

some antacid for her indigestion. During assessment of the patient, you find that

she has had "indigestion" in the mid-chest area for 2 hours. She also complains of

a toothache. She is pale and slightly clammy, with a BP of 248/112, pulse 70, and

RR 22.

17-A. You and a nurse take the patient to the examination room and put her on

the bed. You continue assessing the patient and attach a(n) _____

_____.

17-B. You identify the rhythm on the cardiac monitor as _____

_____; with a heart rate of _____; see Figure 11-37.

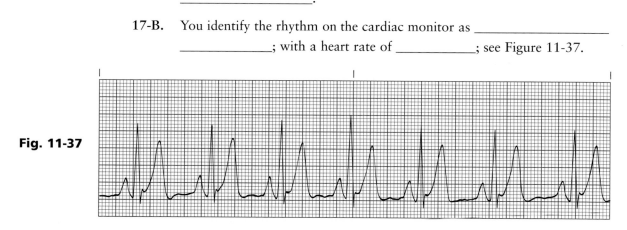

Fig. 11-37

17-C. The physician agrees with your interpretation and orders a chest x-ray

and laboratory blood tests. Following the department's preprinted physi-

cian orders, you initiate the following:

1. _____

2. _____

3. _____

4. _____

17-D.   The physician tells you to continue the MONA protocol, which stands for: (1)_____, (2) _____, (3) _____ and (4) _____.

17-E.   Reassessing the patient, you see the cardiac monitor shows _____ _____ ; with a heart rate of_____; see Figure 11-38. The patient's vital signs are BP 280/156, pulse 50, and RR 18. The patient tells you that her "toothache" is gone but the pain in her chest has improved only slightly.

Fig. 11-38

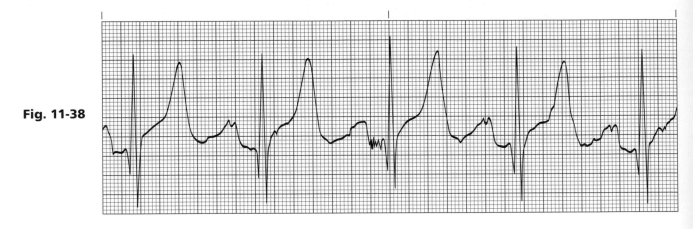

17-F.   The physician orders an infusion of _____ to control the hypertension and pain, while waiting for laboratory confirmation of his diagnosis of an acute MI.

After 10 minutes, the patient's BP is 168/90 and her pain has decreased.

17-G.   The laboratory results help to confirm an acute MI. The physician orders heparin and _____ according to the institution's policies.

The patient is transferred to the care of a cardiologist and admitted to the cardiac care unit.

Case Study 18

A patient is admitted to your unit with a diagnosis of intermittent dizziness.

18-A.   During the initial assessment, you find BP 110/70, pulse 50, and RR 16. You identify the rhythm on the cardiac monitor as _____ _____; with a heart rate of_____, as seen in Figure 11-39.

Fig. 11-39

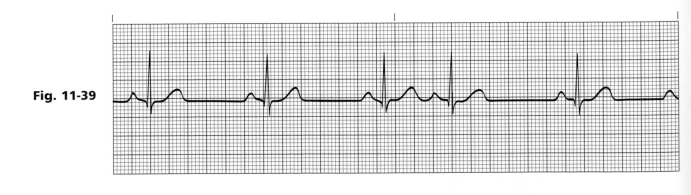

You start oxygen at a flow rate of 2 L/min by nasal cannula and an IV of normal saline according to your department's policies.

18-B. The patient complains of sudden dizziness and slight shortness of breath. The patient's vital signs are now BP 106/72, pulse 180, and RR 24. The cardiac monitor now shows _____; with a heart rate of _____, as seen in Figure 11-40.

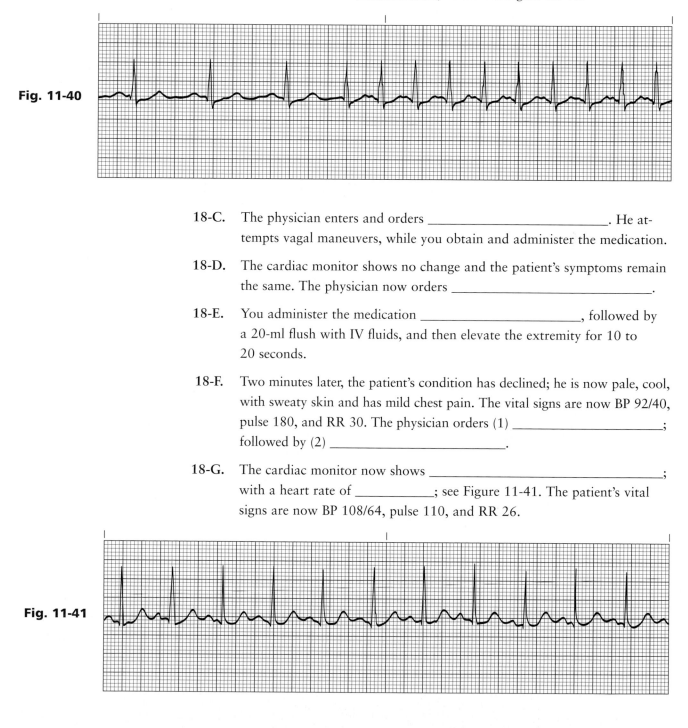

Fig. 11-40

18-C. The physician enters and orders _____. He attempts vagal maneuvers, while you obtain and administer the medication.

18-D. The cardiac monitor shows no change and the patient's symptoms remain the same. The physician now orders _____.

18-E. You administer the medication _____, followed by a 20-ml flush with IV fluids, and then elevate the extremity for 10 to 20 seconds.

18-F. Two minutes later, the patient's condition has declined; he is now pale, cool, with sweaty skin and has mild chest pain. The vital signs are now BP 92/40, pulse 180, and RR 30. The physician orders (1) _____; followed by (2) _____.

18-G. The cardiac monitor now shows _____; with a heart rate of _____; see Figure 11-41. The patient's vital signs are now BP 108/64, pulse 110, and RR 26.

Fig. 11-41

18-H.   The patient's symptoms have improved. He is flushed and has some difficulty breathing. You reassure the patient by explaining that these symptoms are normal and will disappear in a few minutes. After a few minutes, the cardiac monitor now shows _____ ; with a heart rate of _____; see Figure 11-42.

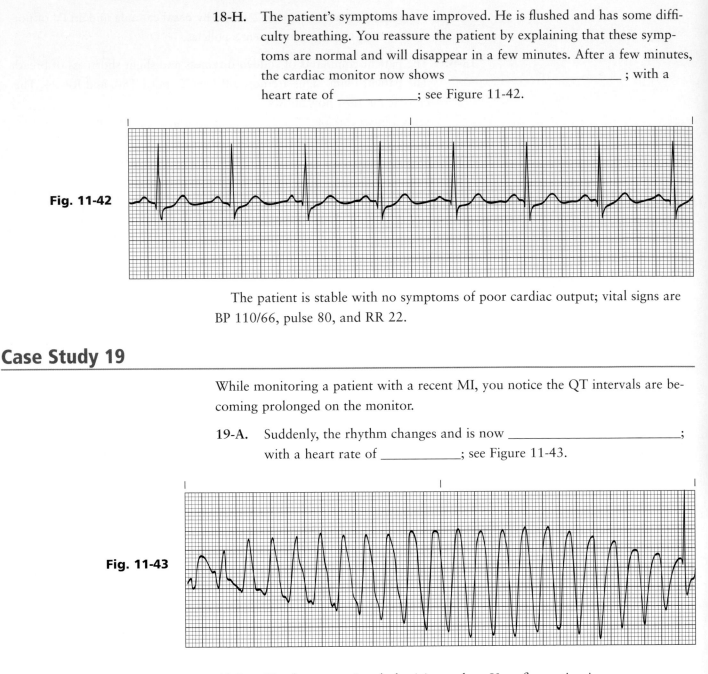

Fig. 11-42

The patient is stable with no symptoms of poor cardiac output; vital signs are BP 110/66, pulse 80, and RR 22.

Case Study 19

While monitoring a patient with a recent MI, you notice the QT intervals are becoming prolonged on the monitor.

19-A.   Suddenly, the rhythm changes and is now _____; with a heart rate of _____; see Figure 11-43.

Fig. 11-43

19-B.   You have preprinted physician orders. Your first action is to _____.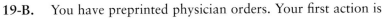

The patient is awake, complaining of some shortness of breath and dizziness, and has pale, cool, and clammy skin. Vital signs are BP 104/48, pulse 220, and RR 26. He has oxygen at a rate of 2 L/min by nasal cannula and an IV of normal saline solution.

19-C.   You increase _____.

19-D.   You administer an infusion of _____. The rhythm now changes.

19-E. You identify the dysrhythmia as _____ ; with a heart rate of _____ ; see Figure 11-44. The patient's symptoms of poor cardiac output have improved slightly, and vital signs are BP 110/52, pulse 40, and RR 22.

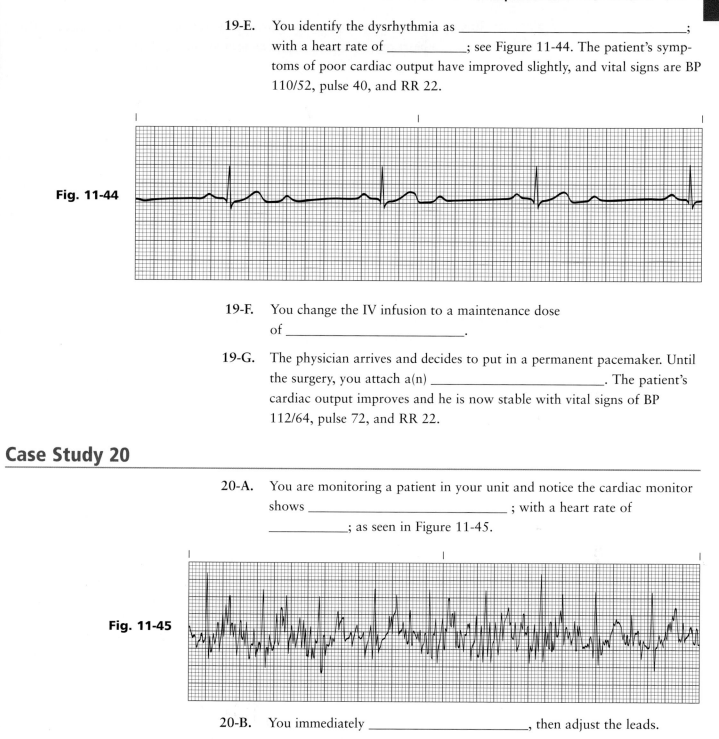

Fig. 11-44

19-F. You change the IV infusion to a maintenance dose of _____ .

19-G. The physician arrives and decides to put in a permanent pacemaker. Until the surgery, you attach a(n) _____ . The patient's cardiac output improves and he is now stable with vital signs of BP 112/64, pulse 72, and RR 22.

Case Study 20

20-A. You are monitoring a patient in your unit and notice the cardiac monitor shows _____ ; with a heart rate of _____ ; as seen in Figure 11-45.

Fig. 11-45

20-B. You immediately _____ , then adjust the leads.

20-C. The cardiac monitor now shows a new rhythm, _____ ; with a heart rate of _____; as seen in Figure 11-46.

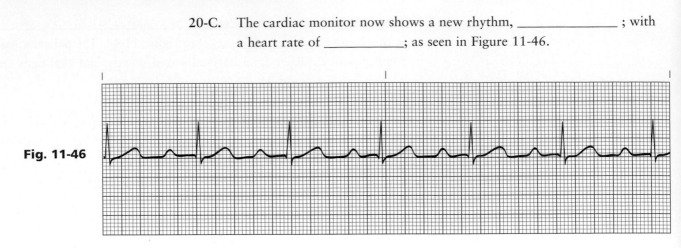

Fig. 11-46

The patient is alert and oriented with no signs of poor cardiac output. Vital signs are BP 118/63, pulse 70, and RR 16.

20-D. You _____of the change in the cardiac rhythm and continue to monitor the patient.

Case Study 21

You are treating a 75-kg patient in the emergency department for a superficial head laceration. During your assessment of the patient, he states that he "blacked out" and hit his head. His vital signs are BP 110/70, pulse 70, and RR 16. He has no signs of poor cardiac output.

21-A. You connect the patient to a cardiac monitor. The rhythm is _____; with a heart rate of _____; see Figure 11-47.

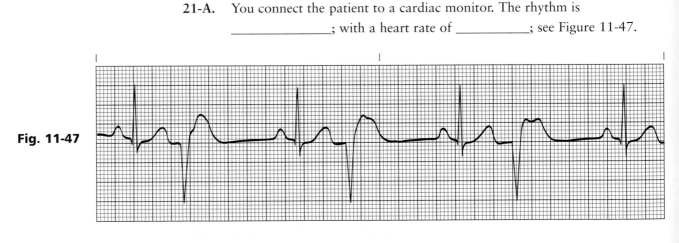

Fig. 11-47

21-B. You notify the doctor. Following the department's preprinted physician orders, you (1) _____ and (2)_____. The physician orders a 12-Lead ECG, blood tests, and (3) _____ _____.

Continuing to assess the patient, you find that his skin is pale, cool and clammy, and vital signs are BP 94/60, pulse 70, and RR 18.

21-C. The cardiac monitor now shows _____ ; with a heart rate of_____; see Figure 11-48.

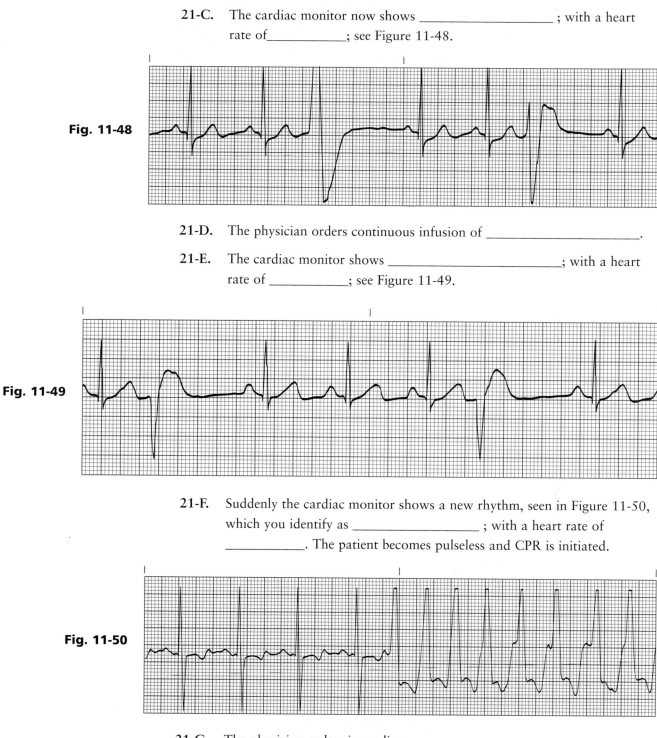

Fig. 11-48

21-D. The physician orders continuous infusion of _____.

21-E. The cardiac monitor shows _____; with a heart rate of _____; see Figure 11-49.

Fig. 11-49

21-F. Suddenly the cardiac monitor shows a new rhythm, seen in Figure 11-50, which you identify as _____ ; with a heart rate of _____. The patient becomes pulseless and CPR is initiated.

Fig. 11-50

21-G. The physician orders immediate _____.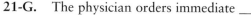

21-H. You reassess the patient, finding vital signs BP 62/40, pulse 40, and RR 14. The dysrhythmia has converted to _____ ; with a heart rate of_____, as seen in Figure 11-51.

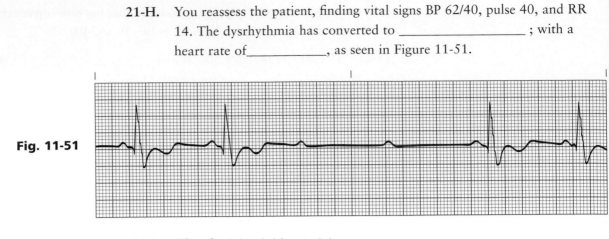

Fig. 11-51

21-I. The physician initiates a(n) _____.

The patient's cardiac output is improved, BP 108/50, pulse 70, and RR 16. He is admitted to the cardiac care unit.

Case Study 22

Your ambulance responds to a call of "man down" in a shopping mall. On the scene, a store manager comes up to you and tells you she has attended CPR and special training classes.

22-A. After seeing the man collapse, she assessed the victim and then applied the _____ when she found he had no pulse.

22-B. After the machine had defibrillated one time, the manager followed the machine's directions and began _____. After several minutes, the man began to breathe on his own and had a pulse.

Your partner has assessed the patient and attached him to a portable cardiac monitor. Vital signs are BP 60/30, pulse 30, and RR 10. The patient is unresponsive and pale.

22-C. The dysrhythmia on the cardiac monitor is _____ ; with a heart rate of _____; see Figure 11-52.

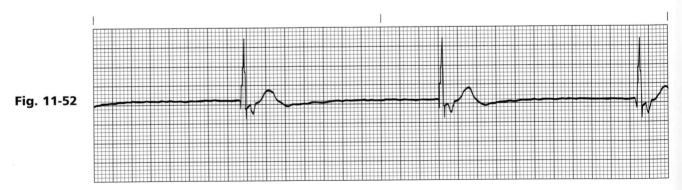

Fig. 11-52

22-D. Using your preprinted physician orders, you immediately begin the following treatments:

1. _____
2. _____
3. _____
4. _____

22-E. The patient now has vital signs of BP 100/52, pulse 50, and RR 14, and the cardiac monitor now shows the new rhythm seen in Figure 11-53 _____ ; with a heart rate of_____.

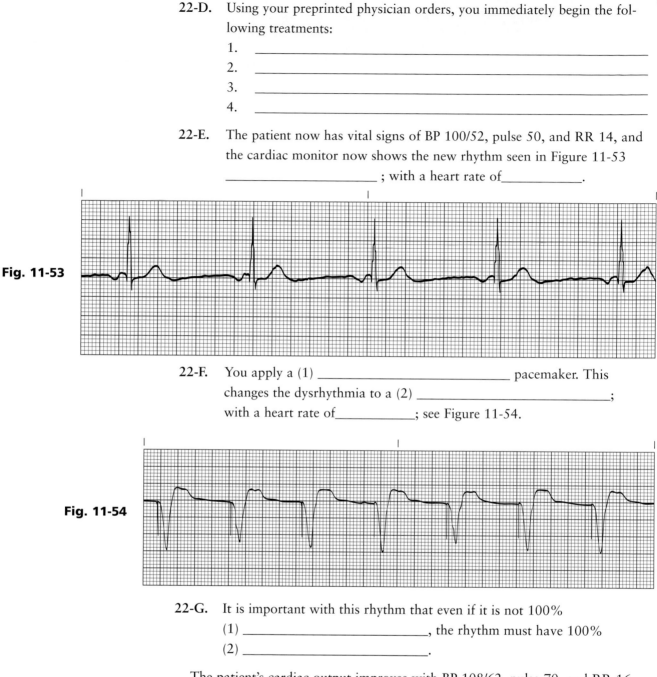

Fig. 11-53

22-F. You apply a (1) _____ pacemaker. This changes the dysrhythmia to a (2) _____; with a heart rate of_____; see Figure 11-54.

Fig. 11-54

22-G. It is important with this rhythm that even if it is not 100%
(1) _____, the rhythm must have 100%
(2) _____.

The patient's cardiac output improves with BP 108/62, pulse 70, and RR 16. You transport him to the hospital for further treatment.

Answer Section

CHAPTER 1

Review Question Answers

1. False
2. True
3. False
4. False
5. Atria; ventricles
6. (in any order)
   a. Endocardium
   b. Myocardium
   c. Epicardium
7. (in any order)
   a. Tricuspid valve
   b. Pulmonic valve
   c. Mitral valve
   d. Aortic valve
8. a. Arteries
   b. Veins
   c. Capillaries
9. b
10. b
11. Alveoli
12. d
13. d
14. d
15. b
16. a. Depolarization occurs as the electrical impulse travels through the cardiac cells, causing potassium to leave the cell and sodium to enter the cell, which causes the cell to become positively charged. This is the phase of contraction.
    b. Repolarization is the recovery stage. The potassium is reentering the cells and the sodium is leaving the inside of the cell. The cells are returning to the ready or negatively charged state.

17. Inferior and superior vena cava → right atrium → tricuspid valve → right ventricle → pulmonic valve → pulmonary arteries → lungs → pulmonary veins → left atrium → mitral valve → left ventricle → aortic valve → aorta → rest of body, including the heart.
18. Sinoatrial (SA) node → intraatrial and internodal pathways → atrioventricular (AV) node → bundle of His → bundle branches (BB) → Purkinje's fibers → ventricular muscle.
19. a. Decreased supply of oxygen in tissue cells, due to decreased blood supply
    b. Death of cardiac tissue, also called myocardial infarction (MI), coronary, or heart attack
    c. Chest pain caused by a decrease in oxygen to the heart muscle; usually relieved by rest or nitroglycerin
    d. Chest pain caused by a decrease in oxygen to the heart muscle, usually not relieved by rest or nitroglycerin; requires emergency evaluation and/or treatment
20. Any four of the following: chest pain; pressure described as a heavy feeling, a dull ache, or a crushing sensation; indigestion not relieved by antacids; pain or pressure that radiates (moves) down the left arm, into the neck, jaw, shoulders, or back; nausea; vomiting; difficulty breathing; shortness of breath; anxiety; a feeling of impending doom; ashen skin; light to extreme sweating; extreme fatigue, confusion or loss of consciousness; symptoms lasting more than 20–30 minutes

Crossword Puzzle Answers

Across

1. VENTRICLE
3. AUTOMATICITY
6. SEPTUM
8. HYPOXIA
9. CC
10. DYSPNEA
14. MURMUR
15. SA
16. PERICARDIAL
17. MYOCARDIUM
20. EXCITABILITY
21. LUNGS
23. ANGINA
25. CONDUCTIVITY
27. POLARIZATION
28. ALVEOLI

Down

2. ISCHEMIA
4. VENA CAVA
5. ATRA
7. CONTRACTILITY
11. SYP
12. VALVE
13. CARDIAC
17. MITRAL
18. HS
19. CYANOSIS
22. AV
24. AORTA
26. M

Word Puzzle Answers

B	E	N	K	L	G	P	E	R	I	C	A	R	D	I	A	L	S	A	C	N	N
F	X	S	M	A	M	N	Y	L	V	G	F	T	L	V	K	I	P	I	M	V	Q
Q	C	A	U	R	L	V	O	P	U	L	M	O	N	A	R	Y	X	T	Q	W	P
G	I	N	T	J	W	V	M	I	K	H	D	M	K	J	N	C	U	O	R	M	J
Y	T	O	P	T	Q	H	E	L	T	T	N	Y	L	Q	Y	P	L	B	P	J	M
T	A	D	E	P	W	R	R	O	K	C	Y	Q	M	X	T	T	L	U	M	Y	L
I	B	E	S	B	K	M	J	N	L	B	R	R	K	U	M	U	R	N	K	Y	H
C	I	L	G	Q	R	W	T	B	R	I	M	A	O	L	N	N	C	D	T	X	E
I	L	M	N	L	X	Q	K	K	Y	X	P	C	F	G	P	O	B	L	N	A	L
T	I	A	I	M	E	H	C	S	I	C	A	A	S	N	N	G	L	E	C	T	B
A	T	H	M	Y	O	C	A	R	D	I	U	M	T	D	I	R	B	B	O	R	A
M	Y	V	R	P	L	J	F	P	D	T	V	R	U	H	Q	D	M	R	R	O	T
O	K	P	D	T	P	N	F	R	Q	P	N	C	B	T	W	Q	W	A	O	A	S
T	V	K	C	Y	H	P	A	T	D	M	T	R	V	L	M	A	J	N	N	K	N
U	L	R	J	H	S	C	K	A	L	I	G	E	J	K	P	M	Y	C	A	Z	U
A	T	T	R	H	N	P	V	W	V	R	N	T	G	N	N	J	L	H	R	X	K
R	L	K	W	K	K	A	N	I	C	T	A	V	N	O	D	E	K	E	Y	J	W
K	B	J	Q	K	C	X	T	E	R	K	G	R	V	W	T	A	Z	S	E	T	G
T	N	B	T	A	W	Y	G	I	A	N	I	G	N	A	Q	K	I	V	N	W	B
K	C	O	N	T	R	A	C	T	I	L	I	T	Y	M	G	K	L	R	X	X	H
V	Z	E	L	N	L	L	K	L	L	D	F	C	M	R	Q	A	L	K	T	N	C
N	V	G	N	H	E	Y	K	C	M	K	N	R	X	R	V	Z	X	C	W	A	M

CHAPTER 2

Review Question Answers

1. True
2. False
3. True
4. True
5. d
6. c
7. d
8. (in any order)
   a. P wave
   b. PR interval
   c. QRS complex
   d. ST segment
   e. T wave
   f. QT interval
   g. Baseline
9. d
10. Less than one half the R to R interval of that complex to the R wave of the following complex
11. Count the number of R waves in 6 seconds, using the indicator lines on the rhythm strip. Multiply the number of R waves by 10 to get the heart rate per minute. **OR**
    Measure 6 inches of strip (1 inch equals 1 second); count the number of R waves on the 6-inch strip; multiply the number of R waves by 10 to get the heart rate. **OR**
    Count the number of R waves in 30 large squares (equals 6 seconds); multiply the number of R waves by 10 to get the heart rate.

12. a. 300 divided by 3 equals 100; 100 is the heart rate; or 3 large squares equals 15 small squares; 1500 divided by 15 equals heart rate of 100.
    b. 300 divided by 4.4 equals 68.18; heart rate approximately 68; or 4 large squares and 2 small squares equals 22 small squares; 1500 divided by 22 equals 68.18 or heart rate approximately 68.
13. (in any order)
    a. Are all PR intervals equal?
    b. Are all PR intervals within normal limits of 0.12−0.20 second?
14. (in any order)
    a. Are QRS complexes present?
    b. Do all QRS complexes look alike?
    c. Is there a QRS complex after each P wave?
    d. Are the R to R intervals equal?
    e. Are all QRS complexes within normal limits of 0.04−0.12 second?
15. d
16. Absolute refractory period occurs when the cardiac cells have depolarized and cannot transmit any electrical stimulus. Relative refractory period occurs when some of the cardiac cells have repolarized to the point where they can be depolarized again, if the electrical stimulus is strong enough.
17. i; f; d; b; j; h; c; e; a.

Rhythm Strip Review Answers

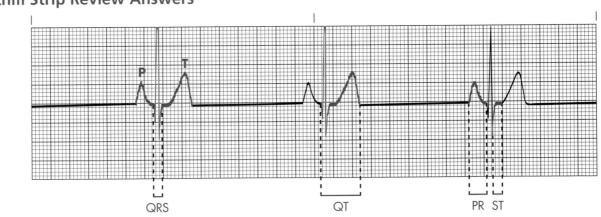

1. Identify P wave, PR interval, QRS complex, ST segment, T wave, and QT interval
   MEASURE PR interval: 0.20   Rhythm: Regular
   QRS: 0.08–0.10   Heart rate: 30
   DESCRIBE: Any abnormal components: Peaked P waves

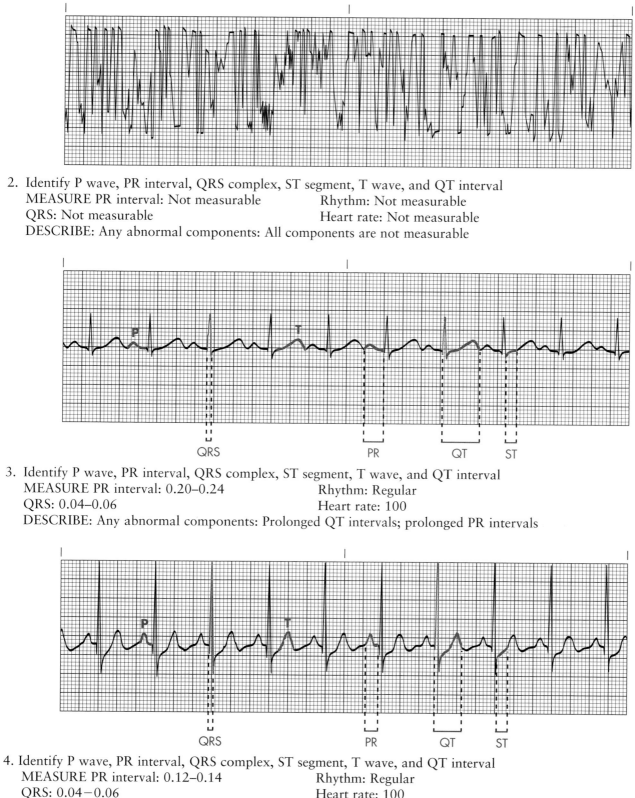

2. Identify P wave, PR interval, QRS complex, ST segment, T wave, and QT interval
   MEASURE PR interval: Not measurable   Rhythm: Not measurable
   QRS: Not measurable   Heart rate: Not measurable
   DESCRIBE: Any abnormal components: All components are not measurable

3. Identify P wave, PR interval, QRS complex, ST segment, T wave, and QT interval
   MEASURE PR interval: 0.20–0.24   Rhythm: Regular
   QRS: 0.04–0.06   Heart rate: 100
   DESCRIBE: Any abnormal components: Prolonged QT intervals; prolonged PR intervals

4. Identify P wave, PR interval, QRS complex, ST segment, T wave, and QT interval
   MEASURE PR interval: 0.12–0.14   Rhythm: Regular
   QRS: 0.04–0.06   Heart rate: 100
   DESCRIBE: Any abnormal components: Depressed ST segments; peaked P waves

Crossword Puzzle Answers

Across:

1. VENTRICULAR
4. T WAVE
8. ARTIFACT
9. DEPRESSED
10. DIPHASIC
11. ELEVATED
17. COMPLEX
18. SMALL
19. PRI
21. ATRIAL
23. P WAVE
24. ELECTRODE

Down:

2. RELAXATION
3. RATE
5. AMPLITUDE
6. QR
7. ISOELECTRIC
12. TELEMETRY
13. GRAPH PAPER
14. PROLONGED
15. REFRACTORY
16. ABSOLUTE
20. RHYTHM
22. LEADS

Word Puzzle Answers

```
P G C D E P O L A R I Z A T I O N M P K J K
L K R H P K R H N T V M Y Z X V R R J Z N T
C L K A J R R M B X L A V R E T N I T Q I X
Q E C G P G I J H J Y R T E M E L E T M F M
R N A T Y H N N F K X Q H R S P L C E W Y Q
S M M W M N P G T Q N L B T R K M K G N V F
C R P L N Z L A L E G G S L L F N V F Q U M
O E L S Q K C X P X R E N I L E S A B Y L K
M F I E L N B I L E G V M H T Y H R R B N R
P R T R M F D D R M R X A M L D G D T Q E M
L A U I L K N E E T M Y B L M E K B H Z R X
E C D W F L E N G H C Q G E R K T J L R A B
X T E D L T T D T N B E V B B A Y K O T B R
N O T A I G C R O F O A L N C E K T Y L L F
F R C E M P E A R R W L N E H P I V V O E Z
Y Y P L M V H K F T T P O M O N D L W V P C
T P Z R A T T A T I G C J R O S T W Q I E V
J E J W C Y M F S K T N E M P F I T R L R L
H R P B W N Z Z W I J R K L L M L A C L I R D
J I W X R L M G J Y C P A B E C T N K I O D
J O T N R D K W M B V J W T L E B G L M D N
T D H C H R J T J B I P H A S I C J R M V N
```

CHAPTER 3

Review Question Answers

1. True
2. True
3. False
4. False
5. True
6. 101–150
7. 0.12
8. Exactly two or more
9. b
10. a
11. c
12. c
13. c
14. Variable ventricular response occurs when the impulse that depolarized the ventricle is conducted from the atria at irregular intervals. This results in changing blocks/ratios, such as 3:1, 4:1, 2:1, etc.
15. SA node to atria (by the intraatrial pathways) and to the AV node (by the internodal pathways), to the bundle of His and bundle branches, to the Purkinje's fibers, to the ventricular muscle cells

16. Upright P wave before each QRS; all P waves look alike; PR interval measuring 0.12–0.20 second; QRS measuring 0.04–0.12 second, follows each P wave; all QRS complexes look alike; upright T waves; QT intervals less than half the R to R intervals; all P to P intervals and R to R intervals are equal; and the heart rate is between 60 to 100 per minute.
17. a. less than 60 impulses per minute
    b. greater than 150 impulses per minute
    c. varies; usually 60–100 impulses per minute
18. a. 250–350 per minute
    b. 350–500 or more per minute
19. The pause of a sinus exit block is exactly two or more cardiac cycles of the underlying rhythm. The pause would fit into exactly two, three, four, or more cardiac cycles of the underlying rhythm. The pause of a sinus arrest is more than two or more cardiac cycles. It will not fit exactly into two, three, or four cardiac cycles of the underlying rhythm.

Rhythm Strip Review Answers

1. PRI: 0.16
   QRS: 0.06–0.08
   Interpretation: Normal Sinus Rhythm
   Rhythm: Regular
   Heart rate: 80

2. PRI: Not measurable
   QRS: 0.04–0.08
   Interpretation: Atrial flutter with a 3:1 block/ratio (atrial flutter rate: 270–280; 3 × 90 = 270)
   Rhythm: Regular
   Heart rate: 90

3. PRI: 0.16–0.20
   QRS: 0.04–0.06
   Interpretation: Sinus tachycardia with prolonged QT intervals
   Rhythm: Regular
   Heart rate: 110

4. PRI: 0.20
   QRS: 0.06–0.08
   Interpretation: Sinus bradycardia with one PAC (4th complex)
   Rhythm: Irregular
   Heart rate: 50

5. PRI: 0.10–0.16
   QRS: 0.06–0.08
   Rhythm: Irregular
   Heart rate (calculated by 3-second method):
       first 3 seconds: 100 (sinus rhythm)
       second 3 seconds: 160 (PAT/PSVT)
   Interpretation: Sinus rhythm to PAT/PSVT (4th complex is a PAC) with prolonged QT intervals

6. PRI: 0.20
   QRS: 0.06–0.08
   Interpretation: Sinus bradycardia with peaked P waves
   Rhythm: Regular
   Heart rate: 40

7. PRI: 0.10–0.12
   QRS: 0.12–Greater than 0.12
   Interpretation: Sinus bradycardia with Wolff-Parkinson-White syndrome; with delta waves; with diphasic T waves
   Rhythm: Regular
   Heart rate: 50

8. PRI: 0.14–0.16
   QRS: 0.08
   Interpretation: Sinus tachycardia with prolonged QT intervals
   Rhythm: Regular
   Heart rate: 110

9. PRI: Not measurable
   QRS: 0.06–0.08
   Interpretation: Controlled atrial fibrillation
   Rhythm: Irregular
   Heart rate: 70 (atrial fibrillation rate: 350–500)

10. PRI: Not measurable
    QRS: 0.06–0.08
    Interpretation: Atrial flutter with varying block/ratio

    Rhythm: Irregular
    Heart rate: 70–80 (atrial flutter rate: 250–350)

11. PRI: Not measurable
    QRS: 0.04–0.06
    Interpretation: Supraventricular tachycardia with depressed ST segments; with prolonged QT intervals

    Rhythm: Regular
    Heart rate: 190

12. PRI: 0.16–0.18
    QRS: 0.04–0.06
    Interpretation: Sinus arrhythmia

    Rhythm: Irregular
    Heart rate: 70

13. PRI: 0.16
    QRS: 0.06
    Interpretation: Sinus bradycardia with depressed ST segments

    Rhythm: Regular
    Heart rate: 40

14. PRI: Not measurable
    QRS: 0.06–0.08
    Interpretation: Controlled atrial fibrillation

    Rhythm: Irregular
    Heart rate: 90 (atrial fibrillation rate: 350–500)

15. PRI: 0.20
    QRS: 0.04–0.06
    Interpretation: Sinus arrest in a sinus rhythm with prolonged QT intervals

    Rhythm: Irregular
    Heart rate: 70

Crossword Puzzle Answers

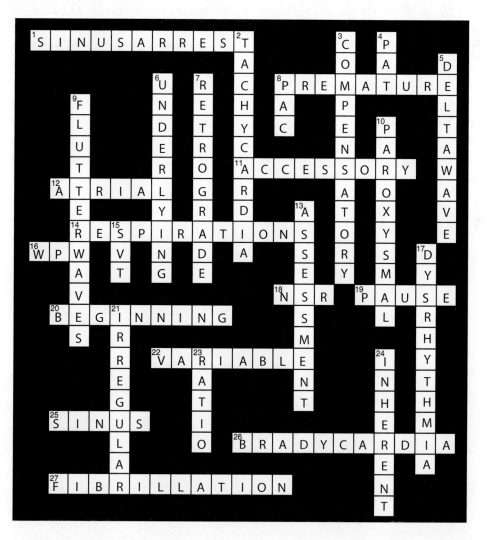

Word Puzzle Answers

```
M G M L D V K N T C A R D I A C C Y C L E Z G R
V Z L M K C O L B T I X E R L P D L F Y B M N H
Y A T R I A L F L U T T E R W M Q H F N F S I H
M B T M N K M T C P X S P F V W L R X M I R R Z
N T X H R N T V S R X L E L M F M Z L N K B E A
R N C T Y A T A C H Y C A R D I A M U G C B V C
C P M Y Q E L W G W K T Q H R F R S M O M N I C
P A E H H D V U T W L L Y P N A A L M M H Q U E
J T D R K O K L C Q V L M K M R S P D N F P Q S
T I I G L N K C N I N G B C R L E U W R B D K S
G E C N R L Y R F J R K K H N N T R N L W B L O
Q N A I L A G R K J V T Y B S Z C L O I J D Z R
R T L Y R I Z P K H G T N A R L J C F M S D C Y
M A L L G R L R N X H F T E R A K V H W T X D P
H S Y R Q T R W B M R O W R V L D T D V T J T A
L S U E L A A C I I R L E A D A Y Y S G Z K A T
T E N D L O T A M Y F S W W V H R P C G R Y P H
N S S N N I K P D U A P X R E M P A A H K V W A
K S T U S I O A L A W W C S J L S R U C R T F A
D M A K R S U Q P Y R L U W M V N R C S K D P Y
K E B F R S R G M M R N P K Z L L J V Z Y P I Z
W N L Y E D R W L X I J N C R K G W N D J L P A
P T E J Z T G P D S D E L T A W A V E K P W F P
R D N O I T A L L I R B I F N T C N T M C W F H
```

CHAPTER 4

Review Question Answers

1. False
2. True
3. False
4. False
5. 40−60
6. d
7. 101−150
8. (in any order)
   a. appearing behind (retrograde P wave)
   b. in a reverse or backwards movement (electrical impulse travels in a retrograde manner from the AV junction throughout the atria)
9. d
10. (in any order)
    a. inverted
    b. buried or hidden
    c. retrograde
11. (in any order)
    a. inverted P wave originates high in the AV junctional area
    b. buried P wave originates in the mid AV junctional area
    c. retrograde P wave originates low in the AV junctional area
12. a
13. P waves vary in size and shape, may originate anywhere in the atria, above the bundle of His; may include junctional complexes. PR intervals vary but are usually less than 0.20 second if present. QRS complexes usually measure less than 0.12 second. P to P intervals and R to R intervals vary so the rhythm is irregular.
14. Junctional tachycardia dysrhythmia has a rate of 101−150 electrical impulses per minute. The rate of an accelerated junctional dysrhythmia is 61−100 electrical impulses per minute.

Rhythm Strip Review Answers

1. PRI: 0.16
   QRS: 0.06–0.08
   Rhythm: Irregular
   Heart rate: 70
   Interpretation: Sinus rhythm with one PJC (7th complex)
2. PRI: Not measurable
   QRS: 0.04–0.06
   Rhythm: Regular
   Heart rate: 30
   Interpretation: Junctional bradycardia dysrhythmia with retrograde P waves
3. PRI: 0.16–0.18
   QRS: 0.04–0.06
   Rhythm: Regular
   Heart rate: 50
   Interpretation: Junctional dysrhythmia with inverted P waves
4. PRI: Not measurable
   QRS: 0.04–0.06
   Rhythm: Regular
   Heart rate: 70
   Interpretation: Accelerated junctional dysrhythmia with hidden P waves
5. PRI: Not measurable
   QRS: 0.08
   Rhythm: Regular
   Heart rate: 110
   Interpretation: Junctional tachycardia dysrhythmia with retrograde P waves; with prolonged QT intervals
6. PRI: 0.14−Not measurable
   QRS: 0.04–0.06
   Rhythm: Irregular
   Heart rate: 40
   Interpretation: Wandering junctional pacemaker dysrhythmia
7. PRI: 0.08−not measurable
   QRS: 0.06–0.08
   Rhythm: Irregular
   Heart rate: 80–90
   Interpretation: Wandering atrial pacemaker dysrhythmia with depressed ST segments

Crossword Puzzle Answers

Across

1. BRADYCARDIA
5. ATRIAL
7. PJC
8. BUNDLE OF HIS
11. ACCELERATED
15. WANDERING
16. AV NODE
17. UNSTABLE

Down

2. INVERTED
3. BURIED
4. TACHYCARDIA
6. JUNCTIONAL
9. SEPTUM
10. QRS COMPLEX
12. RETROGRADE
13. ASSESSMENT
14. INHERENT

Word Puzzle Answers

```
R A P A T H W A Y K H H Z P A C E M A K E R M
T I D N K I P L C J F B Q Y W F M T I F N N M
O D L N L Q N Z P L R W Z M L T L Q M X H K B
R R L V R X X V Z Y Q C R R B V R N H F M G H
X A N R Q N A N E M T Q G Y X E M N T E C K R
E C F O N R J I L R K X T L T R B H Y S M M E
L Y W E I Q S Q D D T I G R L D Q E H U W K K
E H D T H T C C F R L E O R Y M D Z R A T H A
C C J U T K C T O I A G D S Z O M P S P R G M
T B L V T Y A B M R C R M N L T W Y Y H W E E
R T K O M T R A R A P H Y V L O K N D R N N C
I L H S Z Q T G D T Y L A D P W J H L O B J A
C A R B B I H E Q T N T E K A D X W A T U R P
A N R A R Q F H H B T O W X E R H V N A R R G
L O L R T G B M L K B W C T R V B T O S I M N
I I H B B I K Q Q L H A D G L G K I N E V I
M T L P H A Q L W D M R P F K T K K T E D W R
P C T M P F Y F T X E N C T K N K N C P P K E
U N R V T L R B V L B P Q N T X D X N M W N D
L U D L B L N R E N H F J V M L T K U O A M N
S J A V J U N C T I O N M C Z X L N J C V W A
E R P C F C C M W Q K V K P N E D D I H E Z W
L K Q W Q A W W D T Q Q E R U T A M E R P X F
```

CHAPTER 5

Review Question Answers

1. True
2. False
3. False
4. True
5. c
6. b
7. c
8. 0.20

9. Third-degree heart block
10. Longer, QRS complex
11. It has no pattern and may lead to third-degree heart block, or if the block is severe enough, the rate may be too bradycardic to maintain life.
12. (in any order)
   a. Underlying rhythm
   b. Ratio of P waves to each QRS complex
   c. Frequency, or how often the dysrhythmia occurs

Rhythm Strip Review Answers

1. PRI: 0.20–0.32
   QRS: 0.04–0.08
   Rhythm: Irregular
   Heart rate: 50 (atrial rate: 80)
   Interpretation: Second-degree heart block, type I (Mobitz I or Wenckebach), with bradycardic rate

2. PRI: 0.32–0.36
   QRS: 0.04–0.06
   Rhythm: Regular
   Heart rate: 60
   Interpretation: Sinus rhythm with first-degree heart block

3. PRI: 0.22–0.24
   QRS: 0.06
   Rhythm: Regular
   Heart rate: 40 (atrial rate: 70)
   Interpretation: Second-degree heart block, type II (Mobitz II), 2:1 block/ratio, with bradycardic rate

4. PRI: 0.16
   QRS: 0.16–0.20
   Rhythm: Irregular
   Heart rate: 40 (atrial rate: 60)
   Interpretation: Second-degree heart block, type II (Mobitz II), one episode of 3:1 block/ratio, with bradycardic rate, BBB, and depressed (inverted) T waves

5. PRI: 0.20–0.32
   QRS: 0.06–0.08
   Rhythm: Irregular
   Heart rate: 50 (atrial rate: 80)
   Interpretation: Second-degree heart block, type I, (Mobitz I or Wenckebach), with bradycardic rate

6. PRI: 0.24
   QRS: 0.06
   Rhythm: Regular
   Heart rate: 20 (atrial rate: 50)
   Interpretation: Second-degree heart block, type II (Mobitz II), 2:1 block/ratio, with bradycardic rate; peaked P waves

7. PRI: 0.18
   QRS: 0.20
   Rhythm: Irregular
   Heart rate: 30 (atrial rate: 60)
   Interpretation: Second-degree heart block, type II (Mobitz II), varying block/ratio, with bradycardic rate, BBB, and depressed (inverted) T waves

8. PRI: 0.16–0.20
   QRS: 0.16–0.20
   Rhythm: Regular
   Heart rate: 60
   Interpretation: Sinus rhythm with BBB and elevated ST segments; with prolonged QT intervals

9. PRI: Not measurable (No true PRI)
   QRS: 0.12–0.14
   Rhythm: Regular
   Heart rate: 30 (atrial rate: 70; one P wave hidden in first T wave)
   Interpretation: Third-degree heart block with bradycardic rate

10. PRI: 0.24–0.28
    QRS: 0.04
    Rhythm: Regular
    Heart rate: 70
    Interpretation: Sinus rhythm with first-degree heart block

11. PRI: 0.22–0.24
    QRS: 0.08
    Rhythm: Regular
    Heart rate: 20 (atrial rate: 60)
    Interpretation: Second-degree heart block, type II (Mobitz II), 2:1 block/ratio, peaked P waves, with bradycardic rate

12. PRI: Not measurable (No true PRI)
    QRS: 0.12
    Rhythm: Regular
    Heart rate: 30 (atrial rate: 50)
    Interpretation: Third-degree heart block with bradycardic rate; with depressed ST segments

Crossword Puzzle Answers

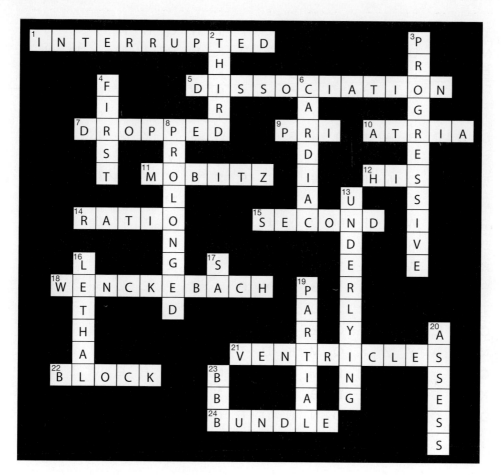

Word Puzzle Answers

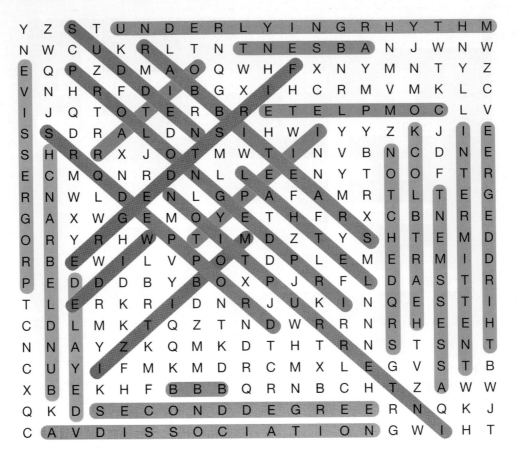

CHAPTER 6

Review Question Answers

1. False
2. True
3. True
4. False
5. False
6. 20
7. The QRS complexes of torsades de pointes begin close to the baseline, and gradually increase and decrease in amplitude, in a twisting, repeating pattern. The QRS complexes of ventricular tachycardia remain more similar in height, without the twisting and turning motion.

8. a. Different sites and different appearances
   b. Two PVCs in a row
   c. Every other complex is a PVC, with at least three episodes in a row.
   d. Every third QRS complex is a PVC
   e. When the R wave of a PVC falls on the T wave of the previous complex
9. In any order: severe heart disease, electrical shock, drug toxicity
10. b
11. d
12. d

Rhythm Strip Review Answers

1. PRI: 0.20–Not measurable
   QRS: 0.06–Greater than 0.12
   Rhythm: Irregular
   Heart rate: 110 overall (V Tach rate is approximately 225)

   Interpretation: Sinus rhythm with run of ventricular tachycardia
2. PRI: Not measurable
   QRS: Not measurable
   Rhythm: Not measurable
   Heart rate: 0 (atrial rate: 0)
   Interpretation: Asystole
3. PRI: 0.16–0.20
   QRS: 0.06–Greater than 0.12
   Rhythm: Irregular
   Heart rate: 80
   Interpretation: Sinus rhythm with unifocal PVCs, occurring in bigeminy (1st, 3rd, 5th, and 7th complexes)
4. PRI: 0.16
   QRS: 0.06–Greater than 0.12
   Rhythm: Irregular
   Heart rate: (calculated by 3-second method)
   first 3 seconds: 60 (sinus rhythm)
   second 3 seconds: 0 (V Fib; atrial rate: 0)
   Interpretation: Sinus rhythm with multifocal PVCs (1st and 6th complexes); R on T phenomenon (6th complex), changing to coarse ventricular fibrillation
5. PRI: 0.20
   QRS: 0.06–Greater than 0.12
   Rhythm: Irregular
   Heart rate: 70
   Interpretation: Sinus rhythm with multifocal PVCs (2nd, 3rd, and 7th complexes), with one multifocal couplet (2nd and 3rd complexes); peaked P waves
6. PRI: Not measurable
   QRS: Greater than 0.12
   Rhythm: Regular
   Heart rate: 310 (atrial rate: 0)
   Interpretation: Torsades de pointes
7. PRI: 0.12
   QRS: 0.04–Greater than 0.12
   Rhythm: Irregular
   Heart rate: 60
   Interpretation: Junctional dysrhythmia (with inverted P waves) with one PVC (3rd complex)
8. PRI: Not measurable
   QRS: Not measurable
   Rhythm: Not measurable
   Heart rate: 0 (atrial rate: 0)
   Interpretation: Fine ventricular fibrillation
9. PRI: Not measurable
   QRS: Greater than 0.12
   Rhythm: Regular
   Heart rate: 30 (atrial rate: 0)
   Interpretation: Idioventricular dysrhythmia
10. PRI: Not measurable
    QRS: Greater than 0.12
    Rhythm: Regular
    Heart rate: 150 (atrial rate: 0)
    Interpretation: Ventricular tachycardia

11. PRI: Not measurable
    QRS: 0.10–Greater than 0.12
    Interpretation: Controlled atrial fibrillation with one PVC (5th complex), and depressed ST segments

    Rhythm: Irregular
    Heart rate: 100 (atrial fibrillation rate: 350–500)

12. PRI: 0.20
    QRS: 0.04–Greater than 0.12
    Interpretation: Sinus rhythm with one multifocal PVC couplet (4th and 5th complexes)

    Rhythm: Irregular
    Heart rate: 70

13. PRI: Not measurable
    QRS: Not measurable
    Interpretation: Coarse ventricular fibrillation

    Rhythm: Not measurable
    Heart rate: 0 (atrial rate: 0)

14. PRI: Not measurable
    QRS: Not measurable
    Interpretation: Ventricular standstill

    Rhythm: Regular
    Heart rate: 0 (atrial rate: 50)

15. PRI: Not measurable
    QRS: Greater than 0.12
    Interpretation: Agonal dysrhythmia

    Rhythm: Not measurable
    Heart rate: 10 (atrial rate: 0)

Crossword Puzzle Answers

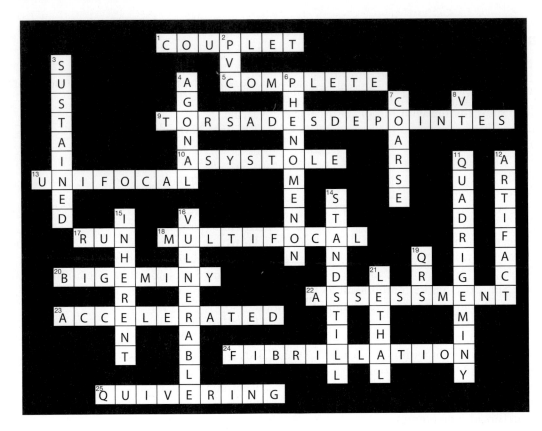

Word Puzzle Answers

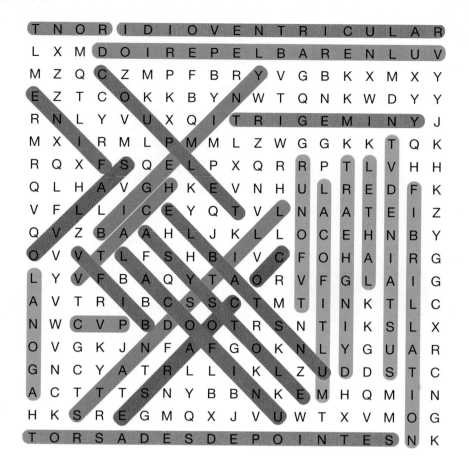

CHAPTER 7

Review Question Answers

1. False
2. True
3. False
4. False
5. False
6. (in any order)
   a. impulse generator
   b. lead wires
   c. electrodes
7. a. 75% capture indicates that one fourth or 25% of the pacer spikes on the rhythm strip are not followed by a QRS complex.
   b. 50% paced indicates that only one half or 50% of the complexes on the rhythm strip are generated by the artificial pacemaker. The other half of the impulses are initiated by the heart.
8. 3
9. d
10. d
11. 3
12. An aberrantly conducted complex is a complex that does not follow the normal pathway of the underlying rhythm and appears different than the normal complexes. It may be smaller than the normal complexes and usually appears as only a single complex.

13. (in any order)
    a. atrial pacemaker stimulates only the atria
    b. ventricular pacemaker stimulates only the ventricles
    c. sequential (dual chamber) pacemaker stimulates both the atria and ventricles in a sequential manner
    d. biventricular pacemaker stimulates both ventricles to depolarize at the same time
14. (in any order)
    a. transcutaneous—applied by means of adhesive pads, which contain electrodes, to either the chest or to the chest and back of the patient.
    b. transvenous—inserted through a large vein by means of a large needle directly into the right atria.
15. (in any order)
    a. fixed rate: set to generate electrical impulses at regular intervals, usually between 70 and 80 impulses per minute.
    b. demand rate: set to generate electrical impulses only when the patient's heart rate falls below a certain point, usually 60 beats per minute.

Rhythm Strip Review Answers

1. PRI: Not measured
   QRS: 0.06–0.08
   Rhythm: Regular
   Heart rate: 70; pacer rate: 70
   Interpretation: Atrial pacemaker with 100% pacing and 100% capture
2. PRI: 0.20
   QRS: 0.06–0.08
   Rhythm: Regular
   Heart rate: 90
   Interpretation: Sinus rhythm with prolonged QT intervals, peaked P waves, and an aberrant beat (5th complex)
3. PRI: Not measured
   QRS: 0.10
   Rhythm: Regular
   Heart rate: 80; pacer rate: 80
   Interpretation: Sequential or biventricular pacemaker with 100% pacing and 100% capture
4. PRI: Not measured
   QRS: 0.10–0.12
   Rhythm: Regular
   Heart rate: 70; pacer rate: 70
   Interpretation: Ventricular pacemaker with 100% pacing and 100% capture;
5. PRI: 0.16–0.18
   QRS: 0.04–0.10
   Rhythm: Irregular
   Heart rate: 120
   Interpretation: Sinus tachycardia with one aberrant beat (10th complex), and prolonged QT intervals
6. PRI: Not measured
   QRS: 0.12
   Rhythm: Regular
   Heart rate: 70; pacer rate: 70
   Interpretation: Sequential or biventricular pacemaker with 100% pacing and 100% capture
7. PRI: Not measured
   QRS: 0.12–0.14
   Rhythm: Regular
   Heart rate: 70; pacer rate: 70
   Interpretation: Ventricular pacemaker with 100% pacing and 100% capture
8. PRI: 0.20
   QRS: 0.04–0.08
   Rhythm: Regular
   Heart rate: 90
   Interpretation: Sinus rhythm with prolonged QT intervals and peaked P waves in the underlying rhythm, and three aberrant beats (1st, 6th, and 7th complexes)

9. PRI: Not measured   Rhythm: Regular
   QRS: Not measurable   Heart rate: 0; pacer rate: 70
   Interpretation: Pacemaker rhythm with 100% pacing and 0% capture
10. PRI: Not measured   Rhythm: Regular
    QRS: 0.04–0.06   Heart rate: 70; pacer rate: 70, 8th pacer spike not counted
    Interpretation: Atrial pacemaker; 100% pacing, 100% capture
11. PRI: 0.20–Not measured   Rhythm: Irregular
    QRS: 0.06–0.22   Heart rate: 60; pacer rate: 30
    Interpretation: Atrial fibrillation with ventricular pacemaker; with 50% pacing and 66% capture
12. PRI: Not measured   Rhythm: Irregular
    QRS: 0.08–0.16   Heart rate: 50; pacer rate: 30
    Interpretation: Sinus bradycardia with a first-degree heart block and ventricular pacemaker; with 60% pacing
       and 100% capture

Crossword Puzzle Answers

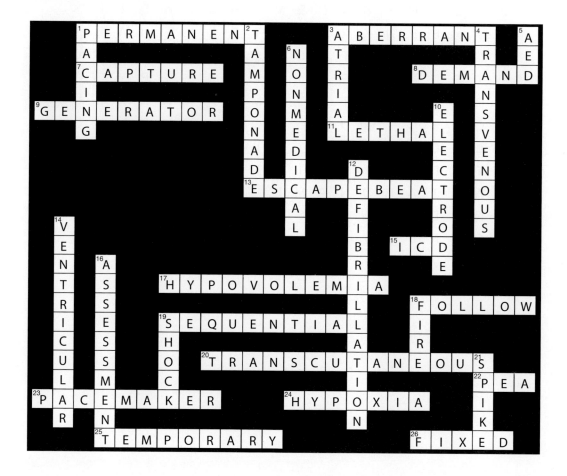

Word Puzzle Answers

```
Z E S C A P E B E A T R M F V K L D M H
F I X E D R A T E Y A V K Y Q V A G K T
E D O R T C E L E L L Z H P Z P I N B R
R N D L T E P Y U B Y R S T A A T I J A
H E N K R F K C S P C U P C B B N C R N
A K K I K D I G E S O Q E K H E E A N S
E L F D P R X R P N E M R Y F R U P N C
K R H Y T X M L E E A L P B H R Q B D U
C L U N K A V V G K A O E V T A E K J T
W L E T N F S X E E V S R S J N S T P A
H V E E P N K R J O N T E Z L T N W E N
Y L N T A A V T L L B E N R Y U R F R E
P T F R H J C E R J G L R X I T P Y C O
O R T Z T A M T K D L M N A K W R X E U
X C N T C I L D T C R Q V L T V D M N S
I L V C A X H F K I M L L P R O K A T G
A T X D E F I B R I L L A T O R R V E F
L W E T A R D N A M E D K R N N Q Z T L
M N Z D F M W P A C E R S P I K E T R Z
R C K N J Z Y R A R O P M E T W N G Z O
```

CHAPTER 10

Rhythm Strip Review Answers

1. PRI: 0.20–0.22   Rhythm: Regular
   QRS: 0.06   Heart rate: 70
   Interpretation: Sinus rhythm with first-degree heart block
2. PRI: 0.16   Rhythm: Irregular
   QRS: 0.06–Greater than 0.12   Heart rate: 80
   Interpretation: Sinus rhythm with one PVC (5th complex)
3. PRI: Not measurable   Rhythm: Not measurable
   QRS: Not measurable   Heart rate: 0 (atrial rate: 0)
   Interpretation: Fine ventricular fibrillation
4. PRI: 0.16   Rhythm: Irregular
   QRS: 0.04   Heart rate: (calculated by 3-second method)
                                                       first 3 seconds: 40 (sinus bradycardia)
                                                     second 3 seconds: 140 (sinus tachycardia)
   Interpretation: Sinus bradycardia changing to sinus tachycardia with prolonged QT intervals
5. PRI: 0.20–0.58   Rhythm: Irregular
   QRS: 0.06–0.08   Heart rate: 50 (atrial rate: 70)
   Interpretation: Second-degree heart block, type I (Mobitz I or Wenckebach), with bradycardic rate and depressed ST segments
6. PRI: 0.08   Rhythm: Regular
   QRS: 0.04–0.06   Heart rate: 220
   Interpretation: Supraventricular tachycardia with depressed ST segments; with prolonged QT intervals
7. PRI: 0.16–0.20   Rhythm: Irregular
   QRS: 0.06–Greater than 0.12   Heart rate: 70
   Interpretation: Sinus rhythm with two unifocal PVCs (R on T phenomenon 4th complex)
8. PRI: Not measurable   Rhythm: Regular
   QRS: 0.06   Heart rate: 30
   Interpretation: Junctional bradycardia dysrhythmia with retrograde P waves
9. PRI: Not measurable   Rhythm: Regular
   QRS: 0.12   Heart rate: 70 (atrial flutter rate: 260–280; 4 × 70 = 280)
   Interpretation: Atrial flutter with 4:1 block/ratio
10. PRI: Not measurable   Rhythm: Regular
    QRS: 0.12– 0.14   Heart rate: 20 (atrial rate: 70; one P wave hidden in
                                                        1st QRS complex)
    Interpretation: Third-degree heart block with bradycardic rate
11. PRI: Not measurable   Rhythm: Regular
    QRS: Greater than 0.12   Heart rate: 30 (atrial rate: 0)
    Interpretation: Idioventricular dysrhythmia
12. PRI: 0.14   Rhythm: Regular
    QRS: 0.04–0.06   Heart rate: 140
    Interpretation: Sinus tachycardia with depressed ST segments and prolonged QT intervals
13. PRI: 0.16–Not measurable   Rhythm: Irregular
    QRS: 0.06–Greater than 0.12   Heart rate: 50
    Interpretation: Junctional dysrhythmia (with inverted P waves) and two unifocal PVCs (1st and 3rd complexes)
14. PRI: Not measurable   Rhythm: Regular
    QRS: Greater than 0.12   Heart rate: 150 (atrial rate: 0)
    Interpretation: Ventricular tachycardia
15. PRI: 0.22–0.24   Rhythm: Regular
    QRS: 0.06   Heart rate: 40 (atrial rate: 70)
    Interpretation: Second-degree heart block, type II (Mobitz II), 2:1 block/ratio, with bradycardic rate
16. PRI: 0.20   Rhythm: Irregular
    QRS: 0.06   Heart rate: 60
    Interpretation: Sinus rhythm with one PAC (2nd complex)

17. PRI: 0.16–Not measurable
    QRS: 0.08–0.10 to Not measurable

    Rhythm: R to R regular; P to P irregular
    Heart rate: (calculated by 3-second method)
       first 3 seconds: 60 (sinus bradycardia; atrial rate: 80)
       second 3 seconds: 0 (ventricular standstill;
       atrial rate: 40)

    Interpretation: Sinus rhythm changing to ventricular standstill

18. PRI: 0.16–Not measurable
    QRS: 0.04–0.06

    Rhythm: Irregular
    Heart rate: 60

    Interpretation: Wandering junctional pacemaker dysrhythmia

19. PRI: 0.20
    QRS: 0.06–Greater than 0.12

    Rhythm: Irregular
    Heart rate: 80

    Interpretation: Sinus rhythm with multifocal PVCs in bigeminy (2nd, 4th, 6th, and 8th complexes)

20. PRI: Not measurable
    QRS: 0.06–0.10

    Rhythm: Regular
    Heart rate: 70 (atrial flutter rate: 280; $4 \times 70 = 280$)

    Interpretation: Atrial flutter with 4:1 block/ratio

21. PRI: Not measured
    QRS: 0.16

    Rhythm: Regular
    Heart rate: 70; pacer rate: 70

    Interpretation: Ventricular pacemaker with 100% pacing and 100% capture

22. PRI: Not measurable
    QRS: 0.06–0.08

    Rhythm: Regular
    Heart rate: 80

    Interpretation: Sinus rhythm with artifact (60-cycle interference)

23. PRI: 0.08–Not measurable
    QRS: 0.06–0.08

    Rhythm: Irregular
    Heart rate: 90

    Interpretation: Wandering atrial pacemaker dysrhythmia with depressed ST segments

24. PRI: 0.20
    QRS: 0.06–0.08

    Rhythm: Irregular
    Heart rate: 80

    Interpretation: Sinus arrest in a sinus rhythm with prolonged QT intervals

25. PRI: 0.16–Not measurable
    QRS: 0.06–Greater than 0.12
       Not measurable

    Rhythm: Irregular
    Heart rate: (calculated by 3-second method)
       first 3 seconds: 100 (sinus rhythm; atrial rate: 80)
       second 3 seconds: 0 (V Fib; atrial rate: 0)

    Interpretation: Sinus rhythm with a PVC (5th complex), R on T phenomenon (5th complex), changing to
       ventricular fibrillation

26. PRI: 0.16–0.48
    QRS: 0.04–0.08

    Rhythm: Irregular
    Heart rate: 50 (atrial rate: 70)

    Interpretation: Second-degree heart block, type I (Mobitz I, Wenckebach) with bradycardic rate

27. PRI: Not measured
    QRS: 0.04–0.06

    Rhythm: Regular
    Heart rate: 70; pacer rate: 70, 8th pacer spike not counted

    Interpretation: Atrial pacemaker with 100% pacing and 100% capture

28. PRI: 0.20
    QRS: 0.06–Greater than 0.12

    Rhythm: Irregular
    Heart rate: 80

    Interpretation: Sinus rhythm with unifocal PVCs (5th and 8th complexes)

29. PRI: Not measurable
    QRS: 0.06–Greater than 0.12

    Rhythm: Irregular
    Heart rate: 90 (atrial fibrillation rate: 350–500)

    Interpretation: Atrial fibrillation with depressed ST segments; with R on T phenomenon (4th complex)
       and run of ventricular tachycardia (4th, 5th, and 6th complexes)

30. PRI: Not measurable
    QRS: Greater than 0.12

    Rhythm: Not measurable
    Heart rate: 10 (atrial rate: 0)

    Interpretation: Agonal dysrhythmia

31. PRI: 0.16–0.20
    QRS: 0.04–0.14

    Rhythm: Irregular
    Heart rate: 110–120

    Interpretation: Sinus tachycardia with prolonged QT intervals; with an aberrantly conducted beat (11th complex)

32. PRI: 0.16–0.18
    QRS: 0.18–0.20

    Rhythm: Regular
    Heart rate: 60

    Interpretation: Sinus rhythm with BBB, elevated ST segments, and prolonged QT intervals

33. PRI: Not measured
    QRS: 0.16

    Rhythm: Regular
    Heart rate: 80; pacer rate: 80

    Interpretation: Sequential or biventricular pacemaker with 100% pacing and 100% capture

34. PRI: 0.32
    QRS: 0.08
    Rhythm: Regular
    Heart rate: 80
    Interpretation: Sinus rhythm with first-degree heart block; prolonged QT intervals; peaked P waves
35. PRI: 0.16–0.18
    QRS: 0.06–Greater than 0.12
    Rhythm: Irregular
    Heart rate: 70
    Interpretation: Sinus rhythm with multifocal PVCs (3rd and 6th complexes); with depressed ST segments
36. PRI: Not measurable
    QRS: 0.04
    Rhythm: Irregular
    Heart rate: 60 (atrial fibrillation rate: 350–500)
    Interpretation: Controlled atrial fibrillation
37. PRI: 0.08–0.10
    QRS: 0.06–0.08
    Rhythm: Regular
    Heart rate: 170
    Interpretation: Supraventricular tachycardia with depressed ST segments, and prolonged QT intervals
38. PRI: 0.16–0.20
    QRS: 0.06–0.08
    Rhythm: Irregular
    Heart rate: 70
    Interpretation: Sinus rhythm with one PJC (6th complex); depressed ST segments
39. PRI: 0.16
    QRS: 0.16–0.20
    Rhythm: Irregular
    Heart rate: 40 (atrial rate: 60)
    Interpretation: Second-degree heart block, type II (Mobitz II), 3:1 block/ratio, with depressed (inverted) T waves, BBB, and a bradycardic rate
40. PRI: 0.16
    QRS: 0.04–Greater than 0.12
    Rhythm: Irregular
    Heart rate: 70
    Interpretation: Sinus rhythm with unifocal PVCs (2nd and 6th complexes)
41. PRI: 0.20
    QRS: 0.06–0.08
    Rhythm: Regular
    Heart rate: 100
    Interpretation: Normal sinus rhythm with prolonged QT intervals
42. PRI: 0.22
    QRS: 0.06–Greater than 0.12
    Rhythm: Irregular
    Heart rate: (calculated by 3-second method)
       first 3 seconds: 80 (sinus rhythm)
       second 3 seconds: 140 (VT); atrial rate: 0)
    Interpretation: Sinus rhythm with peaked P waves; with R on T phenomenon changing into a run of ventricular tachycardia (5th, 6th, 7th, 8th, 9th, and 10th complexes)
43. PRI: 0.18–0.20
    QRS: 0.06–Greater than 0.12
    Rhythm: Irregular
    Heart rate: 90
    Interpretation: Sinus rhythm with two episodes of unifocal PVC couplets (4th and 5th complexes; 8th and 9th complexes)
44. PRI: Not measurable
    QRS: 0.06–0.08
    Rhythm: Regular
    Heart rate: 110
    Interpretation: Junctional tachycardia dysrhythmia (with retrograde P waves); with prolonged QT intervals
45. PRI: 0.16–0.18
    QRS: 0.06–Greater than 0.12
    Rhythm: Irregular
    Heart rate: 80
    Interpretation: Sinus rhythm with unifocal PVCs in bigeminy (1st, 3rd, 5th, and 7th complexes)
46. PRI: 0.16–0.18
    QRS: 0.06
    Rhythm: Irregular
    Heart rate: 50
    Interpretation: Sinus arrhythmia with bradycardic rate
47. PRI: 0.16–0.18
    QRS: 0.04–0.06
    Rhythm: Regular
    Heart rate: 50
    Interpretation: Junctional dysrhythmia with inverted P waves
48. PRI: 0.32–0.36
    QRS: 0.06
    Rhythm: Regular
    Heart rate 50
    Interpretation: Sinus bradycardia with first-degree heart block
49. PRI: 0.16—Not measurable
    QRS: 0.04–0.06
    Rhythm: Irregular
    Heart rate: (by division method)
       first rhythm: 80 (sinus rhythm)
       second rhythm: 160 (PAT/PSVT)
    Interpretation: Sinus rhythm changing to PAT/PSVT with prolonged QT intervals
50. PRI: Not measurable
    QRS: 0.06
    Rhythm: Irregular
    Heart rate: 50
    Interpretation: Wandering junctional pacemaker dysrhythmia with bradycardic rate

51. PRI: 0.12–0.16
    QRS: 0.04–0.06
    Interpretation: Sinus arrhythmia with bradycardic rate

    Rhythm: Irregular
    Heart rate: 50

52. PRI: Not measurable
    QRS: 0.12–0.14
    Interpretation: Third-degree heart block with bradycardic rate

    Rhythm: Regular
    Heart rate: 20 (atrial rate: 70)

53. PRI: Not measurable
    QRS: Not measurable
    Interpretation: Coarse ventricular fibrillation

    Rhythm: Not measurable
    Heart rate: 0 (atrial rate: 0)

54. PRI: Not measurable
    QRS: Greater than 0.12
    Interpretation: Ventricular tachycardia

    Rhythm: Regular
    Heart rate: 140 (atrial rate: 0)

55. PRI: 0.12–Not measurable
    QRS: 0.06
    Interpretation: Wandering atrial pacemaker dysrhythmia

    Rhythm: Irregular
    Heart rate: 90

56. PRI: 0.20
    QRS: 0.06–Greater than 0.12
    Interpretation: Sinus rhythm with multifocal PVCs (1st, 7th, and 8th complexes); one episode of multifocal coupling (7th and 8th complexes)

    Rhythm: Irregular
    Heart rate: 80

57. PRI: Not measurable
    QRS: Not measurable
    Interpretation: Asystole

    Rhythm: Not measurable
    Heart rate: 0 (atrial rate: 0)

58. PRI: 0.20
    QRS: 0.06
    Interpretation: Sinus rhythm with one aberrantly conducted beat (3rd complex) and prolonged QT intervals

    Rhythm: Regular
    Heart rate: 100

59. PRI: Not measurable
    QRS: 0.12–Greater than 0.12
    Interpretation: Controlled atrial fibrillation with one PVC (4th complex); with depressed ST segments

    Rhythm: Irregular
    Heart rate: 100 (atrial fibrillation rate: 350–500)

60. PRI: Not measurable
    QRS: 0.08

    Rhythm: Regular
    Heart rate: 60 (atrial flutter rate: 240–250; $4 \times 60 = 240$)

    Interpretation: Atrial flutter with 4:1 block/ratio

61. PRI: Not measurable
    QRS: Greater than 0.12
    Interpretation: Torsades de pointes

    Rhythm: Regular
    Heart rate: 220–250 (atrial rate: 0)

62. PRI: 0.16–0.20
    QRS: 0.08–0.10
    Interpretation: Sinus bradycardia with depressed ST segments and artifact

    Rhythm: Regular
    Heart rate: 50

63. PRI: Not measurable
    QRS: 0.06–0.08
    Interpretation: Controlled atrial fibrillation with depressed ST segments

    Rhythm: Irregular
    Heart rate: 90 (atrial fibrillation rate: 350–500)

64. PRI: 0.14–0.30
    QRS: 0.06
    Interpretation: Second-degree heart block, type I (Mobitz I, Wenckebach), with bradycardic rate

    Rhythm: Irregular
    Heart rate: 50 (atrial rate: 80)

65. PRI: 0.16–0.20
    QRS: 0.06–0.08
    Interpretation: Sinus rhythm with peaked P waves, one aberrantly conducted beat (7th complex), and artifact

    Rhythm: Irregular
    Heart rate: 90

66. PRI: Not measured
    QRS: 0.06–0.22
    Interpretation: Ventricular pacemaker with 50% pacing and 66% capture, and artifact

    Rhythm: Irregular
    Heart rate: 60; pacer rate: 30

67. PRI: Not measurable
    QRS: Greater than 0.12
    Interpretation: Idioventricular dysrhythmia

    Rhythm: Regular
    Heart rate: 40 (atrial rate: 0)

68. PRI: Not measurable
    QRS: 0.08–0.10
    Interpretation: Sinus rhythm with artifact

    Rhythm: Regular
    Heart rate: 100

69. PRI: Not measurable   Rhythm: Regular
    QRS: 0.08   Heart rate: 100
    Interpretation: Accelerated junctional dysrhythmia with hidden P waves; with elevated ST segments
    and prolonged QT intervals
70. PRI: Not measurable   Rhythm: Not measurable
    QRS: Not measurable   Heart rate: 0 (atrial rate: 0)
    Interpretation: Ventricular fibrillation (fine VF changing to coarse VF, changing back to fine VF)
71. PRI: 0.16   Rhythm: Regular
    QRS: 0.08–0.12   Heart rate: 50
    Interpretation: Sinus bradycardia
72. PRI: Not measurable   Rhythm: Irregular
    QRS: 0.04–0.08   Heart rate: 90 (atrial flutter rate: 250–350)
    Interpretation: Atrial flutter with variable block/ratio and elevated ST segments; with artifact
73. PRI: Not measured   Rhythm: Regular
    QRS: 0.04–0.06   Heart rate: 70; pacer rate: 70
    Interpretation: Atrial pacemaker with 100% pacing and 100% capture
74. PRI: 0.14–0.20   Rhythm: Regular
    QRS: 0.04–0.08   Heart rate: 90
    Interpretation: Sinus rhythm with depressed ST segments; with flat T waves
75. PRI: Not measurable   Rhythm: Regular
    QRS: 0.16   Heart rate: 60
    Interpretation: Junctional dysrhythmia with artifact (possible BBB)
76. PRI: Not measurable   Rhythm: Irregular
    QRS: 0.10–Greater than 0.12 Heart rate: 80
    Interpretation: Sinus rhythm with BBB, two multifocal PVCs (2nd and 4th complexes); with depressed
    ST segments and 60-cycle interference
77. PRI: Not measurable   Rhythm: Regular
    QRS: Greater than 0.12   Heart rate: 160 (atrial rate: 0)
    Interpretation: Ventricular tachycardia
78. PRI: 0.16   Rhythm: Regular
    QRS: 0.08   Heart rate: 70
    Interpretation: Sinus rhythm with elevated ST segments, elevated (peaked) T waves, and peaked P waves
79. PRI: 0.16–0.20   Rhythm: Irregular
    QRS: 0.04–0.08   Heart rate: 90
    Interpretation: Wandering atrial pacemaker dysrhythmia with depressed ST segments
80. PRI: 0.28   Rhythm: Regular
    QRS: 0.08–0.10   Heart rate 90
    Interpretation: Sinus rhythm with first-degree heart block
81. PRI: 0.16   Rhythm: Regular
    QRS: 0.04   Heart rate: 40 (atrial rate: 100)
    Interpretation: Second-degree heart block, type II (Mobitz II), 3:1 block/ratio, with a bradycardic rate
82. PRI: 0.16   Rhythm: Regular
    QRS: 0.06–0.08   Heart rate: 60
    Interpretation: Sinus rhythm with peaked P waves
83. PRI: 0.12–0.14   Rhythm: Regular
    QRS: 0.04–0.06   Heart rate: 100–110
    Interpretation: Sinus tachycardia with depressed ST segments; with prolonged QT intervals
84. PRI: 0.10–0.12   Rhythm: Regular
    QRS: 0.06   Heart rate: 70
    Interpretation: Sinus rhythm with depressed ST segments
85. PRI: Not measurable   Rhythm: Irregular
    QRS: 0.12–Greater than 0.12 Heart rate: 100 (atrial fibrillation rate: 350–500)
    Interpretation: Atrial fibrillation with controlled ventricular response, depressed ST segments,
    and one PVC (7th complex)
86. PRI: 0.20   Rhythm: Irregular
    QRS: 0.06–0.10   Heart rate: 90
    Interpretation: Sinus rhythm with depressed ST segments and one PAC (4th complex); with prolonged QT intervals

87. PRI: 0.16   Rhythm: Regular
    QRS: 0.08   Heart rate: 60
    Interpretation: Sinus rhythm with elevated ST segments; elevated (peaked) T waves and with peaked P waves

88. PRI: Not measurable   Rhythm: Regular
    QRS: Greater than 0.12   Heart rate: 220 (atrial rate: 0)
    Interpretation: Torsades de pointes

89. PRI: Not measurable   Rhythm: Irregular
    QRS: 0.08   Heart rate: 50 (atrial fibrillation rate: 350–500)
    Interpretation: Atrial fibrillation with slow ventricular response

90. PRI: Not measurable   Rhythm: Irregular
    QRS: 0.04–0.06   Heart rate: 100 (atrial flutter rate: 250–350)
    Interpretation: Atrial flutter with varying block/ratio and wandering baseline

91. PRI: 0.12–0.14   Rhythm: Regular
    QRS: 0.08–0.10   Heart rate: 100
    Interpretation: Normal sinus rhythm with prolonged QT intervals

92. PRI: Not measurable   Rhythm: Regular
    QRS: Not measurable   Heart rate: 90 (atrial rate: not measurable)
    Interpretation: Artifact

93. PRI: 0.12–0.16   Rhythm: Regular
    QRS: 0.12   Heart rate: 80
    Interpretation: Sinus rhythm with prolonged QT intervals; with peaked/notched P waves, and artifact

94. PRI: 0.16   Rhythm: Irregular
    QRS: 0.06–0.16   Heart rate: 100
    Interpretation: Sinus rhythm with three aberrantly conducted PACs (1st, 6th, and 10th complexes) and depressed ST segments; prolonged QT intervals; with diphasic T waves; with notched P waves

95. PRI: 0.14–0.16   Rhythm: Regular
    QRS: 0.08–0.10   Heart rate: 80
    Interpretation: Sinus rhythm with notched P waves

96. PRI: 0.14   Rhythm: Regular
    QRS: 0.08   Heart rate: 50
    Interpretation: Junctional dysrhythmia (with inverted P waves) with depressed ST segments and diphasic T waves

97. PRI: Not measurable   Rhythm: Regular
    QRS: 0.06–0.08   Heart rate: 250
    Interpretation: Supraventricular tachycardia with depressed ST segments; with prolonged QT intervals

98. PRI: 0.20   Rhythm: Regular
    QRS: 0.12–0.14   Heart rate: 100
    Interpretation: Sinus rhythm with depressed ST segments; prolonged QT intervals; BBB and diphasic T waves

99. PRI: Not measurable   Rhythm: Regular
    QRS: 0.08   Heart rate: 70
    Interpretation: Accelerated junctional dysrhythmia (with hidden P waves), and depressed ST segments; with flat T waves

100. PRI: Not measurable   Rhythm: Irregular
    QRS: Greater than 0.12−Not measurable   Heart rate: Not measurable (atrial rate: 0)
    Interpretation: Ventricular tachycardia (possible torsades de pointes) changing to fine ventricular fibrillation

101. PRI: 0.14−Not measurable   Rhythm: Irregular
    QRS: 0.10–0.12   Heart rate: 50
    Interpretation: Wandering atrial pacemaker dysrhythmia with bradycardic rate; with diphasic T waves and artifact

102. PRI: Not measurable   Rhythm: (Atrial: regular)
    QRS: 0.10   Heart rate: 10 (atrial rate: 40)
    Interpretation: Ventricular standstill with one escape beat

103. PRI: Not measurable   Rhythm: Irregular
    QRS: Greater than 0.12   Heart rate: 200 (atrial rate: 0)
    Interpretation: Ventricular tachycardia

104. PRI: 0.20–0.40   Rhythm: Irregular
    QRS: 0.08   Heart rate: 60 (atrial rate: 80)
    Interpretation: Second-degree heart block, type I, (Mobitz I, Wenckebach) with elevated ST segments and artifact

105. PRI: Not measurable
 QRS: Not measurable
 Interpretation: Pacemaker rhythm with 100% pacing and 0% capture

Rhythm: Regular
Heart rate: 0; Pacer rate: 70

106. PRI: Not measurable
 QRS: Not measurable
 Interpretation: Coarse ventricular fibrillation

Rhythm: Not measurable
Heart rate: 0 (atrial rate: 0)

107. PRI: 0.10
 QRS: 0.08–0.10
 Interpretation: Sinus rhythm with three PACs (2nd, 4th, and 6th complexes)

Rhythm: Irregular
Heart rate: 70–80

108. PRI: 0.16
 QRS: 0.08–Greater than 0.12
 Interpretation: Sinus rhythm with unifocal PVCs in trigeminy (1st, 4th, 7th, and 10th complexes); with prolonged QT intervals

Rhythm: Regular
Heart rate: 100

109. PRI: Not measurable
 QRS: Not measurable
 Interpretation: Artifact (loose leads, patient movement)

Rhythm: Not measurable
Heart rate: Not measurable

110. PRI: 0.12–0.16
 QRS: 0.04–0.06
 Interpretation: Sinus tachycardia with prolonged QT intervals; with artifact

Rhythm: Regular
Heart rate: 110

111. PRI: Not measurable
 QRS: Greater than 0.12
 Interpretation: Agonal dysrhythmia (possibly changing to asystole)

Rhythm: Not measurable
Heart rate: 10 (atrial rate: 0)

112. PRI: 0.24
 QRS: 0.10
 Interpretation: Second-degree heart block, type II (Mobitz II), 2:1 block/ratio, with a bradycardic rate and artifact

Rhythm: Regular
Heart rate: 40 (atrial rate: 70)

113. PRI: 0.16
 QRS: 0.08–Greater than 0.12
 Interpretation: Sinus rhythm with prolonged QT intervals, multifocal PVCs (2nd and 6th complexes), a run of ventricular tachycardia (8–12 complexes), and one junctional escape beat (13th complex)

Rhythm: Irregular
Heart rate: (overall heart rate: 140)

114. PRI: 0.12–0.16
 QRS: 0.06–0.14
 Interpretation: Sinus tachycardia with two PACs (3rd and 5th complexes), changing to PAT/ PSVT; with depressed ST segments; prolonged QT intervals; with depressed (inverted) T waves

Rhythm: Irregular
Heart rate: (calculated by 3-second method)
 first 3 seconds: 120 (sinus tachycardia)
 second 3 seconds: 180 (PAT/ PSVT)

115. PRI: Not measurable
 QRS: Greater than 0.12
 Interpretation: Ventricular tachycardia (possible torsades de pointes)

Rhythm: Regular
Heart rate: 220 (atrial rate: 0)

116. PRI: 0.10–Not measurable
 QRS: 0.08–0.16
 Interpretation: Supraventricular tachycardia with prolonged QT intervals; with two escape beats (13th and 16th complexes)

Rhythm: Irregular
Heart rate: 170

117. PRI: Not measurable
 QRS: 0.06–0.08
 Interpretation: Sinus tachycardia with depressed ST segments; prolonged QT intervals; with wandering baseline

Rhythm: Regular
Heart rate: 150

118. PRI: 0.12–0.16
 QRS: 0.04–0.06
 Interpretation: Normal sinus rhythm with wandering baseline

Rhythm: Regular
Heart rate: 70

119. PRI: Not measurable
 QRS: 0.06–0.08
 Interpretation: Junctional bradycardia dysrhythmia with retrograde P waves; with depressed ST segments

Rhythm: Regular
Heart rate: 30

120. PRI: 0.14–0.20
 QRS: 0.08–Greater than 0.12

Rhythm: Irregular
Heart rate: (calculated by 3-second method)
 first 3 seconds: 100 (sinus rhythm)
 second 3 seconds: 140 (VT)

 Interpretation: Sinus rhythm with prolonged QT intervals; with diphasic T waves; with R on T phenomenon (5th complex), followed by ventricular tachycardia

121. PRI: 0.20   Rhythm: Irregular
     QRS: 0.04–0.06   Heart rate: 60
     Interpretation: Sinus rhythm with three PACs (2nd, 4th, and 6th complexes)

122. PRI: 0.14–0.16   Rhythm: Irregular
     QRS: 0.04–0.06   Heart rate: 60
     Interpretation: Sinus arrhythmia

123. PRI: Not measurable   Rhythm: Irregular
     QRS: 0.08–Greater than 0.12   Heart rate: 90
     Interpretation: Junctional dysrhythmia (with hidden P waves), with unifocal PVCs in bigeminy
        (2nd, 4th, 6th, and 8th complexes)

124. PRI: Not measurable   Rhythm: Irregular
     QRS: 0.06–0.10   Heart rate: 80 (atrial flutter rate: 250–350)
     Interpretation: Atrial flutter with variable block/ratio

125. PRI: Not measurable   Rhythm: Irregular
     QRS: Not measurable   Heart rate: 0 (atrial rate: 50)
     Interpretation: Ventricular standstill

126. PRI: Not measurable   Rhythm: Not measurable
     QRS: Not measurable–Greater than 0.12   Heart rate: 10 (atrial rate: 0)
     Interpretation: Coarse ventricular fibrillation changing to agonal dysrhythmia

127. PRI: 0.12–Not measurable   Rhythm: Regular
     QRS: 0.06–0.08   Heart rate: 90
     Interpretation: Sinus rhythm with prolonged QT intervals and artifact (possible patient movement)

128. PRI: 0.14–0.16   Rhythm: Irregular
     QRS: 0.06–Greater than 0.12   Heart rate: 50
     Interpretation: Sinus bradycardia with unifocal PVCs in bigeminy (1st, 3rd, and 5th complexes)

129. PRI: 0.16—Not measurable   Rhythm: Irregular
     QRS: 0.04–0.08   Heart rate: 130 (atrial fibrillation rate: 350–500)
     Interpretation: Wandering atrial pacemaker with depressed ST segments; with prolonged QT
        intervals, and a wandering baseline

130. PRI: 0.40–0.48   Rhythm: Regular
     QRS: 0.12–0.16   Heart rate: 50
     Interpretation: Sinus bradycardia with first-degree heart block, depressed ST segments and BBB

131. PRI: Not measurable   Rhythm: Regular
     QRS: 0.10   Heart rate: 40
     Interpretation: Junctional dysrhythmia with hidden P waves

132. PRI: Not measurable–0.16   Rhythm: Regular
     QRS: 0.06   Heart rate: 90
     Interpretation: Sinus rhythm with prolonged QT intervals and artifact

133. PRI: 0.16–0.18   Rhythm: Irregular
     QRS: 0.06–Greater than 0.12   Heart rate: 80
     Interpretation: Sinus rhythm with depressed ST segments and one PVC (3rd complex); with prolonged
        QT intervals

134. PRI: Not measurable   Rhythm: Regular
     QRS: 0.06–0.08   Heart rate: 40
     Interpretation: Junctional dysrhythmia with hidden P waves

135. PRI: 0.16   Rhythm: Regular
     QRS: 0.04–0.06   Heart rate: 70
     Interpretation: Sinus rhythm with depressed ST segments and peaked P waves

136. PRI: Not measurable   Rhythm: Regular
     QRS: 0.04–0.06   Heart rate: 140
     Interpretation: Sinus tachycardia with prolonged QT intervals

137. PRI: Not measurable   Rhythm: Irregular
     QRS: 0.06–0.08   Heart rate: 70 (atrial fibrillation rate: 350–500;
                                                        atrial flutter rate: 250–350)
     Interpretation: Controlled atrial fibrillation changing to atrial flutter with variable block/ratio

138. PRI: Not measured   Rhythm: Regular
     QRS: 0.14–0.18   Heart rate: 70; pacer rate: 70
     Interpretation: Ventricular pacemaker with 100% pacing and 100% capture

139. PRI: 0.18–0.20   Rhythm: Regular
     QRS: 0.10   Heart rate: 70
     Interpretation: Sinus rhythm with elevated (peaked) T waves
140. PRI: Not measurable   Rhythm: Not measurable
     QRS: Not measurable   Heart rate: 0 (atrial rate: 0)
     Interpretation: Fine ventricular fibrillation
141. PRI: 0.18—Not measurable   Rhythm: Irregular
     QRS: 0.06–0.08   Heart rate: 100
     Interpretation: Wandering atrial pacemaker dysrhythmia
142. PRI: 0.20–0.40   Rhythm: Irregular
     QRS: 0.08   Heart rate: 60 (atrial rate: 80)
     Interpretation: Second-degree heart block, type I (Mobitz I, Wenckebach), with elevated ST segments
143. PRI: Not measurable   Rhythm: Not measurable
     QRS: Greater than 0.12—Not measurable   Heart rate: 0 (atrial rate: 0)
     Interpretation: Ventricular tachycardia changing to ventricular fibrillation
144. PRI: 0.16–0.18   Rhythm: Regular
     QRS: 0.06–0.08   Heart rate: 60
     Interpretation: Sinus rhythm with depressed ST segments; with flat T waves
145. PRI: Not measurable   Rhythm: Regular
     QRS: Not measurable   Heart rate: 0 (atrial rate: 70)
     Interpretation: Ventricular standstill
146. PRI: Not measurable   Rhythm: Not measurable
     QRS: Greater than 0.12   Heart rate: 20 (atrial rate: 0)
     Interpretation: Agonal dysrhythmia with artifact (60-cycle interference)
147. PRI: 0.14–0.16   Rhythm: Regular
     QRS: 0.06   Heart rate: 30
     Interpretation: Sinus bradycardia
148. PRI: Not measurable   Rhythm: Not measurable
     QRS: Not measurable   Heart rate: 0 (atrial rate: 0)
     Interpretation: Asystole
149. PRI: Not measured   Rhythm: Regular
     QRS: 0.10   Heart rate: 70; pacer rate: 70
     Interpretation: Sequential or biventricular pacemaker with 100% pacing and 100% capture
150. PRI: Not measurable   Rhythm: Regular
     QRS: Greater than 0.12   Heart rate: 40 (atrial rate: 90; P wave hidden in
                                                  ST segment of 1st and 4th ventricular complexes)
     Interpretation: Third-degree heart block with bradycardic heart rate
151. PRI: 0.12   Rhythm: Regular
     QRS: 0.04–0.06   Heart rate: 120 (calculated using first 3 seconds)
     Interpretation: Sinus tachycardia with prolonged QT intervals
152. PRI: 0.16   Rhythm: Regular
     QRS: 0.04–0.08   Heart rate: 90
     Interpretation: Sinus rhythm with depressed ST segments
153. PRI: Not measurable   Rhythm: Not measurable
     QRS: Not measurable   Heart rate: 0 (atrial rate: 0)
     Interpretation: Coarse ventricular fibrillation
154. PRI: 0.20   Rhythm: Regular
     QRS: 0.04—Greater than 0.12   Heart rate: 60
     Interpretation: Sinus rhythm with one PVC (4th complex)
155. PRI: 0.20–0.36   Rhythm: Irregular
     QRS: 0.04–0.08   Heart rate: 60–70 (atrial rate: 90; P wave hidden in
                                                  1st, 3rd, and 5th T waves)
     Interpretation: Second-degree heart block, type I (Mobitz I, Wenckebach)
156. PRI: 0.12   Rhythm: Regular
     QRS: 0.04–0.08   Heart rate: 180
     Interpretation: Supraventricular tachycardia with prolonged QT intervals

157. PRI: 0.20–0.24   Rhythm: Regular
     QRS: 0.08–0.12   Heart rate: 90
     Interpretation: Sinus rhythm with intermittent first-degree heart block; depressed ST segments,
        and prolonged QT intervals
158. PRI: 0.28   Rhythm: Regular
     QRS: 0.08–0.12   Heart rate: 100
     Interpretation: Sinus rhythm with first-degree heart block
159. PRI: Not measurable   Rhythm: Irregular
     QRS: 0.04–0.08   Heart rate: 70 (atrial fibrillation rate: 350–550)
     Interpretation: Controlled atrial fibrillation with depressed ST segments and flat T waves
160. PRI: Not measurable   Rhythm: Regular
     QRS: Greater than 0.12   Heart rate: 230 (atrial rate: 0)
     Interpretation: Ventricular tachycardia
161. PRI: 0.24   Rhythm: Irregular
     QRS: 0.06 – Greater than 0.12   Heart rate: 90 overall (V Tach rate approximately 140)
     Interpretation: Sinus rhythm with first-degree heart block and a run of V Tach (4th, 5th, 6th, and 7th complexes)
162. PRI: 0.32   Rhythm: Regular
     QRS: 0.16–0.20   Heart rate: 60
     Interpretation: Sinus rhythm with a first-degree heart block; with a BBB, and elevated ST segments
163. PRI: 0.32   Rhythm: Regular
     QRS: 0.08   Heart rate: 90
     Interpretation: Sinus rhythm with first-degree heart block, and depressed ST segments
164. PRI: 0.14–0.16   Rhythm: Regular
     QRS: 0.12   Heart rate: 40 (atrial rate: 80)
     Interpretation: Second-degree heart block, type II (Mobitz II), 2:1 block/ratio, with a bradycardic rate
165. PRI: 0.16—Not measurable   Rhythm: Irregular
     QRS: 0.12   Heart rate: 90 (atrial fibrillation rate: 350–500)
     Interpretation: Controlled atrial fibrillation
166. PRI: 0.20–0.28   Rhythm: Irregular
     QRS: 0.08–0.12   Heart rate: 70 (atrial rate: 80)
     Interpretation: Second-degree heart block, type I (Mobitz I, Wenckebach), with elevated ST
        segments, peaked P waves, and prolonged QT intervals
167. PRI: 0.20   Rhythm: Irregular
     QRS: 0.04–0.08   Heart rate: 80
     Interpretation: Sinus rhythm with one PJC (5th complex), depressed ST segments, and depressed
        (inverted) T waves
168. PRI: 0.28   Rhythm: Regular
     QRS: 0.04–0.06   Heart rate: 40
     Interpretation: Sinus bradycardia with first-degree heart block and elevated (peaked) T waves
169. PRI: 0.12   Rhythm: Irregular
     QRS: 0.06–Greater than 0.12   Heart rate: 70
     Interpretation: Sinus rhythm with depressed (inverted) T waves and unifocal PVCs in bigeminy
        (1st, 3rd, 5th, and 7th complexes)
170. PRI: Not measurable   Rhythm: Regular
     QRS: 0.04   Heart rate: 90
     Interpretation: Accelerated junctional dysrhythmia with retrograde P waves
171. PRI: Not measurable   Rhythm: Regular
     QRS: Greater than 0.12   Heart rate: 100 (atrial rate: 0)
     Interpretation: Accelerated idioventricular dysrhythmia (possible VT)
172. PRI: Not measurable   Rhythm: Regular
     QRS: 0.12 – 0.14   Heart rate: 20 (atrial rate: 60–70; P wave may be
                                                              hidden in 1st ventricular complex)
     Interpretation: Third-degree heart block with bradycardic rate
173. PRI: 0.16–0.18   Rhythm: Regular
     QRS: 0.04   Heart rate: 50
     Interpretation: Junctional dysrhythmia with inverted P waves

174. PRI: Not measurable   Rhythm: Regular
     QRS: 0.04–0.06   Heart rate: 30
     Interpretation: Junctional bradycardia dysrhythmia with retrograde P waves
175. PRI: 0.20   Rhythm: Irregular
     QRS: 0.06–0.08   Heart rate: 70
     Interpretation: Sinus arrhythmia with elevated ST segments
176. PRI: 0.20   Rhythm: Irregular
     QRS: 0.08   Heart rate: 80
     Interpretation: Sinus rhythm with elevated ST segments, one PAC (5th complex), and one PJC (8th complex)
177. PRI: Not measurable   Rhythm: Irregular
     QRS: 0.04–0.06   Heart rate: 100 (atrial fibrillation rate: 350–500)
     Interpretation: Controlled atrial fibrillation with depressed ST segments
178. PRI: Not measurable   Rhythm: Regular
     QRS: 0.10–0.12   Heart rate: 40 (atrial rate: 50; P wave hidden in
                                                                1st T wave)
     Interpretation: Third-degree heart block with bradycardic rate
179. PRI: Not measurable   Rhythm: Regular
     QRS: Greater than 0.12   Heart rate: 170
     Interpretation: Wolff-Parkinson-White syndrome with delta waves (mimicking VT)
180. PRI: Not measurable   Rhythm: Regular
     QRS: Greater than 0.12   Heart rate: 30 (atrial rate: 0)
     Interpretation: Idioventricular dysrhythmia
181. PRI: 0.16–0.20   Rhythm: Irregular
     QRS: 0.06   Heart rate: 60 (calculated by 3-second method)
     Interpretation: Sinus rhythm with PJC (4th complex)
182. PRI: Not measurable   Rhythm: Irregular
     QRS: 0.04–0.06   Heart rate: 170 (atrial fibrillation rate: 350–500)
     Interpretation: Uncontrolled atrial fibrillation with elevated ST segments
183. PRI: 0.16–0.20   Rhythm: Regular
     QRS: 0.04–0.06   Heart rate: 40
     Interpretation: Sinus bradycardia
184. PRI: 0.20—Not measurable   Rhythm: Irregular
     QRS: 0.04–Greater than 0.12   Heart rate: 80 (calculated by 3-second method)
     Interpretation: Sinus rhythm with a PVC (4th complex, escape beat), changing to junctional dysrhythmia
185. PRI: 0.08   Rhythm: Regular
     QRS: Greater than 0.12   Heart rate: 50
     Interpretation: Wolff-Parkinson-White syndrome with bradycardia and delta waves
186. PRI: 0.20–Not measurable   Rhythm: Irregular
     QRS: 0.12–Greater than 0.12   Heart rate: 107–160 (Sinus tachycardia rate: 107 by
                                                                division method; VT rate: 160 by 3-second strip)
     Interpretation: Sinus tachycardia with prolonged QT intervals, changing to ventricular tachycardia
187. PRI: Not measurable   Rhythm: Irregular
     QRS: 0.04–Greater than 0.12   Heart rate: 90 (atrial flutter rate: 250–350)
     Interpretation: Atrial flutter with varying block/ratio; with two PVCs (4th and 7th complexes); with
        elevated ST segments
188. PRI: 0.18–0.20   Rhythm: Irregular
     QRS: 0.06–0.20   Heart rate: 80
     Interpretation: Sinus rhythm with elevated ST segments and aberrantly conducted complexes in
        bigeminy (1st, 3rd, 5th, and 7th complexes); with prolonged QT intervals
189. PRI: Not measurable   Rhythm: Regular
     QRS: 0.08–0.10   Heart rate: 40 (atrial rate: 100; P waves hidden in
                                                                1st and 2nd QRS complexes, and in 3rd T wave)
     Interpretation: Third-degree heart block with elevated (peaked) T waves; with bradycardic rate
190. PRI: Not measurable   Rhythm: Irregular
     QRS: 0.04–0.08   Heart rate: 100 (atrial flutter rate: 250–350)
     Interpretation: Atrial flutter with varying block/ratio

191. PRI: 0.08–0.12
     QRS: 0.08–0.10
     Interpretation: Sinus arrhythmia

     Rhythm: Irregular
     Heart rate: 60

192. PRI: 0.20—Not measured
     QRS: 0.04–Greater than 0.12
     Interpretation: Sinus rhythm with diphasic T waves and one PVC (4th complex), and two ventricular pacer spikes (5th and 6th complexes): 33% pacing and 100% capture

     Rhythm: Irregular
     Heart rate: 70; pacer rate: 20

193. PRI: Not measured
     QRS: 0.20
     Interpretation: Ventricular (possible biventricular) pacemaker with 100% pacing and 100% capture

     Rhythm: Regular
     Heart rate: 70; pacer rate: 70

194. PRI: Not measured
     QRS: 0.08–0.16
     Interpretation: Ventricular pacemaker with 100% pacing and with 60% capture; with bradycardic rate

     Rhythm: Regular
     Heart rate: 50; pacer rate: 50

195. PRI: Not measured
     QRS: 0.16
     Interpretation: Ventricular pacemaker with 100% pacing and 37% capture

     Rhythm: Regular
     Heart rate: 30−0; pacer rate: 70

196. PRI: Not measured
     QRS: 0.08–0.18
     Interpretation: Ventricular pacemaker with 86% pacing and 75% capture

     Rhythm: Regular
     Heart rate: 70; pacer rate: 80

197. PRI: Not measured
     QRS: 0.12–0.18
     Interpretation: Atrial pacemaker with 100% pacing and 86% capture

     Rhythm: Regular
     Heart rate: 60; pacer rate: 70

198. PRI: Not measured
     QRS: 0.16
     Interpretation: Ventricular pacemaker with 100% pacing and 100% capture

     Rhythm: Regular
     Heart rate: 70; pacer rate: 70

199. PRI: Not measured
     QRS: 0.16
     Interpretation: Sequential or biventricular pacemaker with 100% pacing and 100% capture

     Rhythm: Regular
     Heart rate: 70; pacer rate: 70

200. PRI: Not measurable
     QRS: 0.14–Greater than 0.12
     Interpretation: Uncontrolled atrial fibrillation and Wolff-Parkinson-White syndrome with delta waves (mimicking ventricular tachycardia)

     Rhythm: Irregular
     Heart rate: 210 (atrial fibrillation rate: 350–500)

CHAPTER 11

Case Study 1

1-A Sinus tachycardia with depressed ST segments and prolonged QT intervals; HR, 140.
1-B (in any order)
   1. Reassure the patient and listen to her fears. Inform her of the possibility that anxiety and caffeine can cause a rapid heartbeat and palpitations.
   2. Notify the physician.
   3. Continue to monitor the patient.
   4. Consider using relaxation techniques.
1-C Sinus rhythm with prolonged QT intervals and peaked P waves; HR, 100.

Case Study 2

2-A Sinus bradycardia with depressed ST segments; HR, 40.
2-B 1. Assess airway, breathing, and circulation.
   2. Provide oxygen and apply pulse oximetry.
   3. Start an IV infusion.

   4. Request a 12-lead ECG.
   5. Notify the physician.
   6. Administer atropine 0.5 mg IV push.
2-C Atropine 0.5 mg IV push at 3- to 5-minute intervals, until the maximum dose of 3 mg has been given.
2-D Temporary pacemaker (transcutaneous or transvenous).
2-E Epinephrine or dopamine.
2-F Paced rhythm; HR, 70.
2-G 1. 100%.
   2. Paced.

Case Study 3

3-A Sinus rhythm with unifocal PVCs; HR, 70.
3-B Junctional dysrhythmia (with inverted P waves) and unifocal PVCs; HR, 50.
3-C 1. Assess airway, breathing, and circulation.
   2. Provide oxygen and apply pulse oximetry.
   3. Start an IV infusion.
   4. Request a 12-lead ECG.

3-D Administer atropine 0.5 mg IV push.

3-E Sinus rhythm with multifocal PVCs in bigeminy; HR, 80.

3-F Lidocaine 0.5 to 0.75 mg/kg up to 1 to 1.5 mg/kg, IV push.

3-G (in any order)
1. More than 6 PVCs in one minute.
2. Multifocal PVCs.
3. Couplets.
4. R on T phenomenon.
5. Runs of ventricular tachycardia.

Case Study 4

4-A Supraventricular tachycardia with depressed ST segments and prolonged QT intervals; HR, 170.

4-B
1. Assess airway, breathing, and circulation.
2. Provide oxygen and apply pulse oximetry.
3. Start an IV infusion.
4. Attempt vagal maneuvers.
5. Request a 12-lead ECG.
6. Consider sedation.
7. Perform immediate synchronized cardioversion.

4-C Synchronized.

4-D Sinus rhythm with prolonged QT intervals; HR, 70.

Case Study 5

5-A Sinus tachycardia with depressed ST segments; prolonged QT intervals; possible peaked P waves; HR, 100 to 110.

5-B
1. Assess airway, breathing, and circulation.
2. Place the patient in a position of rest.
3. Provide oxygen and apply pulse oximetry.
4. Offer cool fluids to drink, or start an IV infusion.
5. Continue monitoring the patient.

5-C Normal sinus rhythm with prolonged QT intervals; HR, 100.

Case Study 6

6-A Second-degree heart block, type II (Mobitz II), 3:1 block/ratio; HR, 40 (atrial rate: 100 to 120).

6-B
1. Assess airway, breathing, and circulation.
2. Provide oxygen and apply pulse oximetry.
3. Start an IV infusion.
4. Request an ECG.

6-C Third-degree heart block; HR, 40 (atrial rate: 90).

6-D Temporary pacemaker (transcutaneous or transvenous).

Case Study 7

7-A Ventricular tachycardia changing to Ventricular fibrillation; HR, not measurable.

7-B Assess the patient.

7-C
1. Check the telemetry leads and electrodes, change any electrode that is dry, and reconnect any loose leads.
2. Continue monitoring the patient.

Case Study 8

8-A Sinus rhythm with elevated (peaked) T waves; HR, 60 to 70.

8-B Pulseless electrical activity (PEA).

8-C
1. Begin CPR.
2. Provide 100% oxygen by bag-mask device and intubate as soon as possible; apply pulse oximetry.
3. Start an IV/IO infusion.
4. Obtain an ECG, if available.
5. Consider common causes of PEA.
6. Administer epinephrine 1 mg IV/IO push every 3 to 5 minutes or vasopressin 40 units IV/IO (one dose only) to replace the 1st or 2nd dose of epinephrine.
7. Reassess the patient.
8. Consider atropine 1 mg IV/IO push, if monitor shows a heart rate less than 60. May give every 3 to 5 minutes, up to 3 doses, alternating with epinepherine

8-D Cardiac tamponade.

8-E Any three of the following:
1. Hypovolemia; give fluids.
2. Hypoxia; increase ventilations and oxygen.
3. Tension pneumothorax; perform needle decompression.
4. Acidosis; give sodium bicarbonate according to ABG results.
5. Hypokalemia or hyperkalemia; treat according to laboratory results.
6. Drug overdose; treat according to protocol.
7. Cardiac tamponade; pericardiocentesis.
8. Hypothermia; treat according to protocol.
9. Coronary or pulmonary thrombosis; treatment based on patient's condition.
10. Hypoglycemia; treatment based on blood sugar results.
11. Trauma; treatment based on extent of injuries.
12. Cardiac muscle is too damaged to contract; no treatment available.

8-F Second-degree heart block, type I (Mobitz I, Wenckebach); HR, 50 (atrial rate: 80).

8-G Observe the patient for any change in the dysrhythmia or in cardiac output.

Case Study 9

9-A   Torsades de pointes; HR, 220 to 230.

9-B   Any five of the following:
Pale, cool, clammy skin; nausea; vomiting; dizziness, weakness; shortness of breath; sudden decrease in blood pressure; dyspnea; severe chest pain; cyanosis; confusion or disorientation; decreased urinary output; unresponsiveness.

9-C   1.   Continue oxygen and apply pulse oximetry.
2.   Consider sedation, if patient is conscious.
3.   Consider synchronized cardioversion as soon as possible.
4.   Reassess the patient.

9-D   Sinus rhythm with first-degree heart block, prolonged QT intervals and peaked P waves; HR, 80.

Case Study 10

10-A   Second-degree heart block, type I (Mobitz I, Wenckebach) with depressed ST segments; HR, 50 (atrial rate: 70).

10-B   1.   Notify the physician.
2.   Continue to monitor the patient.
3.   Obtain an ECG.

10-C   Second-degree heart block, type II (Mobitz II), 2:1 block/ratio; HR, 40 (atrial rate: 70).

10-D   1.   Increase oxygen and apply pulse oximetry.
2.   Prepare for temporary pacemaker (transcutaneous or transvenous), if available.
3.   Consider atropine 0.5 mg IV push; repeat every 3 to 5 minutes until maximum dosage (3 mg) is given, until pacemaker is available.
4.   Consider epinephrine 2 to 10 mcg/min or dopamine 2 to 10 mcg/min by continuous IV infusion, while waiting for pacemaker.

10-E   Pacemaker rhythm; HR, 70.

10-F   1.   Paced.
2.   Capture.

Case Study 11

11-A   Cardiac output.

11-B   Sinus rhythm with depressed ST segments, a PVC (R on T), and peaked and notched P waves; HR, 80.

11-C   1.   Provide oxygen and apply pulse oximetry.
2.   Start an IV infusion.
3.   Begin "MONA" protocol.
4. Request an ECG.

11-D   Coarse ventricular fibrillation; HR, not measurable.

11-E   1.   Begin CPR; continue CPR until defibrillator is available.
2.   Defibrillate one time and resume CPR immediately.
3.   Administer 100% oxygen by bag-mask device and intubate as soon as possible.

4.   Reassess the patient after 2 minutes of CPR (5 cycles).
5.   Defibrillate one time and resume CPR immediately.
6.   Reassess the patient after 2 minutes of CPR (5 cycles). Administer epinephrine 1 mg IV/IO push every 3 to 5 minutes or vasopressin 40 units IV/IO (one dose only) to replace the 1st or 2nd dose of epinephrine.
7.   Defibrillate one time and resume CPR immediately.
8.   Reassess the patient after 2 minutes of CPR (5 cycles). Administer amiodarone 300 mg IV/IO push; repeat according to protocol until the maximum dose has been given; if lidocaine is used instead, follow the lidocaine protocol.
9.   Continue defibrillation between drugs and CPR.
10. When the patient has a pulse, start an infusion drip of the medication that was successful in ending the V Fib.

11-F   Sinus rhythm with prolonged QT intervals, bundle branch block, peaked and notched P waves; HR, 80.

Case Study 12

12-A   Sinus bradycardia with depressed ST segments, peaked P waves and artifact; HR, 40 to 50.

12-B   Continue to observe the patient and monitor for any changes. It is normal for young adults to have a bradycardic rate during sleep.

Case Study 13

13-A   Sinus rhythm with PVC; HR, 80.

13-B   Sinus rhythm changing to PAT/PSVT; HR, 80 to 220.

13-C   1.   Assess airway, breathing, and circulation.
2.   Provide oxygen and apply pulse oximetry.
3.   Start an IV infusion.
4.   Attempt vagal maneuvers.
5.   Request an ECG.
6.   Consider sedation.
7.   Perform immediate synchronized cardioversion.

13-D   Junctional tachycardia (with retrograde P waves) and prolonged QT intervals; HR, 110.

Case Study 14

14-A   Poor cardiac output.

14-B   Atrial fibrillation with slow ventricular response; HR, 50 (atrial rate: 350 to 500).

14-C   1.   Provide oxygen and apply pulse oximetry, if available.
2.   Start an IV infusion.

3. Obtain an ECG, if available.
4. Administer atropine 0.5 mg IV push every 3 to 5 minutes, until a total of 3 mg has been given.
5. Continue to observe and monitor the patient.
6. Consider temporary pacemaker (transcutaneous or transvenous), if symptoms continue.

14-D Sinus rhythm with R on T phenomenon and a run of ventricular tachycardia; HR, 110 overall.

14-E An antidysrhythmic, such as Lidocaine, Amiodarone, or Procainamide.

Case Study 15

15-A Sinus rhythm with elevated ST segments, elevated (peaked) T waves and peaked P waves; HR, 70.

15-B 1. Provide oxygen and apply pulse oximetry.
2. Start an IV infusion.
3. Request an ECG.
4. Begin "MONA" protocol. Be prepared to administer: aspirin, oxygen, nitroglycerin, and morphine sulfate.

15-C 1. Nitroglycerin at 0.3 to 0.4 mg sublingual (at 5-minute intervals) until 3 doses have been administered.
2. Morphine sulfate at 1 to 5 mg IV over 1 to 5 minutes.

15-D Infusion pump.

15-E Fibrinolytic therapy (or PCI) if available.

15-F Assess and monitor.

Case Study 16

16-A Sinus bradycardia; HR, 40.

16-B 1. Provide oxygen and apply pulse oximetry.
2. Start an IV infusion.
3. Obtain an ECG, if available.
4. Administer atropine 0.5 mg IV push.

16-C Sinus bradycardia with bigeminy of unifocal PVCs; HR, 50.

16-D Repeat atropine 0.5 mg IV push, until a total dose of 3 mg has been given.

16-E Sinus rhythm with one PVC; HR, 80.

16-F Normal sinus rhythm; HR 80.

16-G Normal sinus rhythm; HR 80.

Case Study 17

17-A Cardiac monitor.

17-B Sinus rhythm with elevated ST segments, elevated (peaked) T waves, and peaked P waves; HR, 70.

17-C 1. Provide oxygen and apply pulse oximetry.
2. Start an IV infusion.
3. Request an ECG.
4. Prepare to initiate MONA protocol.

17-D 1. Morphine.
2. Oxygen.
3. Nitroglycerin.
4. Aspirin.

17-E Sinus bradycardia with elevated ST segments, prolonged QT intervals, elevated (peaked) T waves, peaked and notched P waves; HR, 50.

17-F Nitroglycerin 10 to 20 mcg/min, titrated to pain relief and improvement of blood pressure.

17-G Fibrinolytic therapy (or PCI) if available.

Case Study 18

18-A Sinus bradycardia with PAC; HR, 50.

18-B Sinus rhythm changing to PAT/PSVT, with prolonged QT intervals; HR, 80 to 180.

18-C Adenosine 6 mg rapid IV push.

18-D Adenosine 12 mg IV push.

18-E Rapidly.

18-F 1. Sedation.
2. Immediate synchronized cardioversion.

18-G Sinus tachycardia with prolonged QT intervals; HR, 110.

18-H Sinus rhythm with depressed ST segments; HR, 80.

Case Study 19

19-A Torsades de pointes; HR, 220.

19-B Assess the patient.

19-C The oxygen to 100% by using a nonrebreather mask with reservoir, and apply pulse oximetry.

19-D Magnesium sulfate 1 to 2 g in 50 to 100 ml IV fluid titrated over 5 to 60 minutes.

19-E Second-degree heart block, type II (Mobitz II), 2:1 block/ratio; HR, 40 (atrial rate: 70).

19-F Magnesium sulfate 0.5 to 1 g/hr IV, titrated to control torsades de pointes.

19-G Temporary pacemaker (transcutaneous or transvenous).

Case Study 20

20-A Artifact; HR, 90 (atrial rate not measurable).

20-B Assess the patient.

20-C Sinus rhythm with first-degree heart block; HR, 70.

20-D Notify the physician.

Case Study 21

21-A Sinus rhythm with unifocal PVCs in bigeminy; HR, 70.

21-B 1. Provide oxygen and apply pulse oximetry.
     2. Start an IV infusion.
     3. Lidocaine 0.5 to 0.75 mg/kg up to 1 to 1.5 mg/kg, IV push.

21-C Sinus rhythm with depressed ST segments and multifocal PVCs; HR, 70.

21-D Lidocaine.

21-E Sinus rhythm with unifocal PVCs; HR, 70.

21-F Sinus rhythm with prolonged QT intervals, diphasic T waves, and R on T phenomenon progressing to ventricular tachycardia; HR, 120 overall.

21-G Defibrillation.

21-H Second-degree heart block, type II (Mobitz II), with one episode of a 3:1 block/ratio; HR, 40 (atrial rate: 60).

21-I Temporary pacemaker (transcutaneous or transvenous).

Case Study 22

22-A Automated external defibrillator (AED).

22-B CPR.

22-C Junctional bradycardia dysrhythmia with retrograde P waves; HR, 30.

22-D 1. Provide oxygen and apply pulse oximetry.
     2. Start an IV infusion.
     3. Obtain an ECG, if available.
     4. Administer atropine 0.5 mg IV push.

22-E Junctional dysrhythmia with inverted P waves; HR, 50.

22-F 1. Temporary or transcutaneous.
     2. Pacemaker rhythm, HR, 70.

22-G 1. Paced.
     2. Capture.

Glossary

Aberrant Different than normal; may refer to individual complexes or entire rhythm

Aberrantly conducted complexes Single complexes that appear different than the underlying rhythm because they do not follow the same conduction pathway

Absolute bradycardia Cardiac dysrhythmia with a heart rate less than 60 electrical impulses per minute

Absolute refractory period Time in the cardiac cycle when the myocardial cells have not completed repolarization and cannot conduct an electrical impulse; from Q wave to the first half of the T wave

Accelerated idioventricular dysrhythmia Life threatening dysrhythmia that occurs when the electrical impulses originate from a single site in the ventricles at a rate between 41 and 100 impulses per minute

Accelerated junctional dysrhythmia Dysrhythmia that occurs when all the electrical impulses originate from a single site within the atrioventricular junctional area at a rate between 61 and 100 impulses per minute

Accessory pathway Additional or abnormal electrical conduction pathway; example: the bundle of Kent or Kent bundle, is found in Wolff-Parkinson-White syndrome (WPW)

ACE inhibitors Medications that increase cardiac output, lower blood pressure, reduce sodium and water retention (edema)

Acidosis The presence of too much hydrogen in the body, usually caused by an increase in the amount of acid; may result from respiratory problems, kidney failure, or diabetes

Acute Sudden, recent onset of signs and symptoms

Acute coronary syndrome (ACS) Term used to include ischemia, unstable angina, myocardial infarction (MI), and sudden death

Agonal dysrhythmia (dying heart) Ventricular rate less than 20; *see idioventricular dysrhythmia*

Alveoli Tiny grape-like clusters of tissues in the lung, where oxygen and carbon dioxide are exchanged

Amplitude Height of a wave or complex; measured in millivolts (mV)

Anaphylaxis Severe allergic response to a substance, such as drugs or an insect bite; may be fatal; symptoms may include dyspnea, swollen/obstructed airway, shock, hives, or rash

Angina Chest pain caused by a decrease or lack of oxygen to the cardiac muscle; the pain may also be felt in the left arm, jaw, and shoulder; is usually relieved by rest or medication such as nitroglycerin

Antegrade Movement in a forward motion; frequently used with the forward (downward) movement of an electrical impulse from the atria through the ventricles

Antiarrhythmic Medication that acts on the electrical conduction pathway of the heart to prevent or reverse dysrhythmias by slowing the conduction of the electrical impulse, stopping or slowing the reentry pathways, and blocking electrolytes such as potassium

Anticoagulant Drug that prevents or delays the formation of clots

Antipyretic Medication used to reduce fever

Antithrombolytic Medication that helps to prevent the formation of blood clots

Aorta Largest artery in the body

Aortic valve Located between the left ventricle and the aorta

Arrhythmia May be used interchangeably with the term *dysrhythmia*

Arterial blood gas (ABG) Blood test used to measure the amount of oxygen and carbon dioxide in the arterial blood

Artery Blood vessel that carries blood away from the heart; made of smooth muscle

Artifact Abnormality seen on a monitor or in an ECG tracing that does not originate in the heart, such as static electricity, patient movement, or loose leads

Artificial pacemaker Small, battery-operated device that initiates electrical impulses in the heart; may be temporary or permanent

Asystole Absence of electrical activity in the cardiac muscle; also called cardiac standstill

Atria Upper chambers of the heart

Atrial dysrhythmia A rhythm that is initiated from a pacemaker site in the atria, when the sinoatrial (SA) node fails to initiate an electrical impulse

Atrial fibrillation (A Fib) Dysrhythmia that originates from many atrial sites; the atria are making ineffective quivering movements, not actual contractions; only the ventricles are contracting

Atrial flutter Dysrhythmia in which flutter (F) waves are formed instead of P waves; flutter waves are frequently described as having a "saw-toothed" appearance

Atrial rhythm Any rhythm that originates from a pacemaker cell within the atria other than the SA node

Atrioventricular block (AV block) Interruption or block of the electrical conduction pathway at or below the AV junction; example: second-degree heart block, third-degree block, and bundle branch block

Atrioventricular dissociation (AV dissociation) Occurs when the atria and ventricles function independently; also known as third-degree heart block or complete heart block

Atrioventricular node (AV node) Part of the electrical system of the heart; acts as a secondary pacemaker of the heart

Atrium One of the two upper chambers of the heart

Automated external defibrillator (AED) Portable device that identifies lethal dysrhythmias and provides defibrillation when necessary

Automaticity Ability of cardiac pacemaker cells to generate or initiate an electrical impulse

Autonomic nervous system Nerves that maintain the heart and blood vessels in a normal state; divided into the sympathetic and parasympathetic systems

Bag-mask Device that is used to assist with artificial ventilation, and in the delivery of 100% oxygen to patients.

Baseline Imaginary line on the rhythm strip from which all waves and deflections are measured; also known as isoelectric line

Beta-adrenergic blockers (β-blockers) Medications that decrease the rate and force of heart contractions; reduce cardiac ischemia by reducing the heart muscle's need for oxygen; also lower blood pressure, reduce occurrence of dysrhythmias and pain of angina

Bigeminy Every other QRS complex is abnormal (usually premature); a minimum of three occurrences is needed to identify a dysrhythmia with bigeminy

Biphasic (diphasic) Any S-shaped wave that lies both above and below the baseline of the rhythm strip, or moving in two opposite directions

Blood pressure (BP) Measurement of pressure within the blood vessels; measured in millimeters of mercury (mm Hg)

Bolus Rapid infusion of IV fluids or medications; also called IV push

Bradyasystole Pulseless dysrhythmia that appears on the monitor as a bradycardia

Bradycardia (brady) Cardiac dysrhythmia that has a slower than normal heart rate; usually less than 60 electrical impulses per minute

Bronchi Large airway tubes that branch off the trachea and enter the lungs; part of the respiratory system

Bronchioles Small airway tubes that extend from the bronchi into the lobes of the lungs

Bronchus One large airway tube that branches off the trachea and enters one lung

Bundle branches (BB) Part of the electrical conduction system of the heart; located below the bundle of His, leading to the Purkinje's fibers; divided into left and right bundle branches

Bundle branch block (BBB) Dysrhythmia in which the electrical impulse is blocked at one of the bundle branches; the QRS complex has a notched appearance and is usually greater than 0.12 second

Bundle of His Part of the electrical conduction system of the heart; located below the AV junctional area and above the bundle branches

Bundle of Kent (Kent bundle) Additional or abnormal electrical conduction pathway; found in WPW syndrome

Buried P wave The P wave is hidden, or buried, within the QRS complex and therefore not seen

Calcium channel blockers Drugs that decrease the heart rate by slowing conduction of the AV node and by lengthening the refractory periods; drugs that prevent spasms of the coronary arteries by relaxing the smooth muscle of the blood vessels

Caliper Instrument used to measure R to R and P to P intervals on a rhythm strip

Capture Ability of cardiac muscle to respond to an electrical stimulus from an artificial pacemaker and conduct the electrical impulse throughout the cardiac muscle

Cardiac Pertaining to the heart

Cardiac arrest Lack of electrical and/or mechanical activity in the heart; blood is not being pumped throughout the body and the patient does not have a pulse

Cardiac cycle Period from the beginning of one P wave to the beginning of the next P wave ; usually represents the conduction of an electrical impulse for a single heartbeat; includes a P wave, PR interval, QRS complex, ST segment, T wave, and baseline

Cardiac irritability Ability of cardiac cells to respond to an electrical impulse; used interchangeably with excitability

Cardiac output (CO) Amount of blood pumped by the left ventricle in 1 minute

Cardiac tamponade Presence of blood or excess fluid in the pericardial sac that decreases the heart's ability to contract and expand effectively

Cardiomyopathy Enlargement of the heart muscle

Cardiovascular Pertaining to the heart and blood vessels

Cardioversion Procedure that uses controlled electrical currents to correct tachycardic dysrhythmias such as uncontrolled atrial fibrillation, or ventricular tachycardia with a pulse; also known as synchronized cardioversion, or DC (direct current) cardioversion

Cardiovert Process of cardioversion

Chronic Symptoms that begin slowly and last for a long period of time

Circulatory system Body system that includes the heart, lungs, blood vessels, and blood

Clammy Cool, damp skin; a symptom of poor cardiac output

Compensatory pause Pause that follows a premature beat, allowing the underlying rhythm to begin again at its normal rate; may be either complete or incomplete pause

Complex Segment of the rhythm strip that refers to a group of waves; such as the Q, R, and S waves

Component Any part of a cardiac cycle seen on the monitor or rhythm strip; includes the P wave, the PR interval, the QRS complex, the ST segment, the T wave, and/or the QT interval

Conduct Transmit; send; carry an electrical impulse from cell to cell

Conduction system Specialized cardiac cells that transmit an electrical impulse throughout the heart muscle in a sequential manner, from the SA node to the ventricular muscle

Conductivity Ability of cardiac cells to transmit electrical impulses

Congestive heart failure (CHF) Heart disease that occurs when the heart muscle cannot pump enough blood to meet the body's needs; can be right or left sided heart failure; symptoms depend on which side of the heart is involved

Continuous infusion Administration of medication in an intravenous (IV) or intraosseous (IO) solution, at a specific rate

Contractility Ability of cardiac cells to shorten, causing cardiac muscle contraction

Contraction Tightening or squeezing action of a muscle; the contraction of the cardiac muscle pumps blood throughout the body

Coronary Pertaining to the heart; is also used to mean a heart attack or MI

Coronary arteries Arteries that supply oxygenated blood to the heart muscle

Coronary artery disease (CAD) Progressive blockage of one or more coronary arteries, resulting in a decrease of oxygen to the heart muscle

Couplet Two premature complexes occurring in a row; also known as coupling or a pair

Creatinine clearance Blood or urine test to assess kidney function

Cyanosis Bluish or grayish color of the skin, mucous membranes, and/or nail beds; caused by lack of oxygen in the tissue

Deciliter (dL) Measurement of volume in the metric system; 1 dL = 100 ml = 0.1 liter

Defibrillation (shock) Procedure that uses electrical current to correct ventricular fibrillation or pulseless ventricular tachycardia; may also be called unsynchronized cardioversion

Deflection Movement of a wave or complex away from the baseline on a rhythm strip or monitor screen

Delta wave Extra "bump" on the slurred section of a QRS complex; results from the depolarization of the ventricles by way of an accessory pathway before the normal conduction reaches the ventricles; seen in Wolff-Parkinson-White syndrome

Depolarization Conduction of an electrical impulse through the heart muscle; normally causes a cardiac contraction

Depressed wave A wave that is below the baseline

Diaphoresis Extreme sweating; may accompany severe chest pain

Dilate Enlargement or widening of a blood vessel

Diphasic (biphasic) Any S-shaped wave that lies both above and below the baseline of the rhythm strip, or moving in two opposite directions

Dyspnea Difficult or painful breathing

Dysrhythmia Abnormal cardiac rate or rhythm; frequently used interchangeably with the term arrhythmia

Ectopy (ectopic complex) Complex initiated from a site other than the SA node

Electrical impulse Electrical stimulus generated by pacemaker cells in the myocardium, which causes depolarization of the myocardial cells; normally initiated by the SA node; may also be generated by an artificial pacemaker

Electrocardiogram (ECG) Printed record of the conduction of electrical impulses of the heart

Electrode Conduction pad that connects the patient to a telemetry monitor or an ECG machine; also the tip of an artificial pacemaker lead wire

Electrolyte Chemical found in the blood and body fluids, such as sodium (Na^+) and potassium (K^+), which aid in the conduction of electricity

Electrophysiology Study of the ability of cells and tissue to use electrical currents

Embolism Substance such as a blood clot that moves through the circulatory system, until it becomes lodged against the wall of a smaller blood vessel

Endocardium Lines the heart chambers and the heart valves

Endotracheal tube Specialized tube inserted through the mouth, into the trachea; used to administer oxygen; used to administer some medication during treatment for cardiac arrest

Epicardium Thin, protective membrane that covers the outside of the heart

Escape beat Complex initiated from a site other than the SA node; usually is the heart's attempt to maintain a normal rate or rhythm; is also the complex that ends the pause of a sinus exit block

Excitability Ability of cardiac cells to respond to an electrical impulse; used interchangeably with irritability

Fibrillation Uncontrolled, uncoordinated, and ineffective quivering movements of cardiac muscle

Fibrinolytic agents May also be called reperfusers; drugs that dissolve clots in the coronary arteries that cause ischemia and infarction; may reduce the number of deaths from myocardial infarction

First-degree heart block Dysrhythmia caused by a delay in the conduction system between the atria and the bundle of His; PR intervals measure greater than 0.20 second

Flutter wave (F wave) Wave formed instead of a P wave during a rapid, flutter dysrhythmia

"Funny looking beats" (FLBs) Informal term for complexes that do not follow the usual pattern

Generate Initiate; begin an electrical impulse

Glycoprotein IIb/IIIa inhibitors Medications that stop or slow the ability of platelets to form clots

Gram (g, gm) Measurement of weight used in the metric system; frequently used in drug dosages; 1 gram = 1000 milligrams

Heart Muscular organ that pumps blood to the body cells

Heart block Partial or complete interruption in the normal cardiac electrical conduction system

Heart/lung circulation Transportation of blood from the body cells through the heart and lungs, and back to the body cells

Heart rate (HR) Number of times the ventricles beat in 1 minute; pulse or heartbeat

Hypercalcemia Greater than normal amounts of calcium in the blood

Hyperkalemia Greater than normal amounts of potassium in the blood

Hypersensitivity Term used to indicate an allergy to a substance, usually a medication

Hypertension Blood pressure measurement above normal

Hypertensive crisis Sudden, severe increase in blood pressure above 200/120 mm Hg, which does not respond to routine blood pressure medications

Hypomagnesemia Less than normal amounts of magnesium in the blood

Hypotension Blood pressure measurement below normal

Hypovolemia Decreased amount of blood in the heart chambers and blood vessels; caused by severe dehydration or blood loss

Hypoxia Lack of oxygen at the cell level of the body tissues

Idioventricular dysrhythmia Dysrhythmia in which the atria, AV junction, bundle of His, and bundle branches are no longer functioning; only the ventricular muscle is attempting to function; HR 20 to 40

Implantable cardioverter defibrillator (ICD) Surgically implanted pacemaker/defibrillator that can identify and treat some rapid lethal dysrhythmias, such as ventricular tachycardia; also known as automatic implantable cardioverter defibrillator (AICD)

Incompatible One substance that cannot be mixed with another; for example, sodium nitroprusside is incompatible with saline solutions

Infarction Death of tissue; as in myocardial infarction

Infiltration Occurs when an IV catheter slips out of a vein and solution infuses into the surrounding tissue

Infusion pump Device that regulates the rate of administration and dosage of IV/IO medications or fluids

Inherent Normal, natural, or inborn; for example, the inherent heart rate of the atria is 60 to 100 beats per minute

Initiate Generate or start an electrical impulse

Intermittent heart block Interruption of the electrical impulse, occurs suddenly and without warning, completely blocking the conduction of the impulse to the ventricles

Internodal pathways Multiple electrical conduction pathways between the SA node and the AV node

Interval Period of time used to measure the distance between waves or complexes on the rhythm strip, such as PR interval or P to P interval

Intraatrial pathways Multiple electrical conduction pathways between the right and left atria

Intraosseous (IO) Administration of medication or fluids into bone marrow

Intravenous (IV) Administration of medication or fluids into a vein

Inverted P wave Upside down P wave before the QRS complex

Irritability Ability of cardiac cells to respond to an electrical impulse; used interchangeably with excitability

Ischemia Decreased amount of oxygen available to the tissue cells, due to decreased blood supply

Isoelectric line Imaginary line on the rhythm strip from which all waves and deflections are measured; also known as the baseline

Joules Measurement of electrical current used in either cardiac defibrillation (unsynchronized cardioversion) or synchronized cardioversion

Junctional bradycardia dysrhythmia Junctional dysrhythmia in which the heart rate is less than 40 electrical impulses per minute

Junctional dysrhythmia Dysrhythmia occurring when the electrical impulses are generated by a site in the AV junctional area; inherent heart rate is 40 to 60 impulses per minute

Junctional tachycardia dysrhythmia Junctional dysrhythmia with a heart rate between 101 and 150 electrical impulses per minute

Kilogram (kg) Measurement of weight used in the metric system; 1 kg = 2.2 pounds

Lead Identifies different types of electrode placement, such as Lead I or Lead II for cardiac monitoring

Lead wire (lead) A wire that connects the electrode to a monitor or telemetry unit; also wire leading from a pacemaker generator to the heart chambers

Lethal Death producing

Life threatening Dysrhythmia that causes a severely decreased cardiac output, which may progress to death

Loading dose Term used interchangeably with initial dose of medication

Loss of capture QRS complex does not follow a pacemaker spike; myocardium does not respond to the electrical stimulus from the artificial pacemaker, and does not depolarize (contract)

Lungs Two organs that remove carbon dioxide from the blood, replacing it with oxygen

Medically unstable Patient's condition in which any combination of the following signs and symptoms of poor cardiac output occurs: pale, cool, clammy skin; nausea/vomiting (N/V); shortness of breath (SOB); sudden decrease in blood pressure; chest pain, or change in level of consciousness

Microgram (mcg) Measurement of weight used in the metric system; used in drug dosages; 1 mcg = 0.001 milligram; 1000 mcg = 1 milligram

Milligram (mg) Measurement of weight used in the metric system; frequently used in drug dosages; 1 mg = 0.001 gram; 1000 mg = 1 gram

Milliliter (mL) Measurement of liquid volume used in the metric system; 1 mL = 0.001 liter; 1 liter = 1000 mL (approximately 1 quart)

Millimeter (mm) Measurement of distance used in the metric system; 1 mm is equal to one small horizontal square on rhythm strip graph paper; as a measurement of time, 1 mm = 0.04 second

Millivolt (mV) Measurement of amplitude; 0.1 mV equals one small vertical square on the rhythm strip graph paper

Mitral valve Heart valve located between the left atrium and the left ventricle

Mobitz I Progressive heart block that occurs when the atrial impulse is interrupted at the AV junction; also called second-degree heart block, type I or Wenckebach

Mobitz II Intermittent interruption in the electrical conduction system at or below the AV junction; occurs suddenly and without warning; also called second-degree heart block, type II or classic

MONA (morphine, oxygen, nitroglycerin, aspirin) Treatment protocol for acute coronary syndrome

Monitor Television-like screen that shows the conduction of electrical impulses, as they travel through the electrical conduction pathway of the heart

Multifocal (polymorphic) Complexes that originate from different pacemaker sites and look different from each other; usually refers to premature ventricular complexes

Murmur Abnormal sound made by blood flowing through a valve that is not functioning correctly

Myocardial infarction (MI) Death of part of the cardiac muscle caused by a blockage in one or more of the coronary arteries; also called heart attack, coronary, or acute coronary syndrome (ACS)

Myocardium Middle layer of cardiac muscle

Narrow complex tachycardia Any dysrhythmia in a tachycardic rate, with QRS complexes measuring 0.04 to 0.12 second

Needle decompression Removal of air from the pleural sac, using a specialized needle

Nodal Term that has been used to mean AV junctional area

Noncompensatory pause Pause in the rhythm that measures less than two times the R to R intervals of the underlying rhythm

Normal sinus rhythm (NSR) Normal conduction rhythm; electrical impulses are generated by the SA node at an inherent heart rate of 60 to 100 impulses per minute

Normal electrical conduction pathway Sinoatrial (SA) node to atrioventricular (AV) node, through the bundle of His, bundle branches, through the Purkinje's fibers, ending in the ventricular muscle

NSTEMI (Non-ST Elevation Myocardial Infarction) Part of treatment protocol for myocardial infarction

Oxygen (O_2) Gas necessary for cell life; drug used to increase oxygen available to tissue cells; decreases shortness of breath and pain caused by ischemia

P to P interval Measurement of time from one P wave to the following P wave

P wave Small wave seen before the QRS; it represents the depolarization of both the right and left atria

Pacemaker Cardiac cells that initiate an electrical impulse, causing cardiac depolarization (contraction); the SA node is the normal pacemaker of the heart; also refers to an artificial pacemaker

Pacemaker cells Any cardiac cell that is capable of initiating an electrical impulse

Pacer Abbreviated term for an artificial pacemaker

Pacer spike Vertical line seen on the rhythm strip that represents the electrical impulse from an artificial pacemaker

Pacing Use of artificially generated electrical impulses that follow the electrical conduction system of the heart, and usually stimulate the cardiac muscle to contract; also refers to the percent of complexes initiated by an artificial pacemaker

Palpitations Sensation of being able to feel own heart beating or "skipping beats"; frequently associated with rapid heart rates ("racing heart") or premature complexes

Parasympathetic nervous system Nerves that decrease the rate of cardiac contractions, usually after stress or emergencies, allowing the body to restore energy

Paroxysmal Sudden onset of a rapid cardiac dysrhythmia

Paroxysmal atrial tachycardia (PAT) Dysrhythmia with a sudden onset; the electrical impulses are generated at a rate greater than 150 impulses per minute; the current term for this dysrhythmia is paroxysmal supraventricular tachycardia (PSVT)

Paroxysmal supraventricular tachycardia (PSVT) Dysrhythmia with a rate greater than 150 electrical impulses per minute; originates suddenly from the atria or AV junctional area

Percutaneous coronary intervention (PCI) Treatment methods of opening blocked coronary arteries; includes the use of balloon angioplasty, laser, and the insertion of coronary stents (devices used to hold open a coronary artery)

Perfusion Movement of blood through a specific organ or part of the body, such as the cells of the heart muscle

Pericardial sac Tough, loose-fitting, fibrous sac that contains the heart

Pericardiocentesis Removal of extra fluid or blood from pericardial sac by a physician, using a needle and syringe; also known as "needle aspiration"

Peripheral Pertaining to the arms and legs

Permanent pacemaker Artificial pacemaker that is surgically implanted under the patient's skin

Platelets Blood cells that aid in the clotting of blood

Pleural sac Protective sac that surrounds each lung

Polarization Cardiac ready state; the cells are ready to receive an electrical impulse

Poor cardiac output Patient condition in which the heart is not pumping enough blood for the body to function properly; any combination of the following symptoms may be seen: pale, cool, and clammy skin; difficulty breathing; sudden decrease in blood pressure; chest pain, or change in level of consciousness

Potassium (K⁺) Chemical found in the body that aids in the conduction of electricity through the cardiac cells

PR interval (PRI) Time required for an electrical impulse to travel through the atria and AV junction; measured from the beginning of the P wave to the beginning of the QRS complex

Premature atrial complex (PAC) Atrial complex that occurs earlier than the next expected complex of the underlying rhythm

Premature junctional complex (PJC) Complex initiated from the junctional area that occurs earlier than the next expected complex of the underlying rhythm

Premature ventricular complex (PVC) Complex initiated from an area below the AV junction that occurs earlier than the next expected complex of the underlying rhythm

Preprinted physician's orders Term for physician's standing orders

Progressive heart block Interruption of the electrical impulse that becomes longer with each impulse, until it is completely blocked and does not reach the ventricles

Pulmonary Pertaining to the lungs

Pulmonary edema Abnormal amount of fluid in the alveoli and other lung tissues, causing rapid, difficult breathing; usually caused by congestive heart failure (CHF)

Pulmonary thrombosis Blockage of an artery in the lungs

Pulmonic valve Valve between the right ventricle and the pulmonary artery

Pulse Wave of pressure caused by the pumping action of the left ventricle that can be counted; usually defined as heart beats per minute; heart rate (HR)

Pulseless electrical activity (PEA) Dysrhythmia that occurs when there is electrical activity in the heart, but the cardiac muscle does not contract in response to the electrical stimulus; the patient does **not** have a pulse

Pulse oximetry Device used to measure the percentage of oxygen saturation in the red blood cells; a reading of 93% or greater is usually considered normal

Purkinje's fibers Muscular fibers found in the ventricles; part of the electrical conduction system of the heart

QRS complex Group of one Q, R, and S wave that represents the depolarization of both the right and left ventricles

QT interval Time required for the depolarization and repolarization of ventricular muscle cells; measured from the beginning of the Q wave to the end of the T wave

Quadrigeminy Every fourth QRS complex is abnormal (usually premature); should have a minimum of three occurrences to be identified

R on T phenomenon Occurs when the R wave of a premature ventricular complex falls on the T wave of the preceding complex; can lead to a lethal dysrhythmia

R to R interval Measurement of time from one R wave to the next R wave

"Rabbit ears" Informal term used to describe notched appearance of the widened QRS complexes in bundle branch blocks

Radiofrequency catheter ablation Procedure used in Wolff-Parkinson-White syndrome to destroy the abnormal pathway in the electrical conduction system

Rate Number of electrical impulses conducted in 1 minute

Refractory Does not respond as expected; difficult to manage with usual treatment

Refractory period Time between the end of a contraction and the return of the cardiac cells to the ready state; divided into absolute and relative refractory periods

Relative refractory period Time during the cardiac cycle when cardiac cells have repolarized to the point that some cells can be stimulated to contract again, if the stimulation is strong enough; from the last half of the T wave to the end of the T wave

Reperfusion Process of opening blocked arteries in order to reestablish the flow of blood; can be done with medications or surgical procedures

Repolarization Cardiac recovery phase; the cells are returning to the ready state

Responsiveness Term used in assessment of patient condition, such as responsive to painful stimulation or lack of responsiveness; used interchangeably with consciousness

Retrograde Occurs after or behind; traveling in a reverse or backward direction

Retrograde P waves Inverted P wave that is seen after the QRS complex

Rhythm The regularity of the appearance of the complex components

Run of ventricular tachycardia (run of VT) Group of three or more premature ventricular contractions in a row; usually has duration of less than 30 seconds

Salvo Run of ventricular tachycardia; may also be called a burst of PVCs

Second-degree heart block, type I Progressive heart block that occurs when the atrial impulse is interrupted at the AV junction; also called Wenckebach or Mobitz I

Second-degree heart block, type II Intermittent interruption in the electrical conduction system at or below the AV junction; occurs suddenly and without warning; also called Mobitz II or classical

Septum Thick, muscular wall that separates the right and left chambers of the heart

Shock Physical condition caused by poor cardiac output; also used as an informal term for cardiac defibrillation

Sick sinus syndrome (SSS) Term used in the past to describe a sinus rhythm with a pause; currently used for any dysrhythmia caused by a disruption in the atrial electrical conduction pathway

Sinoatrial node (SA node) Part of the electrical conduction system of the heart; normal pacemaker of the heart located in the upper right atrium

Sinus arrest Dysrhythmia that occurs when the SA node fails to initiate an electrical impulse; therefore the atrium does not depolarize, causing a pause in the cardiac rhythm

Sinus arrhythmia Dysrhythmia that occurs when the heart rate changes with respirations; meets all criteria of normal sinus rhythm except it is NOT regular

Sinus bradycardia Dysrhythmia that occurs when all electrical impulses originate from the SA node, but at a rate slower than 60 impulses per minute

Sinus exit block Dysrhythmia that occurs when the SA node initiates an electrical impulse that is blocked and not conducted to the atria, creating a pause in the cardiac rhythm; the pause is ended by an escape beat

Sinus rhythm Any cardiac rhythm that originates from the SA node; heart rate is usually between 60 and 100 electrical impulses per minute

Sinus tachycardia Dysrhythmia that occurs when all electrical impulses originate from the SA node, but at a rate of 101 to 150 impulses per minute

Sodium (Na⁺) Chemical found in the body that aids in the conduction of electricity through the cells

Spasm Sudden, temporary contraction or shortening of a muscle; a spasm in a coronary artery can cause a partial blockage of blood flow to the heart muscle

Spike Vertical line seen on the rhythm strip that represents the electrical impulse from an artificial pacemaker; also known as pacer spike

Stable No serious signs or symptoms of poor cardiac output

Stable angina Chest pain that usually starts with physical exertion and is relieved by rest

STEMI (ST Elevation Myocardial Infarction) Part of the treatment protocol for myocardial infarction

Stroke volume (SV) Amount of blood pumped by the left ventricle with each contraction or beat; usually about 70 ml

ST segment Wave component that starts at the end of the S wave and stops at the beginning of the T wave

Subcutaneous administration Injection of a medication into the tissue below the skin, usually at a 45- to 60-degree angle

Sublingual administration Placing a tablet or spray such as nitroglycerin under the tongue, allowing the medication to be dissolved and absorbed

Supraventricular tachycardia (SVT) Dysrhythmia that has all the characteristics of paroxysmal atrial tachycardia, but the onset is not seen; general term describing any rapid dysrhythmia (heart rate greater than 150) originating from above the bundle of His

Sympathetic nervous system Nerves that prepare the body to react in times of stress or emergencies by increasing the heart rate and force of cardiac contractions

Symptomatic Showing signs of poor cardiac output; *see medically unstable*

Synchronized cardioversion Procedure used to correct unstable rapid dysrhythmias using electrical current timed to discharge or "fire" only on the R wave, avoiding the relative refractory period

Systolic blood pressure Pressure in the arteries measured during ventricular contractions

T wave Complex component that represents repolarization of the ventricles

Tachycardia Dysrhythmia in which the heart rate is faster than normal; usually greater than 100 beats per minute

Telemetry System of electrodes, leads, monitors, and graph paper that receives and displays cardiac electrical impulses

Tension pneumothorax Presence of air in the pleural space around a lung; usually caused by an injury to the chest wall; may cause respiratory arrest if not treated

Third-degree heart block Dysrhythmia in which both the atria and the ventricles are beating independently; functioning as two separate hearts; also known as complete heart block or complete AV dissociation

Thrombolytic therapy Drugs used to dissolve clots in coronary arteries; may reduce the number of deaths from MI; currently used term is fibrinolytic therapy

Thrombosis Development of a blood clot within a blood vessel

Titrate Small adjustment of IV fluids or medications to improve vital signs, treat dysrhythmias, or relieve pain

Torsades de pointes Dysrhythmia that resembles VT; has increasing and decreasing amplitude along the baseline; usually occurs in rhythms with a prolonged QT interval

Toxicity Condition of harmful physical changes, resulting from amounts of a substance that would usually not cause problems

Trachea Round airway tube, which is about 4.5 inches long, extending from the larynx (voice box) to the bronchi; part of the respiratory system

Transmit Conduct or carry electrical impulses through the cardiac muscle; usually using normal conduction pathways

Tricuspid valve Valve located between the right atria and right ventricle

Trigeminy Every third QRS complex is abnormal (usually premature); should have a minimum of three occurrences to be identified as trigeminy

UA/NSTEMI (Unstable Angina with Non-ST Elevation Myocardial Infarction) Part of the treatment protocol for myocardial infarction

Underlying rhythm Basic cardiac rhythm in which dysrhythmias or abnormal complexes can be identified

Unifocal (monomorphic) Complexes that originate from a single pacemaker site and look alike; usually refers to premature ventricular complexes

Unstable See medically unstable or poor cardiac output

Unstable angina Chest pain that is not relieved with rest or nitroglycerine; usually lasts longer than thirty minutes

Unsynchronized cardioversion Term meaning defibrillation

Vagal stimulation Stimulation of the vagus nerve in order to decrease heart rate by using physical maneuvers, such as Valsalva maneuver or carotid massage

Valsalva maneuver Forceful bearing down, as if trying to have a bowel movement; sometimes used to treat PAT/PSVT

Valves Flap-like structures in the heart that are composed of endocardial tissue; they open and close in response to the pumping action of the myocardium, preventing the backflow of blood

Vasoconstriction Decreased size in the diameter of a blood vessel

Vasodilation Increased size in the diameter of a blood vessel

Vein Blood vessels that carry blood back to the heart

Vena cava Superior and inferior; largest veins in the body

Venous Pertaining to the veins

Ventilations Use of a bag-mask to assist in the patient's breathing

Ventricles Lower right and left chambers of the heart

Ventricular dysrhythmia Cardiac rhythm that is initiated from a pacemaker cell in the ventricles when the sinoatrial node, atrial sites, and the atrioventricular junction fail to initiate an electrical impulse; HR 20 to 40

Ventricular fibrillation (V Fib) Dysrhythmia that originates from many ventricular sites; the ventricles make ineffective, quivering movements, not actual contractions; the patient does **not** have a pulse

Ventricular muscle Part of the electrical conduction system of the heart with specialized tissue containing pacemaker cells; the muscle of the left ventricle is thicker since it pumps blood throughout the entire body

Ventricular rate Number of times the left ventricle contracts in 1 minute; should equal the pulse rate

Ventricular rupture Tear or break in the ventricular muscle; usually caused by a myocardial infarction or trauma, such as a gunshot wound or stabbing

Ventricular standstill Dysrhythmia that occurs when no ventricular activity exists, only atrial complexes; the patient does **not** have a pulse

Ventricular tachycardia (VT) Dysrhythmia that contains more than three premature ventricular complexes in a row; duration of more than 30 seconds; also called sustained ventricular tachycardia; HR usually greater than 100

Venturi mask Mask that mixes pure oxygen with room air to provide a flow of oxygen at specific concentrations

Voltage Measurement of electrical force

Vulnerable period The cardiac cells have repolarized to the point that some cells can again be stimulated to depolarize again, if the stimulus is strong enough; also known as the relative refractory period

Wandering atrial pacemaker dysrhythmia Dysrhythmia originating from at least three different sites above the bundle of His

Wandering junctional pacemaker dysrhythmia Dysrhythmia that originates from at least three different sites within the AV junctional area

Wenckebach Progressive heart block that occurs when the atrial impulse is interrupted at the AV junction; also called second-degree heart block, type I or Mobitz I

Wide complex tachycardia Any dysrhythmia in a tachycardic rate, with QRS complexes measuring greater than 0.12 second

Wolff-Parkinson-White syndrome (WPW) Dysrhythmia involving additional or accessory pathways in the electrical conduction system; an upright P wave, shortened PR interval, and delta waves are seen

Abbreviation List

ABG	Arterial blood gas
ACS	Acute coronary syndrome
AED	Automated external defibrillator
A Fib	Atrial fibrillation
AICD	Automatic implantable cardioverter defibrillator
AIVR	Accelerated idioventricular rhythm
AV	Atrioventricular
BB	Bundle branch
BBB	Bundle branch block
BID	Twice a day; usually given every 12 hours
BMV	Bag-mask-ventilator
BP	Blood pressure
Brady	Bradycardia
CAD	Coronary artery disease
CHF	Congestive heart failure
CO	Cardiac output
CPR	Cardiopulmonary resuscitation
CVA	Cerebral vascular accident
D_5NS	Dextrose 5% in normal saline
D_5W	Dextrose 5% in water
dL	Deciliter
ECG	Electrocardiogram
F wave	Flutter wave
FLBs	Funny looking beats
g, gm	Gram
HR	Heart rate
hr	Hour
ICD	Implantable cardioverter defibrillator
IO	Intraosseous
IV	Intravenous
K^+	Potassium
kg	Kilogram
L	Liter
L/min	Liters per minute
mcg	Microgram
mEq	Milliequivalent
mg	Milligram
mg/kg	Milligram per kilogram of body weight
MI	Myocardial infarction
min	Minute

mL	Milliliter
ml/min	Milliliters per minute
mm	Millimeter
mm Hg	Millimeters of mercury
MONA	Morphine, oxygen, nitroglycerin, aspirin
mV	Millivolt
Na^+	Sodium
NS	0.9% normal saline
NSR	Normal sinus rhythm
NSTEMI	Non–ST Elevation Myocardial Infarction
N/V	Nausea and vomiting
O_2	Oxygen
PAC	Premature atrial complex
PAT	Paroxysmal atrial tachycardia
PCI	Percutaneous coronary intervention
PEA	Pulseless electrical activity
PJC	Premature junctional complex
PO	Per os (by mouth)
PRI	PR interval
PSVT	Paroxysmal supraventricular tachycardia
PVC	Premature ventricular complex
QT	Interval between beginning of Q wave and end of T wave
RR	Respiratory rate
SA	Sinoatrial
SOB	Shortness of breath
SSS	Sick sinus syndrome
STEMI	ST Elevation Myocardial Infarction
SV	Stroke volume
SVT	Supraventricular tachycardia
Tach	Tachycardia
TID	Three times a day; usually given every 8 hours
UA/NSTEMI	Unstable Angina with Non–ST Elevation Myocardial Infarction
VF, V Fib	Ventricular fibrillation
VR	Ventricular rate
VT, V Tach	Ventricular tachycardia
WPW	Wolff-Parkinson-White syndrome

Reference List

ACLS Instructor Manual. (2006). Dallas: American Heart Association.

ACLS Provider Manual. (2006). Dallas: American Heart Association.

American Heart Association Guidelines for CPR and ECC. (2005). Dallas: American Heart Association.

BLS for Healthcare Providers Manual. (2006). Dallas: American Heart Association.

BLS for Instructors Manual. (2006). Dallas: American Heart Association.

Conover, M.B. (2003). *Understanding Electrocardiography* (8th ed.). St. Louis: Mosby.

Handbook of Emergency Cardiovascular Care for Healthcare Providers. (2006). Dallas: American Heart Association.

Herbert-Ashton, M. (2006). Living with an implantable cardiac device. *RN,* 69:7, 43-46.

ISMP's List of Error-Prone Abbreviations, Symbols, and Dose Designations. (2006). Retrieved October 1, 2006, http://www.ismp.org.

The Joint Commission List of "Do Not Use" Abbreviations. Retrieved January 3, 2008, http://www.jointcommission.org/PatientSafety/DoNotUseList/.

Mosby's Dictionary of Medicine, Nursing, and Health Professions (7th ed.). (2006). St. Louis: Mosby.

Nurse's Drug Looseleaf (9th ed.). (2005). New Cumberland, PA: Blanchard & Loeb Publishers.

Nursing 2004 Drug Handbook. (24th ed.). (2004). Springhouse, PA: Lippincott Williams and Wilkins.

Permanent Pacemaker. Nursing 2006, 51. Retrieved August 18, 2006, http://www.nursing2006.com.

Sifton, D.W. (2005). *Physician's Desk Reference.* (59th ed.). Montvale: Medical Economics Production Company.

Skidmore-Roth, L. (2007). *Mosby's Nursing Drug Reference.* St. Louis: Mosby.

Index

Heart Rate Review

Some rhythms that are similar to one another can be identified specifically by the heart rate associated with them. This quick-reference may be used to speed that process. For example, junctional dysrhythmia, and junctional bradycardia are similar to one another; the main difference is heart rate. Readers presented with a strip belonging to this type of rhythm can use the Heart Rate Review and quickly select the correct rhythm without needing to search for each individual rate.

NSR:	HR: 60-100
Sinus Brady:	HR: less than 60
Sinus Tach:	HR: 101-150
PAT/PSVT:	HR: greater than 150; must see the beginning
SVT:	HR: greater than 150 (151-250); do not see the beginning
A Flutter:	VR: 60-100; atrial rate: 250-350
A Flutter with slow ventricular response:	VR: less than 60; atrial rate: 250-350
A Flutter with rapid ventricular response:	VR: 101-150; atrial rate: 250-350
A Fib (controlled):	VR: 60-100; atrial rate: 350-500
A Fib with slow ventricular response:	VR: less than 60; atrial rate: 350-500
A Fib with rapid ventricular response:	VR: 101-150; atrial rate: 350-500
Uncontrolled A Fib:	VR: greater than 150; atrial rate: 350-500
Junctional Dysrhythmia:	HR: 40-60
Junctional Brady:	HR: less than 40
Accelerated Junctional Dysrhythmia:	HR: 61-100
Junctional Tachycardia:	HR: 101-150
Torsades de pointes:	VR: greater than 150; atrial rate: 0
V Tach:	VR: 101-250; atrial rate: 0
Accelerated Idioventricular Dysrhythmia:	VR: 41-100; atrial rate: 0
Idioventricular Dysrhythmia:	VR: 21-40; atrial rate: 0
Agonal Dysrhythmia:	VR: 10-20; atrial rate: 0
Ventricular Standstill:	VR: 0; atrial rate: usually 60-100
V Fib:	HR: 0
Asystole:	HR: 0

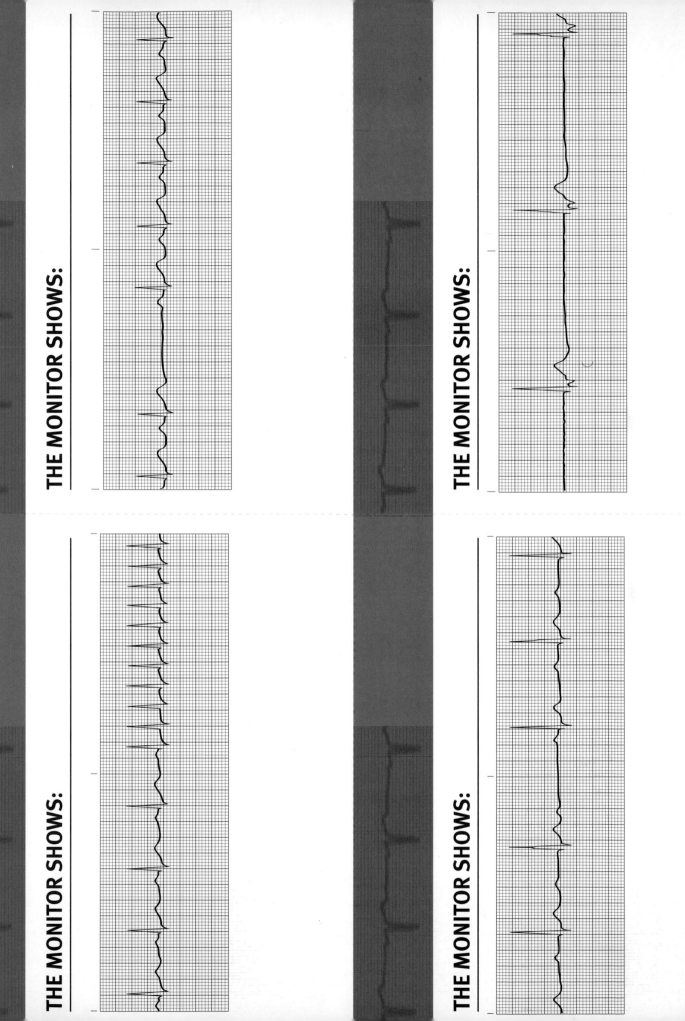

THE MONITOR SHOWS:

THE MONITOR SHOWS:

THE MONITOR SHOWS:

THE MONITOR SHOWS:

RHYTHM IDENTIFICATION

Sinus Exit Block in a **Sinus Rhythm**

Pause equal to exactly two or more complete cardiac cycles of the underlying rhythm;

heart rate: 70

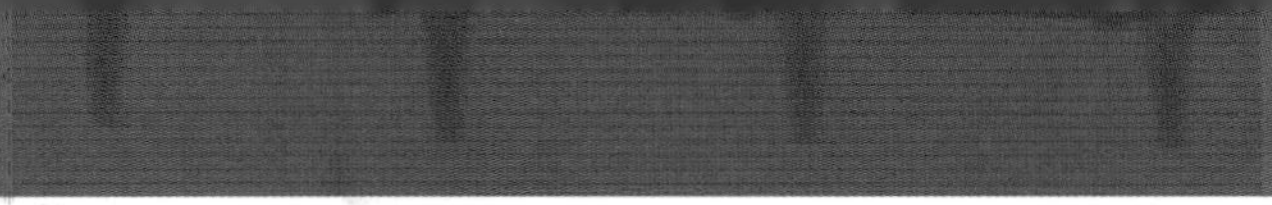

RHYTHM IDENTIFICATION

Junctional Bradycardia Dysrhytmia

A junctional rhythm with a heart rate less than 40;

Retrograde P waves;

heart rate: 30

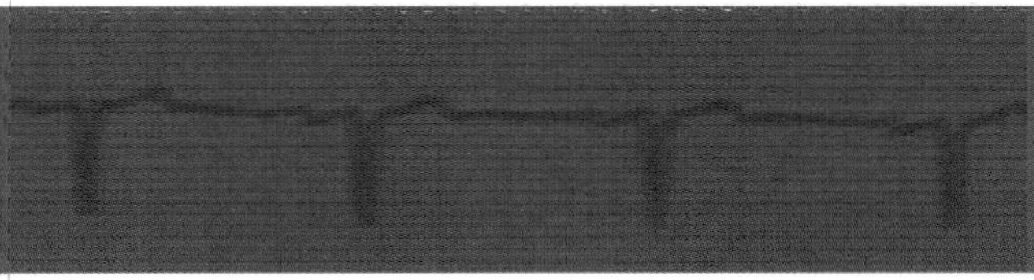

RHYTHM IDENTIFICATION

Paroxysmal Atrial Tachycardia (PAT) **or Paroxysmal Supraventricular Tachycardia** (PSVT)

Beginning of the PAT/PSVT **must** be seen;

HR **must** be greater than 150;

Normal sinus →→→ PAT/PSVT

heart rate: 80 →→ heart rate: 220

RHYTHM IDENTIFICATION

Second-Degree Heart Block, Type I (Mobitz I, Wenckebach)

Progressively longer PR intervals, followed by a dropped QRS;

pattern is then repeated;

ventricular rate: 50

atrial rate: 60

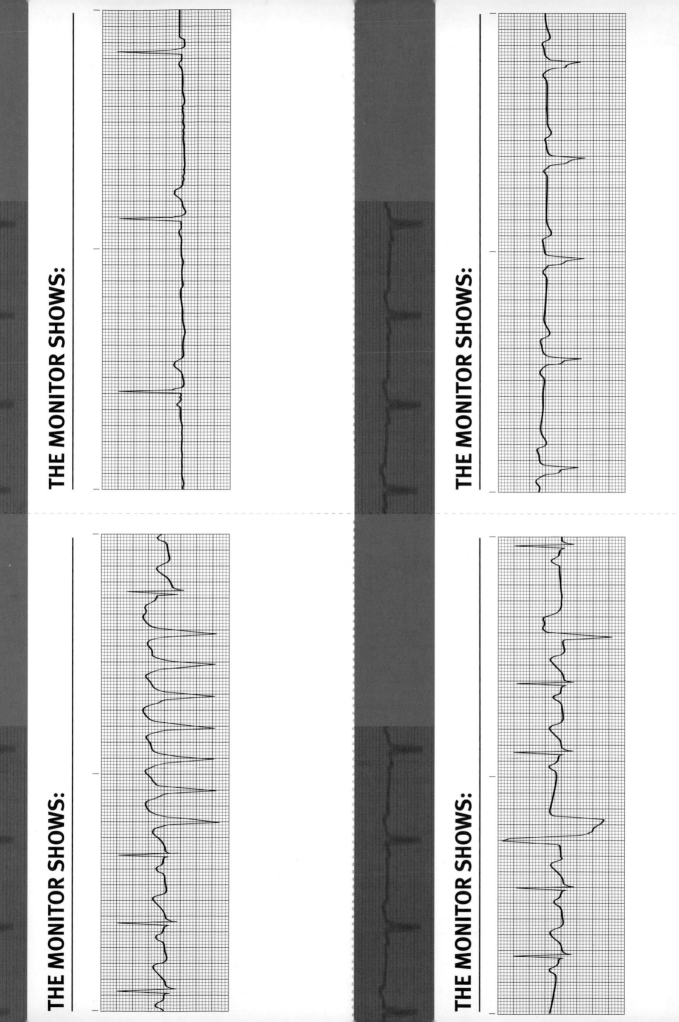

THE MONITOR SHOWS:

THE MONITOR SHOWS:

THE MONITOR SHOWS:

THE MONITOR SHOWS:

RHYTHM IDENTIFICATION

Sinus Bradycardia

A sinus rhythm with a heart rate less than 60;
heart rate: 30

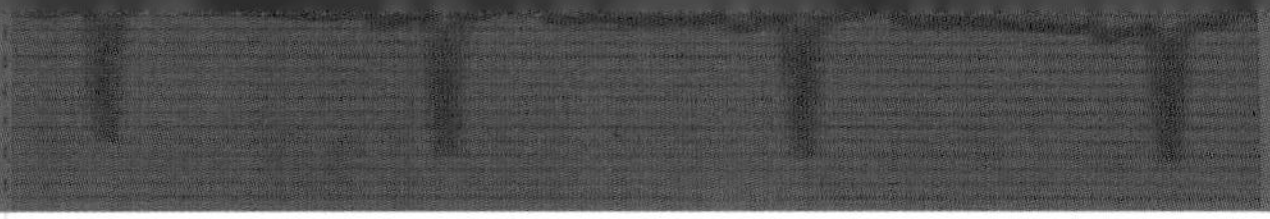

RHYTHM IDENTIFICATION

Run of Ventricular Tachycardia in a Sinus Rhythm

More than 3 PVCs in a row;
duration less than 30 seconds;
overall heart rate: 110 (V Tach rate is approximately 150)

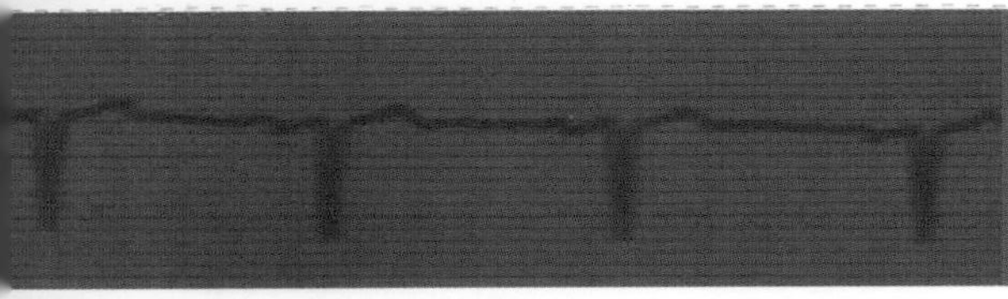

RHYTHM IDENTIFICATION

Sinus Bradycardia with WPW Syndrome

Shortened PRI; slurred QRS;
Delta wave present
heart rate: 50

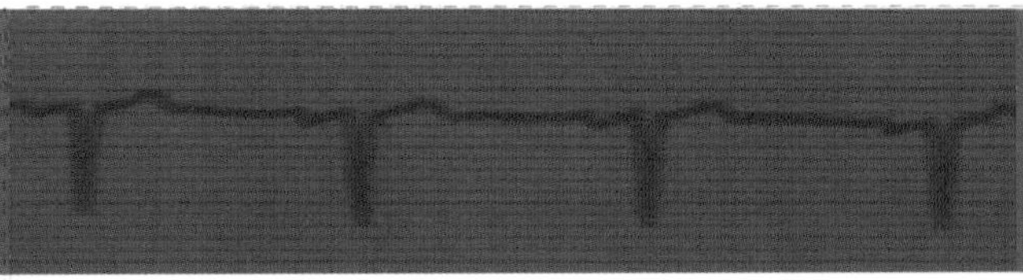

RHYTHM IDENTIFICATION

Multifocal PVCs in a Sinus Rhythm

Complex occurs earlier than expected;
originates from below the bundle of His;
PVCs look different, (QRS greater than 0.12 seconds)
heart rate: 70 (includes both PVCs)

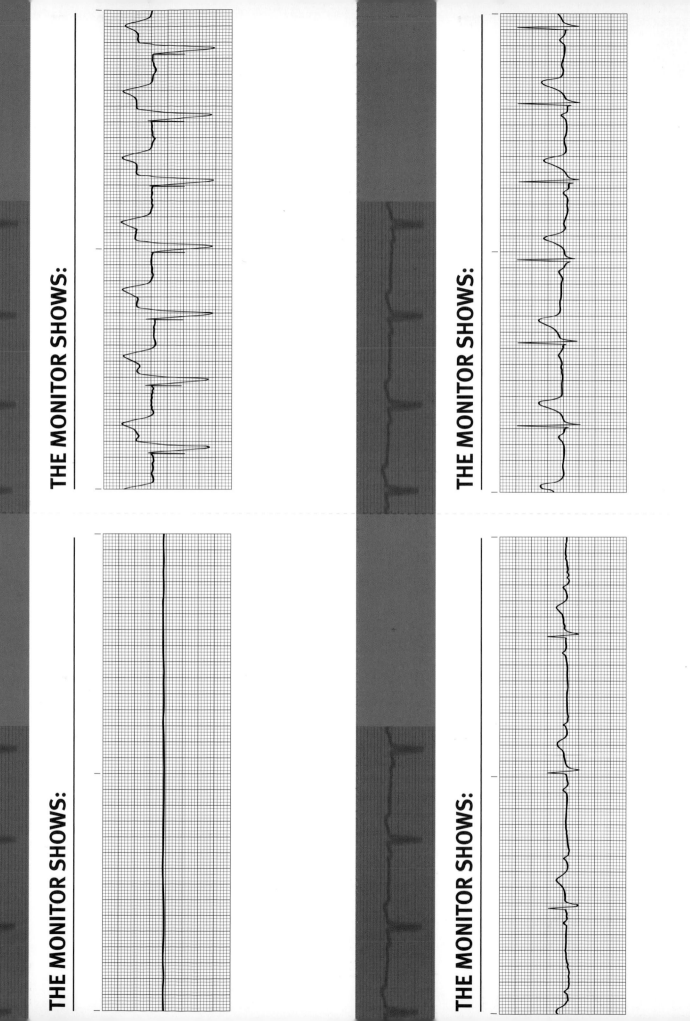

THE MONITOR SHOWS:

THE MONITOR SHOWS:

THE MONITOR SHOWS:

THE MONITOR SHOWS:

RHYTHM IDENTIFICATION

Pacemaker Rhythm

100% paced;
100% capture;
heart rate: 70

RHYTHM IDENTIFICATION

Asystole

No electrical activity seen;
must be confirmed in 2 different leads
ventricular rate: 0
atrial rate: 0

RHYTHM IDENTIFICATION

Normal Sinus Rhythm

P, PRI, QRS, rate, rhythm are all within normal limits;
heart rate: 60

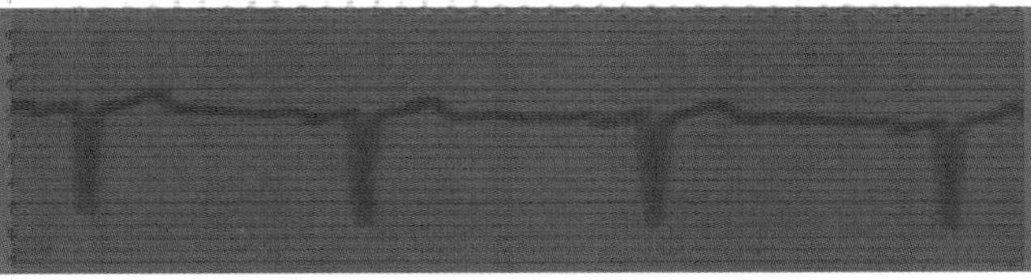

RHYTHM IDENTIFICATION

Second-Degree Heart Block, Type II (Mobitz II)

Bradycardic rate;
2 P waves for each QRS, 2:1 block/ratio;
PR intervals do not become progressively longer;
ventricular rate: 30
atrial rate: 70

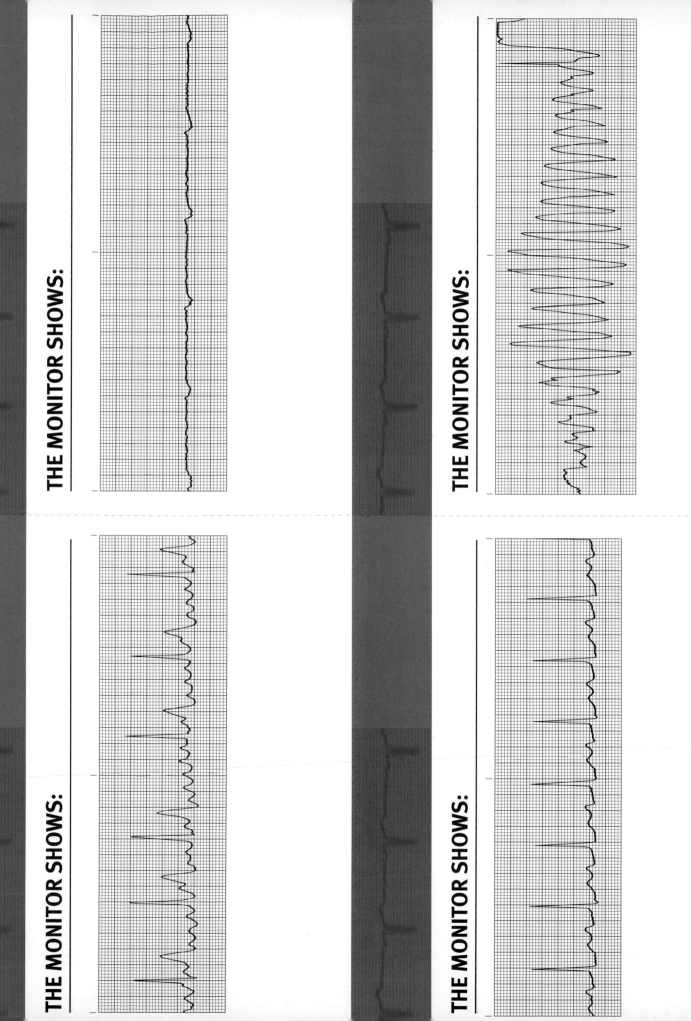

THE MONITOR SHOWS:

THE MONITOR SHOWS:

THE MONITOR SHOWS:

THE MONITOR SHOWS:

RHYTHM IDENTIFICATION

Ventricular Standstill

No QRS after P wave;
ventricular rate: 0
atrial rate: 60

RHYTHM IDENTIFICATION

Torsades de Pointes

QRS increases and decreases in amplitude;
usually occurs in rhythms with prolonged QT intervals;
ventricular rate: 240 to 250
atrial rate: 0

RHYTHM IDENTIFICATION

Atrial Flutter with Variable Ventricular Response

Sawtooth F waves;
ventricular rate: 60;
atrial rate: 250-350

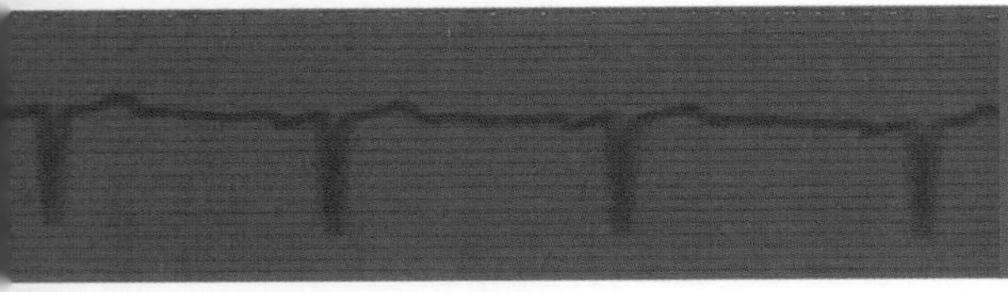

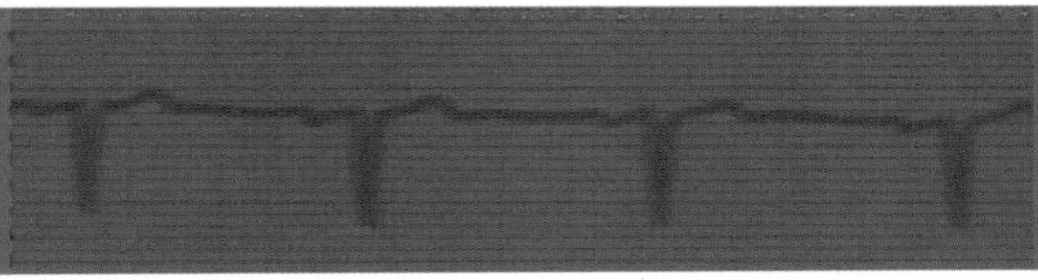

RHYTHM IDENTIFICATION

Sinus Rhythm with a First-Degree Heart Block

Prolonged PR interval (greater than 0.20 second);
heart rate: 70-80

THE MONITOR SHOWS:

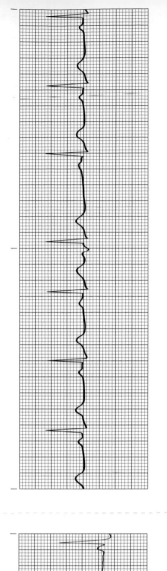

THE MONITOR SHOWS:

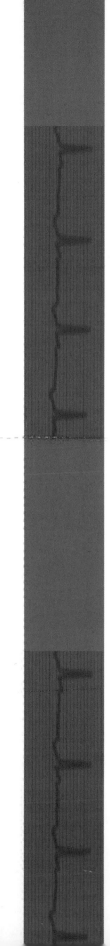

THE MONITOR SHOWS:

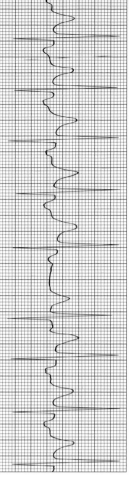

THE MONITOR SHOWS:

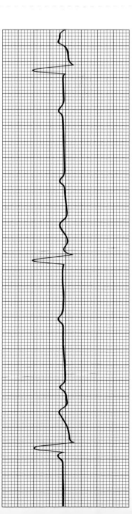

RHYTHM IDENTIFICATION

Premature Junctional Complex (PJC) **in a Sinus Rhythm**

Occurs earlier than expected;
originates from junction;
inverted P wave;
narrow QRS in premature complexes;
heart rate: 70 (includes one PJC)

RHYTHM IDENTIFICATION

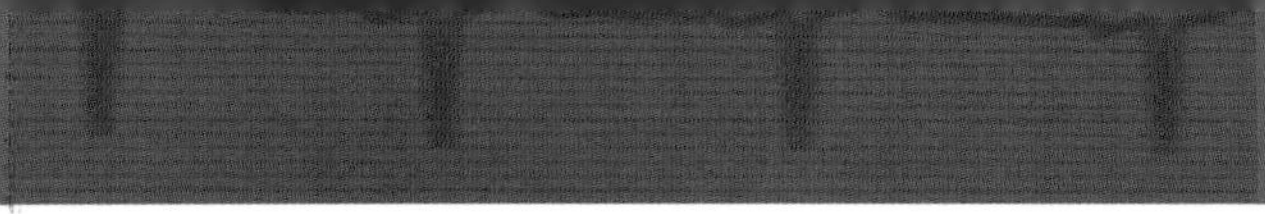

Wandering Atrial Pacemaker Dysrhythmia

Complexes originate from at least three sites in SA node, atria, and/or AV junctional area;
heart rate: 80-90

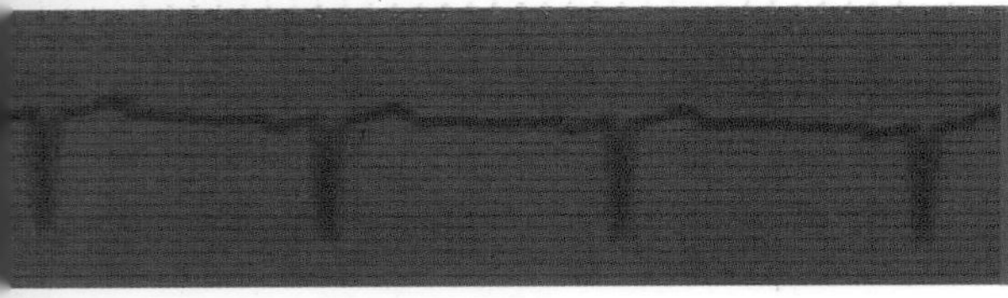

RHYTHM IDENTIFICATION

Premature Atrial Complex (PAC) **in a Sinus Rhythm**

Occurs earlier than expected;
originates from atria;
heart rate: 90 (includes one PAC)

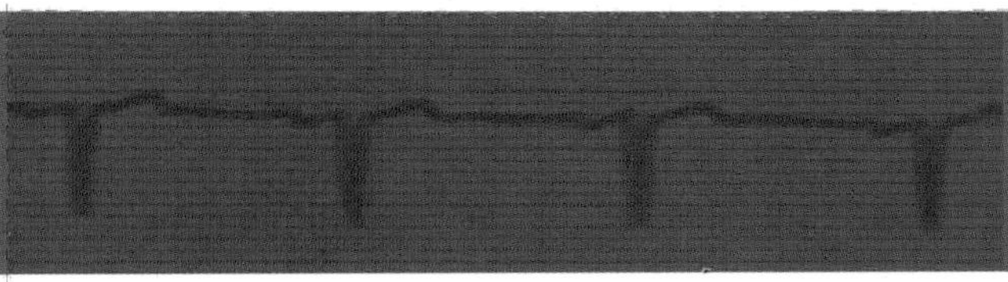

RHYTHM IDENTIFICATION

Third-Degree Heart Block

Atria and ventricles function independently;
no relationship between P waves and QRS complexes;
apparently irregular PR intervals;
ventricular rate: 30
atrial rate: 70

THE MONITOR SHOWS:

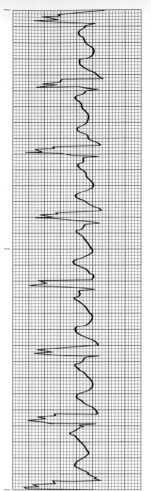

THE MONITOR SHOWS:

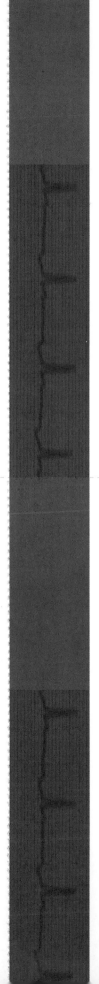

THE MONITOR SHOWS:

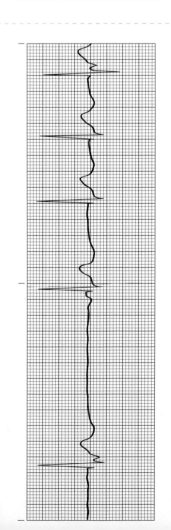

THE MONITOR SHOWS:

RHYTHM IDENTIFICATION

Sinus Rhythm with Bundle Branch Block

Notched QRS, (greater than 0.12 second);
heart rate: 80

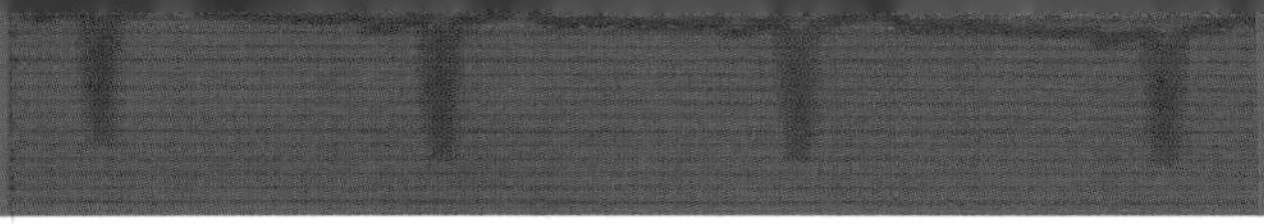

RHYTHM IDENTIFICATION

Sinus Tachycardia

Sinus rhythm with heart rate between 101 and 150;
heart rate: 150

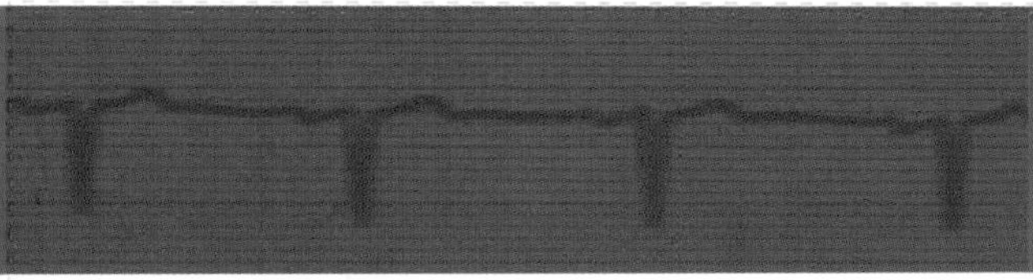

RHYTHM IDENTIFICATION

Wandering Junctional Pacemaker Dysrhythmia

Originates from 3 or more junctional sites;
heart rate: 50

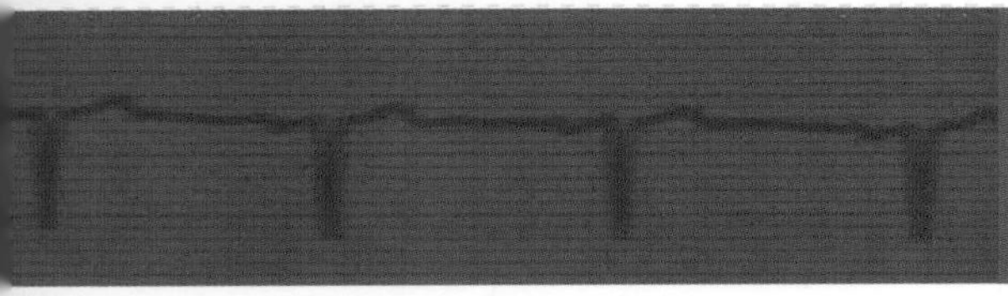

RHYTHM IDENTIFICATION

Ventricular Tachycardia

QRS greater than 0.12 second;
no visible P waves;
ventricular rate: 230-240
atrial rate: 0

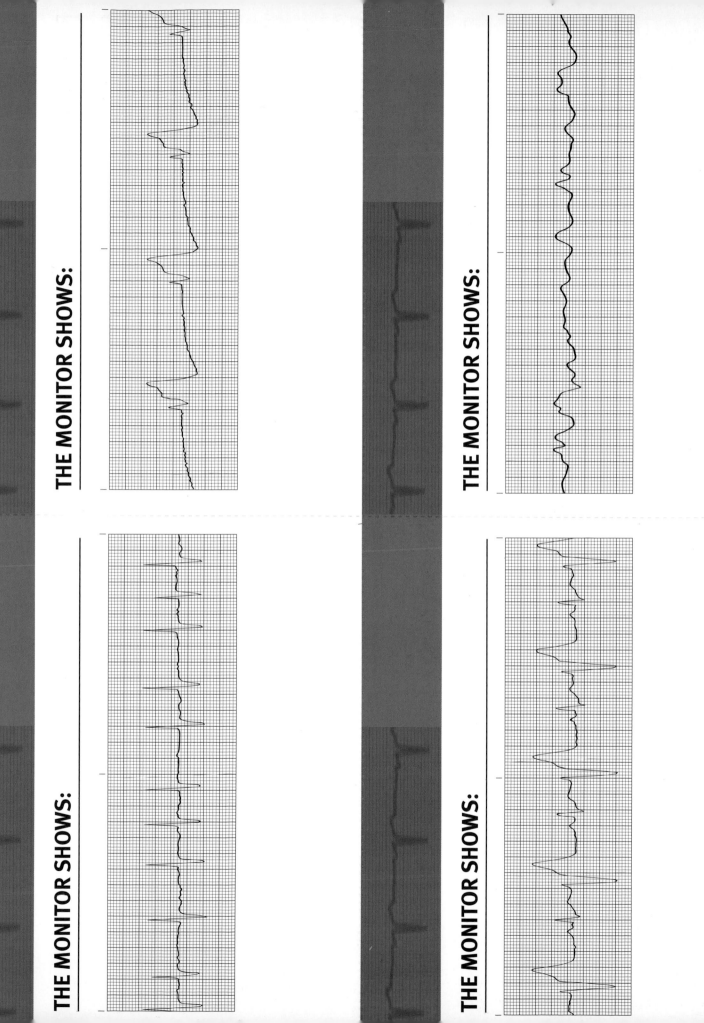

THE MONITOR SHOWS:

THE MONITOR SHOWS:

THE MONITOR SHOWS:

THE MONITOR SHOWS:

RHYTHM IDENTIFICATION

Idioventricular Dysrhythmia

No P waves;
QRS wide and bizarre, greater than 0.12 second;
ventricular rate between 20 and 40;
ventricular rate: 40
atrial rate: 0

RHYTHM IDENTIFICATION

Ventricular Fibrillation (Coarse)

No P waves;
no QRS complexes;
ventricular rate: 0
atrial rate: 0

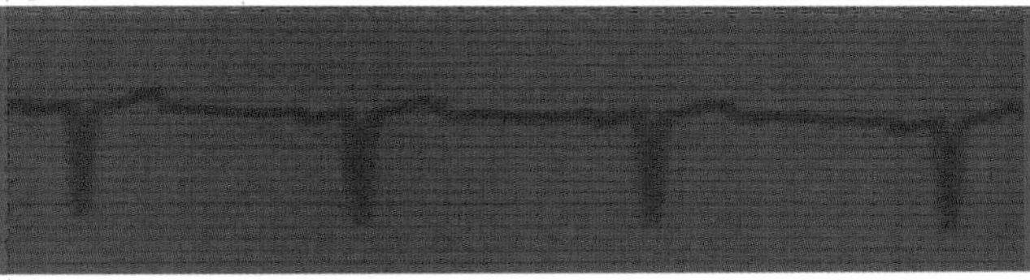

RHYTHM IDENTIFICATION

Atrial Fibrillation with Rapid Ventricular Response

Irregular rhythm;
no recognizable P wave;
ventricular rate: 110
atrial rate: 350-500

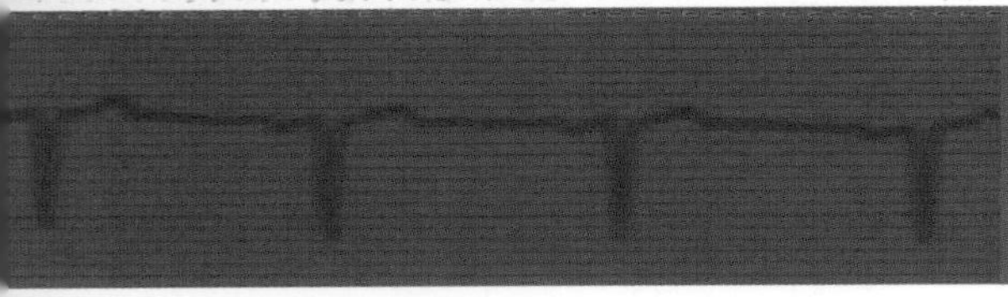

RHYTHM IDENTIFICATION

Unifocal PVCS in Bigeminy in a Sinus Rhythm

PVC occurs earlier than expected;
originates from below the bundle of His;
PVCs look alike;
every other complex is a PVC;
heart rate: 90 (includes all PVCs)

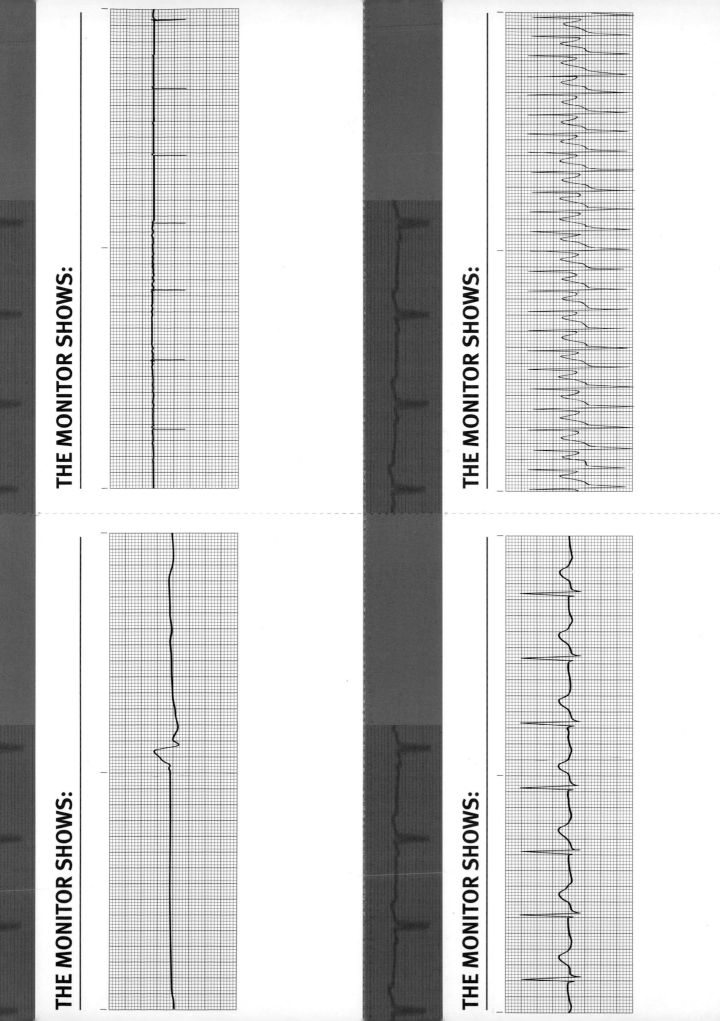

THE MONITOR SHOWS:

THE MONITOR SHOWS:

THE MONITOR SHOWS:

THE MONITOR SHOWS:

RHYTHM IDENTIFICATION

Pacemaker Rhythm with Loss of Capture

100% paced;
0% capture;
no pulse;
no cardiac electrical activity;
pacer rate: 70
heart rate: 0

RHYTHM IDENTIFICATION

Supraventricular Tachycardia (SVT)

Beginning or end of dysrhythmia is not seen;
narrow QRS complexes;
rate greater than 150;
heart rate: 250

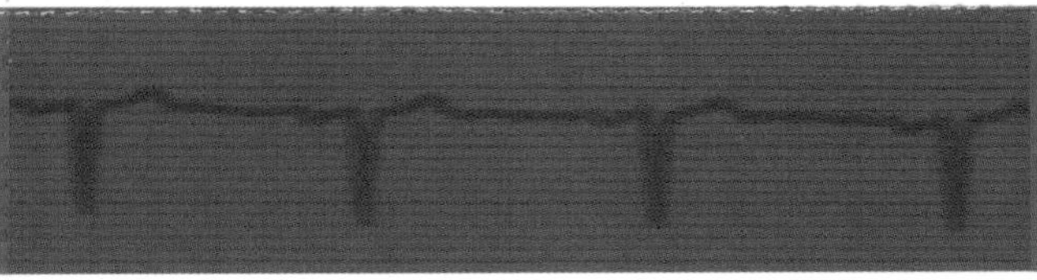

RHYTHM IDENTIFICATION

Agonal Dysrhythmia (Dying Heart)

No P waves;
QRS wide and bizarre, greater than 0.12 second;
heart rate less than 20;
usually no pulse;
ventricular rate: 10
atrial rate: 0

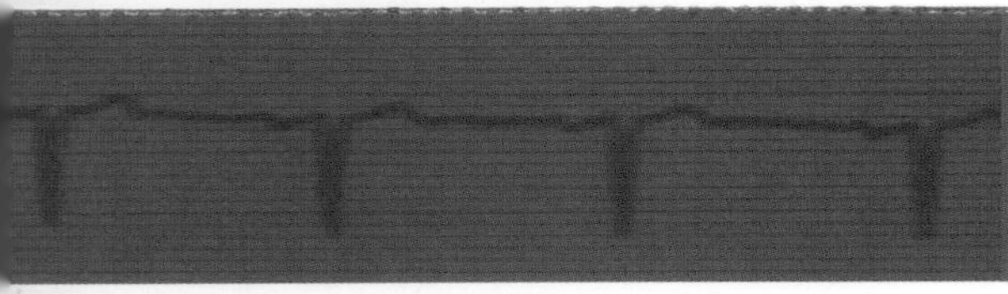

RHYTHM IDENTIFICATION

Accelerated Junctional Dysrhythmia

Rate between 61 and 100;
hidden P waves;
heart rate: 70

ACE Inhibitors
(Captopril, Enalapril, Enalaprilat, Lisinopril, Ramipril)

Action: Increases cardiac output; lowers blood pressure; reduces sodium and water retention (edema).

Indications: To improve left ventricular function; reduce death rate after acute MI; to treat high blood pressure.

Adenosine

Action: Decreases HR by depressing SA node and AV junctional activity.

Indications: To treat PAT/PSVT or SVT.

Aspirin
(Acetylsalicylic Acid)

Action: Decreases platelet formation of clots against the inside of arterial walls.

Indications: "MONA" protocol for acute MI; preventive measure for MI, stroke, and angina.

Amiodarone

Action: Decreases HR; slows conduction; prolongs effective refractory period.

Indications: To treat VT, V Fib, or pulseless VT.

Dosage: 6 mg rapid IV push over 1 to 3 seconds; repeat at 12 mg rapid IV push if no response in 1 to 2 minutes; may repeat once more at 12 mg rapid IV push, if no response in 1 to 2 minutes; immediately follow each dose with a 20 ml flush of IV solution and elevation of extremity.

Precautions: Side effects: flushing, dyspnea, hypotension, mild chest pain lasting 1 to 2 minutes; may also have short episodes of bradycardia, asystole, or abnormal beats; PAT/PSVT and SVT may recur due to short acting effects of this medication. Use with caution: in the elderly. Contraindications: hypersensitivity, atrial flutter, A Fib, WPW syndrome. Do not mix with aminophylline, dipyridamole, or carbamazepine.

Dosage: V Fib/pulseless VT: 300 mg IV/IO push; if no response within 3 to 5 minutes, repeat once at 150 mg IV push. **Stable VT with a pulse:** 150 mg IV over 10 minutes; if no response, repeat 150 mg IV once. If dysrhythmia is controlled, begin a continuous infusion at 1 mg/min for 6 hours, followed by 0.5 mg/min for 18 hours; up to a total dose of 2.2 g in 24 hours.

Precautions: May cause: bradycardia, hypotension, prolonged QT intervals. Use with caution: CHF, kidney, liver, and lung disease. Contraindications: hypersensitivity, pregnancy, or second- and third-degree heart blocks. Use only in D₅W solution, with an in-line filter and in a glass bottle. Do not shake. May cause hypotension for several months; may cause scarring of lung tissue or thyroid problems.

Dosage: Captopril: Initial dose: 6.25 mg, PO; advance to 25 mg TID, then 50 mg TID, as tolerated. **Enalapril:** initial dose: 2.5 mg PO; titrate to 20 mg PO, BID. **Enalaprilat:** initial dose: 0.625 mg IV over 5 min, then 1.25 mg to 5 mg IV every 6 hours. **Lisinopril:** 5 mg PO within 24 hours of symptom onset; then 5 mg PO after 24 hours; then 10 mg PO g after 48 hours; then 10 mg PO daily. **Ramipril:** initial dose: 2.5 mg PO; titrate to 5 mg PO BID, as tolerated.

Precautions: Use with caution: dialysis, diabetes and kidney disease. Contraindications: pregnancy, hypersensitivity, hypotension, potassium level over 5 mEq/L. Start after blood pressure has stabilized and completion of reperfusion therapy. IV Enalaprilat: contraindicated in STEMI.

Dosage: Chew 160 to 325 mg PO immediately in acute MI.

Precautions: May cause: nausea, GI bleeding, ringing in the ears, heartburn, dizziness, and wheezing. Use with caution: liver or kidney disease, asthma, pregnancy, ulcer disease, or in patients taking warfarin (Coumadin). Contraindications: hypersensitivity or bleeding disorders. Do not use enteric coated tablets.

Beta-Adrenergic Blockers

(Atenolol, Esmolol Hydrochloride, Labetalol, Metoprolol Tartrate, and Propranolol Hydrochloride)

Action: Decreases heart rate by slowing SA node and AV junctional conduction; reduces hypertension and cardiac ischemia; may reduce V Fib after MI.

Indications: To treat recurring VT and V Fib; to slow ventricular response to tachycardias with normal QRS complexes; to treat severe hypertension, after emergency treatment of acute MI.

Atropine Sulfate

Action: Increases heart rate; increases SA node automaticity and improves AV junctional conduction.

Indications: To correct symptomatic bradycardia; asystole; PEA; to increase heart rate in bradycardic rhythm with PVCs.

Calcium Chloride

Action: Increases myocardial contractility.

Indications: To maintain normal calcium levels; to treat increased potassium levels or calcium channel blocker toxicity.

Calcium Channel Blockers

(Diltiazem Hydrochloride; Verapamil Hydrochloride)

Action: Decreases heart rate by slowing AV junctional conduction and prolonging refractory periods; decreases hypertension by dilating coronary arteries.

Indications: To treat PAT/PSVT, SVT, and rapid ventricular response to atrial flutter and A Fib; to treat hypertension or angina.

Dosage: Atenolol: 5 mg IV over 5 minutes; repeat dose after 10 minutes. **Esmolol:** initial dose: 0.5 mg/kg IV over 1 minute, followed by a four minute infusion at 0.05 mg/kg per minute. Titrate to a maximum dose of 0.3 mg/kg per minute, to a total of 200 mcg/kg. **Labetalol:** 10 mg to 20 mg IV push over 1 to 2 minutes. May either repeat or double the dose every 10 minutes to a maximum dose of 150 mg, or follow initial bolus dose with an IV infusion of 2 to 8 mg/min. **Metoprolol:** 5 mg slow IV push, over 2 to 5 minutes, repeated at 5 minute intervals to a total dose of 15 mg. **Propranolol:** give 1 to 3 mg divided into 3 equal doses, slow IV push. Give no more than 1 mg/min, at 2 to 3 minute intervals.

Precautions: May cause: bradycardia, AV conduction delays, and hypotension. **Use with caution:** pregnancy and kidney disease. **Contraindications:** hypersensitivity, heart blocks, CHF, cocaine induced ACS, WPW syndrome, bronchospasm, bradycardia or hypotension. Do not mix with furosemide, sodium bicarbonate, or use with calcium channel blockers.

Dosage: Symptomatic bradycardia: 0.5 mg IV; repeated in 3 to 5 minute intervals to a total dose of 3 mg. Asystole/PEA: 1 mg IV/IO; repeated in 3 to 5 minutes to a total dose of 3 mg.

Precautions: May cause: tachycardia; may increase ischemia. **Use with caution:** pregnancy, in the elderly, MIs, and ACS. **Contraindications:** hypersensitivity, second-degree heart block, Type II or third-degree heart block.

Dosage: 500 to 1000 mg diluted in equal amounts of NS, IV slowly at 0.5 to 1 ml/min.

Precautions: Rapid administrations may cause bradycardia, spasms of coronary and cerebral arteries. **Use with caution:** pregnancy; digitalis; kidney or lung disease. **Contraindications:** hypersensitivity; hypercalcemia; digitalis toxicity; V Fib; kidney stones; sodium bicarbonate. Not routinely used in cardiac arrest.

Dosage: Diltiazem: 0.25 mg/kg IV over 2 minutes followed by infusion; may repeat in 15 minutes at 0.35 mg/kg over 2 minutes; if no response after 15 minutes, start IV infusion of 5 to 15 mg/hr, titrated to heart rate. **Verapamil:** 5 to 10 mg IV over 2 min, may repeat dose 30 minutes after first dose, if needed.

Precautions: May cause: brief episode of hypotension and/or bradycardia. **Use with caution:** pregnancy; reduce dose and slow the infusion rate in the elderly. **Contraindications:** hypersensitivity; do not use in WPW syndrome, wide complex tachycardias (VT), hypotension (if systolic blood pressure is less than 90 mm Hg), severe CHF, Sick Sinus Syndrome, or acute MI. Do not use with second- or third-degree AV block, unless a temporary pacemaker is available.

Digitalis Glycoside
(Digoxin; Lanoxin)

Action: Increases myocardial contractility improving cardiac output; decreases heart rate and AV junctional conduction.

Indications: To treat atrial flutter, atrial fib, PAT/PSVT, SVT; to treat CHF.

Clopidogrel Bisulfate

Action: Anticoagulant

Indications: Antiplatelet therapy when aspirin is not tolerated.

Dobutamine Hydrochloride

Action: Increases myocardial contractility improving cardiac output and coronary artery blood flow.

Indications: To treat short-term heart failure.

Digoxin Immune FAB
(ovine) (Digibind, DigiFab)

Action: Corrects digoxin toxicity.

Indications: To treat elevated digitalis blood levels if patient is symptomatic or has life threatening dysrhythmias; CHF; shock; hyperkalemia (potassium level greater than 5.5 mEq/L).

Digitalis Glycoside

Dosage: Loading dose: 10 to 15 mcg/kg IV, in three divided doses.

Precautions: May cause: AV blocks, bradycardias, or VT. Use with caution: acute MI, pregnancy, amiodarone or in the elderly. **Contraindications:** hypersensitivity; heart rate less than 60 beats/min; digitalis toxicity; torsades de pointes, second- or third-degree heart block, VT, V Fib, or WPW syndrome. Avoid cardioversion if patient taking digitalis, unless condition is life threatening; then use 10 to 20 joules settings.

Clopidogrel Bisulfate

Dosage: Initial dose: 300 mg PO, then 75 mg PO daily. Give as soon as possible to MI patients with UA/NSTEMI, if not contraindicated.

Precautions: May cause: nausea, vomiting, heartburn, GI bleeding. Use with caution: pregnancy; kidney or liver disease. **Contraindications:** hypersensitivity; ulcer disease; active bleeding.

Dobutamine Hydrochloride

Dosage: 2 to 20 mcg/kg/min IV infusion; titrated so heart rate does not increase more than 10%. Use with infusion pump.

Precautions: May cause: headache, nausea, vomiting, chest pain, changes in BP, tachycardias, PVCs or increased ischemia. **Use with caution:** pregnancy; hypertension. May increase AV conduction in atrial fib, causing rapid ventricular response. **Contraindications:** hypersensitivity to drug and sulfites. Do not mix with aminophylline, verapamil, digoxin, heparin or sodium bicarbonate. Do not use in patients with systolic BP less than 100 mmHg who are in shock, or in shock caused by known poisons or drugs.

Digoxin Immune FAB

Dosage: Chronic toxicity: 3 to 5 vials (120 to 200 mg); each vial binds 0.6 mg digoxin. **Acute toxicity:** 10 vials (400 mg); may require up to 20 vials (800 mg). Dosage varies with amount of digoxin taken.

Precautions: May cause: CHF, ventricular rate increase, atrial fib, hypokalemia. Use with caution: pregnancy, in the elderly; cardiac or kidney disease, or sheep protein allergy. **Contraindications:** hypersensitivity; mild digoxin toxicity. Do not mix with any other medication.

Epinepherine Hydrochloride

Actions: Increases myocardial automaticity and contractility, improving cardiac output, heart rate, BP; increases coronary and cerebral blood flow.

Indications: To treat cardiac arrest: V Fib, pulseless VT, asystole, PEA; to treat severe bradycardia or hypotension not responding to other therapies; to treat anaphylaxis (**severe allergic reaction**).

Dopamine Hydrochloride

Action: Increases myocardial contractility and heart rate, improving cardiac output; constricts arteries and veins increasing BP.

Indications: To treat: symptomatic hypotension, not caused by hypovolemia; to treat symptomatic bradycardia.

Flumazenil

Action: Complete or partial reversal of sedative effects of benzodiazepines.

Indications: Severe sedation from benzodiazepine overdose.

Fibrinolytic Agents

"Clot Busters"; Alteplase (Activase), Tissue Plasminogen Activator (t-PA); Reteplase (Retavase); Streptokinase (Streptase); Tenecteplase (TNKase)

Action: Breaks down blood clots in blood vessels, decreasing cardiac ischemia and infarction; may reduce number of deaths from MI.

Indications: To treat symptoms and ECG findings of STEMI, within 12 hours of symptom onset, if no contraindications exist. Consider percutaneous coronary intervention (PCI) if available.

Epinepherine Hydrochloride

Dosage: IV or IO: 1 mg (1: 10,000 dilution) IV or IO, every 3 to 5 minutes as needed. **Continuous infusion:** 1 mg (1:1000) mixed with 500 ml of D₅W or NS solution (2 mcg per ml), at a rate of 1 mcg/min, titrated as needed. Use with infusion pump. Start continuous infusion **only** when patient has pulse.

Precautions: May cause: increased ischemia; ventricular ectopies. Use **with caution:** hypertension; pregnancy; in the elderly. **Contraindications:** hypersensitivity. Do not mix with sodium bicarbonate.

Dopamine Hydrochloride

Dosage: 2 to 20 mcg/kg/min IV infusion; titrated to BP and heart rate. Use with infusion pump. Discontinue dopamine slowly.

Precautions: May cause: nausea, vomiting, ischemia, supraventricular and ventricular dysrhythmias. Monitor BP and HR frequently; check IV site frequently for infiltration. **Use with caution:** pregnancy and in the elderly. **Contraindications:** hypersensivity; V Fib or tachycardias. Do not mix with sodium bicarbonate.

Flumazenil

Dosage: 0.2 mg IV over 15 seconds; repeat at 0.3 mg IV over 30 seconds, if consciousness does not occur; may repeat every minute until patient becomes conscious or a total of 1 mg in 5 minutes or 3 mg in 1 hour is given.

Precautions: May cause: nausea, vomiting, dizziness, blurred vision, hypertension, seizures, or chest pain. **Use with caution:** pregnancy, in the elderly, liver or kidney disease, or seizure disorders. **Contraindications:** hypersensitivity to drug or long term use of benzodiazepines; tricyclic antidepressant overdose; patients being given benzodiazepines for life threatening conditions. Monitor for recurrent respiratory depression.

Fibrinolytic Agents

Dosage: Varies with specific fibrinolytic agent; follow manufacturer's directions or the policies of your institution and specific directions of the physician.

Precautions: May cause: active bleeding and decreased clot formation. Patients must meet specific criteria before use. **Use with caution:** pregnancy. **Contraindications:** hypersensitivity; bleeding disorders, recent surgery, major trauma, or recent cerebral bleeding. All patients receiving fibrinolytic therapy should also receive 160 to 325 mg of chewable aspirin as soon as possible, if no contraindications exist. May require heparinization after fibrinolytic therapy.

Furosemide
(Lasix)

Action: Removes excessive fluid from tissues; increases urine formation.

Indications: To treat CHF; pulmonary edema; cerebral edema after MIs; hypertensive emergencies.

Glucagon

Action: Relaxes smooth muscles; raises blood glucose level.

Indications: To treat calcium channel blocker or beta-adrenergic blocker toxicity.

Glycoprotein IIb/IIIa Inhibitors
(Abciximab; Eptifbatide; Tirofiban)

Action: Platelet inhibitor.

Indications: ACS with NSTEMI or UA/NSTEMI.

Heparin Unfractionated
(UFH)

Action: Anticoagulant; prevents or delays formation of clots.

Indications: Acute MI (STEMI; NSTEMI).

Dosage: Initial dose: 3 mg IV slowly, followed by an IV infusion at 3 mg/hr, as needed.

Precautions: May cause: nausea, vomiting, or high blood glucose levels.
Contraindications: hypersensitivity.

Dosage: 20 to 40 mg IV, over 1 to 2 minutes; if no response, double the dose to 40 to 80 mg IV over 1 to 2 minutes. Start at 40 mg IV for new onset pulmonary edema without hypovolemia.

Precautions: May cause: severe dehydration, hypotension, hypovolemia, electrolyte imbalance, high blood glucose levels, and damage to hearing. Use with caution: pregnancy, diabetes, severe kidney or liver disease, dehydration. Contraindications: hypersensitivity to sulfonamides; hypovolemia; severely decreased electrolyte levels.

Dosage: Initial bolus: 60 to 70 units/kg with maximum dose of 4,000 units. Continuous infusion: 12 units/kg/hr with maximum dose of 1000 units/hr for patients weighing more than 70 kg. Follow the heparin protocol of your institution. Use an infusion pump.

Precautions: May cause: active bleeding, bleeding disorders, GI bleeding, or hypertension. **Use with caution:** pregnancy, in the elderly, diabetes. **Contraindications:** recent surgery; hypersensitivity; severe hypertension; liver or kidney disease; low platelet count.

Dosage: Abciximab: MI: 0.25mg IV over 5 minutes, then 0.125 mcg/kg/min IV infusion for 12 hours. **PCI:** 0.25 mg/kg IV 10 to 60 minutes before procedure; then 0.125 mcg/kg/min IV infusion for 12 hours. Use with heparin. **Eptifibatide: ACS:** 180mcg/kg (maximum dose 22.6mg) IV over 1 to 2 minutes; then IV infusion at 2 mcg/kg/min up to 72 hr, with maximum rate of 15 mg/hr; **PCI:** 180 mcg/kg IV immediately before PCI; start IV infusion 2 mcg/kg/min for 18 to 24 hours, repeat 180 mcg/kg IV bolus 10 minutes after initial dose. **Tirofiban: ACS or PCI:** 0.4 mcg/kg/min IV for 30 minutes; then 0.1 mcg/kg/minute IV infusion for 48 to 96 hours.

Precautions: Use with caution: pregnancy, in the elderly and patients with abnormal creatinine clearance levels. **Contraindications:** hypersensitivity; active bleeding, bleeding disorders, platelet count below 150,000 mm^3, or trauma or surgery within 30 days. **NOTE:** Check package insert for current indications, dosage, and duration of therapy since optimal treatment therapy has not been established.

Heparin Low Molecular Weight Heparin

(LMWH): Enoxaparin, (Lovenox)

Action: Anticoagulant; inhibits or delays formation of clots.

Indications: ACS, STEMI, NSTEMI.

Ibutilide

Action: Decreases heart rate by slowing AV junctional conduction and prolonging refractory periods.

Indications: To treat rapid ventricular response in atrial flutter and atrial fibrillation, of less than 48 hour duration.

Inamrinone

(Amrinone)

Action: Increases cardiac contractility improving cardiac output; relaxes and dilates blood vessel walls decreasing blood pressure.

Indications: CHF that has not responded to other drug therapy.

Intravenous (IV) or Intraosseous (IO) Fluids

Actions: Replaces lost body fluids; provides IV or IO access for medication administration; dilutes and delivers IV or IO medications.

Indications: Hypovolemia; IV or IO medication administration access.

Ibutilide

Dosage: Adults more than 60 kg: 1 mg (10 ml) IV infusion over 10 minutes. May repeat dose after 10 minutes at same rate. **Adults less than 60 kg:** 0.01 mg/kg IV infusion over 10 minutes. May repeat dose after 10 minutes at same rate.

Precautions: May cause: VT or Torsades de Pointes, monitor during use and for 6 hours afterwards; keep defibrillator available. **Use with caution:** in the elderly, and with heart blocks. **Contraindications:** hypersensitivity.

Heparin (LMWH)

Dosage: Enoxaparin NSTEMI protocol: 1 mg/kg subcutaneous BID; 1st dose may be preceded by 30 mg IV bolus. **Enoxaparin STEMI protocol:** used with fibrinolytic therapy: 30 mg IV bolus; then 1 mg/kg subcutaneous BID until hospital discharge.

Precautions: May cause: active bleeding or hypertension. **Use with caution:** in pregnancy, in the elderly, severe hypertension, blood disorder, liver or kidney disease. **Contraindications:** hypersensitivity to pork products or heparin; recent surgery; platelet count below 100,000/mm³; elevated creatinine blood level. Do not use in conjunction with epidural therapy.

IV/IO Fluids

Dosage: 1000 ml of NS or LR; **IV:** access into vein via needle or specialized catheter. **IO:** access to bone marrow of specific areas of arms, legs, sternum, or pelvic bones via an adult IO device. **Hypovolemia:** 300 ml/hr or more. **Medication access:** usually 60 ml/hr or less. **Continuous infusion:** rate varies since fluids are titrated to the patient's needs.

Precautions: **Use with caution:** in the elderly, chronic lung problems, CHF, and brain injury. Monitor insertion site for infiltration of solution. Check for incompatibilities of various medications with saline or dextrose fluids.

Inamrinone

Dosage: 0.75 mg/kg slow IV push; may repeat in 30 minutes, if needed; then maintenance dose of 5 to 10 mcg/kg/min IV infusion, titrated to BP. Use with infusion pump.

Precautions: May cause: stomach upset, fever, liver or kidney problems, decreased platelet count, cardiac ischemia, increased ventricular irritability and/or dysrhythmias. **Use with caution:** pregnancy or in the elderly. **Contraindications:** hypersensitivity to drug or sulfites; acute MI. Do not use with fusosemide, sodium bicarbonate, or dextrose. Reduce dose by 50% to 75% for creatinine clearance less than 10 ml/min.

Isoproterenol Hydrochloride
(Isuprel)

Action: Increases force and rate of myocardial contractions, improving cardiac output and systolic BP.

Indications: Torsades de pointes that does not respond to magnesium sulfate; used for symptomatic bradycardia unresponsive to atropine, until temporary pacing can be established.

Lidocaine Hydrochloride
(Xylocaine)

Action: Decreases automaticity, helping to decrease ventricular dysrhythmias.

Indications: To control ventricular dysrhythmias such as PVCs; VT; alternative treatment for pulseless VT or V Fib.

Magnesium Sulfate

Action: Reduces ventricular dysrhythmias that may follow an MI (decreased magnesium levels may cause V Fib and may also prevent VT from responding to treatment).

Indications: Treatment of choice in torsades de pointes; may be used in V Fib or pulseless VT, or digoxin toxicity; magnesium sulfate should be used whenever magnesium levels are decreased.

Milrinone

Actions: Improves cardiac output by increasing strength of cardiac contractions; decreases BP by relaxing and dilating blood vessel walls.

Indications: Congestive heart failure that has not responded to other drug therapy.

Dosage: 1 to 1.5 mg/kg IV/IO, repeated at 5 to 10 minute intervals in doses of 0.5 to 0.75 mg/kg IV, until a total of 3 mg/kg has been given; if the ventricular ectopy has been suppressed and the patient has a pulse, begin a continuous infusion at 1 to 4 mg/min. **NOTE:** If underlying rhythm is bradycardic, consider giving atropine before Lidocaine.

Precautions: Signs of toxicity include numbness in hands or feet, decreased hearing, drowsiness, slurred speech, confusion, or muscle twitching. In severe cases of toxicity, seizures may occur; large doses of lidocaine may cause bradycardia, heart block, or AV conduction dysrhythmias. **Use with caution:** pregnancy and in the elderly. **Contraindications:** hypersensitivity; in patients with WPW syndrome or severe heart block.

Dosage: Initial bolus: 50 mcg/kg IV over 10 minutes. Maintenance dose: 0.375 to 0.750 mcg/kg/min for 2 to 3 days. Use with infusion pump.

Precautions: May cause: stomach upset, fever, or decrease of platelet count; may cause increased ischemia and ventricular irritability. Monitor for dysrhythmias. **Use with caution:** atrial flutter, atrial fib, liver or kidney disease, pregnancy, and in the elderly. **Contraindications:** hypersensitivity to this drug or sulfites; acute MI, or cardiac valve disease. Do not use with furosemide or procainamide.

Dosage: Continuous infusion: 2 to 10 mcg/min, titrated to patient's BP and pulse. **Torsades de pointes:** titrate to increase the HR of the underlying rhythm (causing the QT intervals to shorten), until the torsades de pointes is resolved. Must be used with infusion pump.

Precautions: Use with extreme caution. Do not use with other tachycardic dysrhythmias or cardiac arrest. Use with caution: pregnancy and in the elderly. **Contraindications:** hypersensitivity or sulfite allergies. Do not mix with aminophylline or sodium bicarbonate. Do not use with epinephrine (may cause V Fib or VT).

Dosage: **Torsades de pointes without a pulse or hypomagnesemia:** 1 to 2 g diluted in 10 ml IV fluid over 5 to 20 minutes, IV/IO. **Torsades de pointes with a pulse:** loading dose of 1 to 2 g in 50 to 100 ml IV fluid, over 5 to 60 minutes. Follow with 0.5 to 1 g/hr IV, titrating dosage to control torsades de pointes.

Precautions: May cause: flushing, sweating, slight bradycardia, and hypotension. **Use with caution:** kidney failure and in pregnancy. **Contraindications:** hypersensitivity. Should be diluted in IV fluid.

Naloxone Hydrochloride

Action: Unknown; may replace narcotics at narcotic receptor sites.

Indications: Respiratory depression or unconsciousness due to known or suspected narcotic overdose.

Nitroprusside Sodium
(Sodium Nitroprusside)

Actions: Dilates and relaxes smooth muscle of blood vessel walls: decreasing BP, increasing cardiac output, relieving chest pain by reducing ischemia.

Indications: Hypertensive emergencies that do not respond to other medications; acute CHF.

Morphine Sulfate

Action: Narcotic analgesic that provides chest pain relief.

Indications: Part of "MONA" protocol for MIs.

Nitroglycerin

Action: Relieves cardiac chest pain and hypertension by relaxing and dilating smooth muscle in blood vessels, including the coronary arteries.

Indications: To treat cardiac chest pain, hypertension, CHF; part of "MONA" protocol for acute MI.

Naloxone Hydrochloride

Dosage: 0.4 to 2 mg IV titrated until respirations improve; may repeat dose every 2 to 3 minutes; up to 6 to 10 mg within 10 minutes. Respiratory rate increases within 1 to 2 minutes. Do not mix with other medications.

Precautions: May cause: narcotic withdrawal (nausea, vomiting, anxiety, abdominal cramping, hypertension). **Use with caution:** increased cardiac irritability, pregnancy or seizure disorders. **Contraindications:** hypersensitivity to drug or sulfite allergies. May need to repeat doses. Monitor for recurring respiratory depression.

Morphine Sulfate

Dosage: 1 to 5 mg IV over 1 to 5 minutes, titrated to pain relief; may repeat at 5 to 15 min intervals.

Precautions: May cause: hypotension, respiratory depression. **Use with caution:** pregnancy, liver or kidney disease, or in the elderly. **Contraindications:** hypersensitivity or asthma.

Nitroprusside Sodium

Dosage: 50 mg diluted in 250 ml D₅W; **initial dose:** 0.25 to 0.3 mcg/kg per minute, titrated every 3 to 5 minutes until desired BP, up to 10 mcg/kg/min. Reconstitute with D₅W solution. Use with infusion pump.

Precautions: BP may drop quickly; monitor vital signs every 2 to 3 minutes. May cause: headache, nausea, vomiting, abdominal cramping, and severe hypotension. **Use with caution:** pregnancy, liver or kidney disease, and in the elderly. **Contraindications:** hypersensitivity. Do **not** use with bacteriostatic water, saline solution or mix any other medications or preservatives with nitroprusside solution. Protect solution from light by covering IV bottle with foil or dark plastic; follow your institution's policy regarding covering IV tubing.

Nitroglycerin

Dosage: Sublingual (under the tongue): one tablet (0.3 or 0.4 mg); repeat at 5 minute intervals, if necessary; maximum 3 tablets. **Spray: (do not shake)** 0.4 mg under or on the tongue by metered-dose canister, waiting 10 seconds before swallowing; repeat at 5 minute intervals if necessary, until maximum of 3 sprays. **IV infusion:** initial dose of 10 to 20 mcg/min, titrated to pain and hypertension relief. May increase by 5 to 10 mcg/min, every 5 to 10 minutes as needed. Use with infusion pump.

Precautions: May cause: headache, nausea, vomiting, severe hypotension (monitor vital signs frequently). **Use with caution:** pregnancy, liver or kidney disease, or IV use in the elderly. **Contraindications:** systolic BP less than 90 mm Hg; hypersensitivity or nitrite allergy; use of medications for erectile dysfunction. Do not mix with other medications. Absorbed by plastic, use glass bottle and polyethylene tubing.

Norepinephrine Bitartrate

Action: Constricts blood vessels and increases BP, heart rate, and the force of cardiac contractions.

Indications: Acute and severe hypotension not caused by hypovolemia.

Oxygen
(O$_2$)

Action: Increases oxygen available to all tissue cells; helps to reduce shortness of breath; may help to decrease ischemia.

Indications: For all patients with respiratory distress, SOB, chest pains, dysrhythmias, decreased cardiac output, and in all cardiopulmonary arrests; part of "MONA" protocol for acute MI.

Procainamide Hydrochloride

Action: Suppresses ventricular and atrial ectopy; decreases cardiac excitability and automaticity.

Indications: To control a wide variety of dysrhythmias.

Sodium Bicarbonate

Action: Reduces acidosis.

Indications: Metabolic acidosis; prolonged cardiac arrest; cardiotoxicity with some drug overdoses; hyperkalemia.

Dosage: For alert patients with mild distress: 1 to 6 L/min delivered by nasal cannula. For patients with moderate respiratory distress: 4 to 12 L/min by Venturi mask, at 24% to 50%. For patients with severe respiratory distress: 6 to 10 L/min of 100% oxygen, delivered by a partial rebreather mask at 35% to 60%, or non-rebreather mask with reservoir at 6 to 15 L/min for 60% to 100%. **During CPR:** give by bag-mask device or endotracheal tube at 15 L/min at 100%. Pulse oximetry may be helpful in oxygen titration.

Precautions: Flammable; do **not** use in presence of flames, sparks, or during cardioversion and defibrillation. **Use with caution:** in alert patients with chronic lung disease. Should be used at 100% in all resuscitation attempts. Pulse oximetry may be inaccurate with low cardiac output or anemia.

Dosage: 0.5 to 1 mcg/min IV (only route), titrate infusion to patient's BP, to a maximum dose of 30 mcg/min. Use only with D_5W or D_5NS.

Precautions: May cause: BP to drop very rapidly, monitor vital signs every 2 to 3 minutes. **May also cause:** myocardial ischemia, monitor patient's rhythm continuously for dysrhythmias. **Use with caution:** pregnancy and in the elderly. **Contraindications:** hypersensitivity; V Fib, dysrhythmias with rapid heart rates, or hypertension. Do not mix with aminophylline, lidocaine, sodium bicarbonate, or plain normal saline. Assess IV site frequently as infiltration may cause death of tissue around the IV site.

Dosages: 1 mEq/kg IV; repeat based on arterial blood gas results. Flush IV with 20 ml NS solution **before** and **after** administering medication to reduce possibility of drug interactions.

Precautions: Monitor electrolytes, kidney function and arterial blood gases. **Use with caution:** pregnancy, CHF, and in the elderly. **Contraindications:** hypersensitivity or respiratory acidosis. Do **not** mix with any other medications.

Dosage: 20 mg/min IV until any of the following occur:
(1) The dysrhythmia is suppressed.
(2) The patient becomes hypotensive.
(3) The QRS complex widens by 50% of its original width.
(4) A total of 17 mg/kg has been given.

If necessary, 50 mg/min IV up to 17 mg/kg IV can be given, until any of the above symptoms occur. A continuous IV infusion at a rate of 1 to 4 mg/min should be started if the ventricular dysrhythmia has been suppressed and the patient has a pulse.

Precautions: May cause: hypotension if administered too quickly; decrease maintenance dose if patient has kidney failure. **Use with caution:** bradycardia or pregnancy. **Contraindications:** hypersensitivity; prolonged QT intervals; torsades de pointes; myasthenia gravis; systemic lupis; second- or third-degree heart block. Monitor BP closely.